Genomics

Editor

STEPHEN D. KRAU

NURSING CLINICS
OF NORTH AMERICA

www.nursing.theclinics.com

Consulting Editor
STEPHEN D. KRAU

December 2013 • Volume 48 • Number 4

ELSEVIER

1600 John F. Kennedy Boulevard • Suite 1800 • Philadelphia, Pennsylvania, 19103-2899

http://www.theclinics.com

NURSING CLINICS OF NORTH AMERICA Volume 48, Number 4
December 2013 ISSN 0029-6465, ISBN-13: 978-0-323-26110-4

Editor: Kerry Holland
Developmental Editor: Susan Showalter

Nursing Clinics of North America (ISSN 0029-6465) is published quarterly by Elsevier Inc., 360 Park Avenue South, New York, NY 10010-1710. Months of issue are March, June, September, and December. Periodicals postage paid at New York, NY and additional mailing offices. Subscription price per year is, $150.00 (US individuals), $400.00 (US institutions), $275.00 (international individuals), $488.00 (international institutions), $220.00 (Canadian individuals), $488.00 (Canadian institutions), $85.00 (US students), and $135.00 (international students). To receive student/resident rate, orders must be accompanied by name of affiliated institution, date of term, and the signature of program/residency coordinator on institution letterhead. Orders will be billed at individual rate until proof of status is received. Foreign air speed delivery is included in all *Clinics* subscription prices. All prices are subject to change without notice. **POSTMASTER:** Send address changes to *Nursing Clinics*, Elsevier Health Sciences Division, Subscription Customer Service, 3251 Riverport Lane, Maryland Heights, MO 63043. **Customer Service: Telephone: 1-800-654-2452** (U.S. and Canada); **1-314-447-8871 (outside U.S. and Canada). Fax: 1-314-447-8029. E-mail: journalscustomerservice-usa@elsevier.com** (for print support) and **journalsonlinesupport-usa@elsevier.com** (for online support).

Nursing Clinics of North America is covered in *EMBASE/Excerpta Medica, MEDLINE/PubMed (Index Medicus), Social Sciences Citation Index, Current Contents, ASCA, Cumulative Index to Nursing, RNdex Top 100,* and Allied Health Literature and International Nursing Index (INI).

Printed in the United States of America.

Contributors

CONSULTING EDITOR

STEPHEN D. KRAU, PhD, RN, CNE
Associate Professor, Vanderbilt University Medical Center, School of Nursing, Nashville, Tennessee

EDITOR

STEPHEN D. KRAU, PhD, RN, CNE
Associate Professor, Vanderbilt University Medical Center, School of Nursing, Nashville, Tennessee

AUTHORS

MARIA ADAMIAN, ACNP-BC, CRNA, FAAPM
Doctoral Student, Graduate School of Health Sciences, Seton Hall University, South Orange, New Jersey

ELIZABETH K. BANCROFT, RN, PhD
Senior Research Nurse in Oncogenetics, The Royal Marsden NHS Foundation Trust and The Institute of Cancer Research, Sutton, Surrey, United Kingdom

LAURA CURR BEAMER, DNP, AOCNP, APNG
Assistant Professor, School of Nursing & Health Studies, College of Health & Human Sciences, Northern Illinois University, DeKalb, Illinois; PhD Candidate, College of Nursing, University of Utah, Salt Lake City, Utah

CHITO A. BELCHEZ, MSN, RN-BC
Clinical Assistant Professor, School of Nursing, The University of Kansas Medical Center, Kansas City, Kansas

BASHIRA ADDULLAH CHARLES, PhD, RN
PostDoctoral Fellow, Center Research Genomics & Global Health, National Human Genome Research Institute, National Institutes of Health, Bethesda, Maryland

PEI-YING CHUANG, PhD, MSN, RN
Assistant Professor, School of Nursing, University of Texas Health Science Center at Houston, Houston, Texas

ASHLEY ERIN CLARK, MSN, RN
Delta Mu-STTI, Doctoral Student, Yale University, School of Nursing, Orange, Connecticut

SANDRA DAACK-HIRSCH, PhD, RN
Associate Professor, The University of Iowa College of Nursing, Iowa City, Iowa

JULIA EGGERT, PhD, GNP-BC, AOCN®
Mary Cox Professor, Doctoral Coordinator Healthcare Genetics, School of Nursing, Health, College of Education and Human Development, Clemson University, Clemson; Advanced Practice Nurse Geneticist, Cancer Risk, Screening Program, Bon Secours St. Francis Hospital, Greenville, South Carolina

BETTY ELDER, PhD, RN
Associate Professor, School of Nursing, Wichita State University, Wichita, Kansas

SUSAN FLAVIN, MSN, RN
Alpha-1 Community Research Partnership, Medical University of South Carolina, Charleston, South Carolina

EZRA C. HOLSTON, PhD, RN
Assistant Professor, College of Nursing, The University of Tennessee – Knoxville, Knoxville, Tennessee

CHING HSIU HSIEH, EdPhD, RN
Assistant Professor, Department of Nursing, Chang Gung University of Science and Technology, Putzu City, Taiwan, Republic of China

ROXANNE HURLEY, MS, RN
Clinical Associate Professor, Associate Dean of Undergraduate Studies, College of Nursing, University of North Dakota, Grand Forks, North Dakota

SADIE P. HUTSON, PhD, RN, WHNP, BC
Associate Professor, College of Nursing, The University of Tennessee – Knoxville, Knoxville, Tennessee

BARBARA JACKSON, PhD
Associate Professor, Munroe-Meyer Institute, University of Nebraska Medical Center, Omaha, Nebraska

JAMILA KEITH
Alpha-1 Community Research Partnership, Medical University of South Carolina, Charleston, South Carolina

PEG KERR, PhD, RN
Associate Professor, Department Head, Department of Nursing, University of Dubuque, Dubuque, Iowa

STEPHEN D. KRAU, PhD, RN, CNE
Associate Professor, Vanderbilt University Medical Center, School of Nursing, Nashville, Tennessee

LAURI LINDER, PhD, APRN, CPON
Assistant Professor, College of Nursing, University of Utah; Clinical Nurse Specialist, Cancer Transplant Service Line, Primary Children's Hospital, Salt Lake City, Utah

MARY KAY NISSEN, ARNP-BC, MSN, COHN-S
Assistant Professor, Department of Nursing, Briar Cliff University, Sioux City, Iowa

MARGARET PIERCE, DNP, FNP-BC
Assistant Professor, College of Nursing, The University of Tennessee – Knoxville, Knoxville, Tennessee

overview of the pathophysiology, symptoms, complications, diagnostic testing, and treatment. The silent presentation of HCM presents unique diagnostic challenges and complicates prompt identification. Diagnostic testing and management strategies for the care of a person with HCM are discussed. HCM has individualized presentation and therefore requires individualized therapy.

Since 2003, genetics and genomics information has led to exciting new diagnostics, prognostics, and treatment options in oncology practice. Profiling of cancers offers providers insight into treatment and prognostic factors. Germline testing provides an individual with information for surveillance or therapy that may help them prevent cancer in their lifetime and options for family members as yet untouched by malignancy. This offers a challenge for oncology nurses and other oncology health care providers to become comfortable with incorporating education about genetics/genomics into their clinical practice and patient education.

Patients with rare chronic disorders and their caregivers increasingly form communities to support and exchange social experiences. Because up to 10% of the United States population is affected by one of 5000 to 6000 rare disorders, efforts to understand the individuals and affected communities are important. This study was conducted using community-based participatory research approaches within a community of patients and caregivers living with alpha-1 antitrypsin (AAT) deficiency. Patient populations at some risk for lung transplant include individuals who smoked cigarettes and patients who underwent liver transplant in infancy and later adulthood due to accumulation of misfolded AAT within hepatocytes.

Biobanks function as vital components in genetic research, which often requires large disease-based or population-based biospecimens and clinical data to study complex or rare diseases. Genetic biobanks aim to provide resources for translational research focusing on rapidly moving scientific findings from the laboratory into health care practice. The nursing profession must evolve as genetic biobanking practices advance. Nursing involvement in genetic biobanking practices comes with a distinct set of educational, ethical, and practice competencies. In response to these growing competency standards, nursing science developed a conceptual framework and continues to study ethical considerations to guide genetic biobanking initiatives.

Contents

ERICA YU, PhD, RN, ARNP
Assistant Professor, Department of Acute and Continuing Care, School of Nursing, The University of Texas Health Science Center at Houston, Houston, Texas

JIM QUILL
Alpha-1 Community Research Partnership, Medical University of South Carolina, Charleston, South Carolina

JENNIFER E. SANNER, PhD, RN
Assistant Professor, Department of Nursing Systems, School of Nursing, The University of Texas Health Science Center at Houston, Houston, Texas

LUCINDA SHORE, MS
Alpha-1 Community Research Partnership, Medical University of South Carolina, Charleston, South Carolina

MARVIN SINEATH
Alpha-1 Community Research Partnership, Medical University of South Carolina, Charleston, South Carolina

CHARLIE STRANGE, MD
Alpha-1 Community Research Partnership, Medical University of South Carolina, Charleston, South Carolina

KIM SUBASIC, BSN, MS, PhD
Assistant Professor, Department of Nursing, University of Scranton, Scranton, Pennsylvania

JACQUELYN Y. TAYLOR, PhD, PNP-BC, RN, FAAN
Delta Mu, STTI, Associate Professor and Robert Wood Johnson Foundation, Nurse Faculty Scholar Alumna, Yale University, School of Nursing, Orange, Connecticut

MALINI UDTHA, PhD
Research Coordinator, Department of Nursing Systems, School of Nursing, The University of Texas Health Science Center at Houston, Houston, Texas

REBA UMBERGER, PhD, RN, CCRN
Assistant Professor, College of Nursing, The University of Tennessee – Knoxville, Knoxville, Tennessee

DEIRDRE WALKER
Alpha-1 Community Research Partnership, Medical University of South Carolina, Charleston, South Carolina

BARBARA WARNER
Alpha-1 Community Research Partnership, Medical University of South Carolina, Charleston, South Carolina

SARA WIENKE, MS, CGC
Alpha-1 Community Research Partnership, Medical University of South Carolina, Charleston, South Carolina

PAMELA HOLTZCLAW WILLIAMS, JD, PhD, RN
Associate Professor, Nursing Science Department, College of Nursing, Medical University of South Carolina, Charleston, South Carolina; College of Nursing, University of Arkansas for Medical Sciences, Little Rock, Arkansas

BOHUA WU, MD
Student, Healthcare Genetics Doctoral Program, School of Nursing, Health, College of Education and Human Development, Clemson University, Clemson, South Carolina

Epigenetic changes to the genome are biochemical alterations to the DNA that do not change an individual's genome but do change and influence gene expression. The nursing profession is qualified to conduct and integrate epigenetic-focused nursing research into practice. This article discusses current epigenetic nursing research, provides an overview of how epigenetic research relates to nursing practice, makes recommendations, and provides epigenetic online resources for nursing research. An overview of major epigenetic studies in nursing (specific to childbirth studies, preeclampsia, metabolic syndrome, immunotherapy cancer, and pain) is provided, with recommendations on next steps.

Rapid advances in knowledge and technology related to genomics cross health care disciplines and touch almost every aspect of patient care. The ability to sequence a genome holds the promise that health care can be personalized. Health care professionals are faced with a gap in the ability to use the rapidly expanding technology and knowledge related to genomics in practice. Yet, nurses are key to bridging the gap between genomic discoveries and the human experience of illness. This article presents a case study documenting the experience of five nursing schools/colleges of nursing as they work to integrate genetics and genomics into their curricula.

Although knowledge about the impact of cytochrome p450 on individual variations in drug response has been known for decades, the transition to clinical practice has not evolved. Nurses who administer and prescribe medications have a responsibility to their patients to understand the responses to medications that are mediated by this family of enzymes. An overview of the variations seen in drug responses based on genetics is presented with discussion focusing on the current prescriptive practices and limitations in clinical drug trials.

To provide the best patient care related to medication administration and prescription, an understanding of the specific enzymes is essential. Enzymes affect the metabolizing of most medications that nurses administer and that nurse practitioners and physicians prescribe on a regular basis. More specifically, the most important p450 enzymes in drug metabolism are cytochrome p450 (CYP) 1A2, the CYP2C family, CYP2D6, and CYP3A4. In addition, the enzymes are instrumental in the body's reaction to environmental factors, some of which are carcinogens.

The most important considerations related to understanding cytochrome p450 enzymes is the appreciation that all drug effects vary among individuals and, although there are multiple causes of these variations, drug effects are strongly influenced by genes. Nurses who administer and monitor, or prescribe, these medications can only be safe if there is understanding of these processes. The same enzyme may display a variety of functions and alterations, which can range from ultrarapid activity to no activity. Foods given with medications also can affect the metabolism of the medication. Each cytochrome p450 subfamily is instrumental in the metabolism of numerous drugs.

NURSING CLINICS OF NORTH AMERICA

NOW AVAILABLE FOR YOUR iPhone and iPad

Preface

Genomics

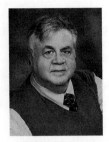

Stephen D. Krau, PhD, RN, CNE
Editor

The science behind genomics, variation, and implications for health has been known for several decades. Since completion of the Human Genome Project in 2003 and continuing initiatives in genomic research, the practice of nursing and medicine has been undergoing rapid change.[1,2] Only recently have the information and science transitioned to a prominent place in clinical practice. Although somewhat embryonic, the impact and potential impact of genomics on health are so evident that it is clearly going to be a major arena of science and education for health care providers. The relevance of genomic variation to health, implications for risk factors for rare and common diseases, and treatment modalities has been demonstrated. This issue is designed to illuminate the applications of genomic discoveries in a variety of nursing practice areas. Currently genomic discoveries are influencing diagnoses, treatment, and prevention at a rapid pace, with hopes that we will improve health care outcomes worldwide.

As one the largest professional health care groups, nurses are vital in the effort to improve outcomes and understand how genomics will affect health care. To this end genetics and genomic literacy are essential for all nurses. Some of the information is being used by nurses who might not even know it. For example, it is not rare that a nurse will instruct a patient to avoid certain foods or beverages while taking certain medications, such as grapefruit juice. Although the nurse may understand that there is an effect grapefruit juice has on the medication, it is the pharmacogenomic science that reveals that grapefruit juice in some patients impacts variant cytochrome p450 enzymes, resulting in overmedication due to enhanced bioavailability, or undermedication due to decreased bioavailability when the two are combined.

Genetic variations among us impact how we metabolize which medications and at what rate they are metabolized. This contributes to a huge potential for variant outcomes for the patient, such that due to genetic variations, we could be overmedicating the patient, undermedicating the patient, or completely using the wrong medication for that patient, despite the compelling clinical drug trials.

Nurs Clin N Am 48 (2013) xiii–xiv
http://dx.doi.org/10.1016/j.cnur.2013.09.006
0029-6465/13/$ – see front matter © 2013 Published by Elsevier Inc.

nursing.theclinics.com

The field of epigenetics, which is the area that studies genetic variations as the result of something other than underlying DNA sequencing, is expanding. This introduces a strong potential for some salient influences over health care outcomes. The field of biobanking is expanding and is fraught with legal and ethical implications discussed in this issue.

It is hoped that this issue will provide some foundational information for nurses who wish to obtain a broader yet more in-depth understanding on genomics and its impact on the patient, health care in general, and future treatment modalities. Although some of the information has been available for a few decades, the field continues to grow. As genomics and its multilevel implications expand into clinical practice, it is essential that nurses continue to keep informed and up to date with information to provide patients with optimal care and to make valuable contributions to the health care team.

Stephen D. Krau, PhD, RN, CNE
Vanderbilt University Medical Center
School of Nursing
461 21st Avenue South
Nashville, TN 37240, USA

E-mail address:
steve.krau@vanderbilt.edu

REFERENCES

1. Jenkins J, Grady PA, Collins FS. Nurses and the genomic revolution. J Nurs Scholarsh 2005;37(2):98–101.
2. Fweero WG, Guttmacher AE, Collins FS. Genomic medicine—an updated primer. N Engl J Med 2010;361(21):2001–11.

Nursing Genomics
Practice Implications Every Nurse Should Know

Reba Umberger, PhD, RN, CCRN*, Ezra C. Holston, PhD, RN,
Sadie P. Hutson, PhD, RN, WHNP, BC, Margaret Pierce, DNP, FNP-BC

KEYWORDS

• Genomics • Genetics • Ethics • Technology • Nursing practice • Nursing education

KEY POINTS

• Genetics/genomics should not be considered a specialty discipline in nursing, as it affects every point along the health to illness continuum.
• Rapid technological advances in whole-genome sequencing will cause an inevitable increase in the use of genomic information in clinical patient care. This shift will have a profound effect on disease prevention, screening, diagnosis, prognosis, treatment selection, and treatment efficacy.
• Nurse clinicians, scientists, and educators in the twenty-first century will be challenged to become proficient in genetic competencies to provide the best available evidenced-based care to patients.
• Expanding the understanding of genetics/genomics comes with many related ethical, legal, and social issues.

It is essential for nurses to recognize the impact that genetics and genomics have on their practice as both genetic science and the nursing discipline move forward in the twenty-first century. This article is divided into 3 sections: an historical context of genetics/genomics, a review of genomics applications, and the implications for genomics in nursing practice. Each section provides foundational knowledge about this rapidly evolving field that is vital for student and practicing nurses.

HISTORICAL CONTEXT

From the beginning of recorded history, humans have noted the effects of genetics. As early as 5000 years ago, Babylonians described birth defects among their population.

Funding Sources: None.
Conflicts of Interest: None.
The University of Tennessee – Knoxville, College of Nursing, 1200 Volunteer Boulevard, Knoxville, TN 37996-4180, USA
* Corresponding author.
E-mail address: rumberge@utk.edu

The Talmud, an ancient Jewish holy text, noted the inheritance of hemophilia. More than 2000 years ago, people began to breed animals and plants for specific characteristics, such as speed for horses and hardiness for plants.[1,2] The science of modern genetics began in 1865 when Gregor Mendel, known as the father of genetics,[3,4] explained the concepts of dominant and recessive traits in his work with garden peas. Although Mendel did not know about deoxyribonucleic acid (DNA) or genes, his descriptions of the traits of the offspring of garden peas that were fertilized with pollen from plants with specific characteristics continues to be an accurate portrayal of the basic concepts of inheritance.

In 1869, Friedrich Miescher noted the presence of a weak acid in white blood cells that was later determined to be DNA.[5] The late nineteenth century saw 2 important developments in genetics. First, scientists began to understand the importance of the fusion of the male and female cells' nuclei during fertilization. Second, chromosomes were first seen under the microscope. By the early twentieth century the scientific community had accepted that every time a cell divided, chromosomes split into two identical pieces with one becoming part of each daughter cell. The belief that these chromosomes contained the genes first described by Mendel was documented in 1903.[5]

The era of modern genetics is widely recognized to have begun with the discovery of DNA, described in 1953 by James Watson and Francis Crick as a double-stranded helix of nucleotides, which can replicate because of each strand's identical structure. Although the exact mechanism was not understood, their experiments demonstrated that genes produced proteins for living organisms.[6,7] The developments of prenatal chromosome analysis, chromosome banding, and DNA sequencing followed quickly.[8] The first drugs produced by genetic engineering, somatostatin in 1977 and insulin in 1979, paved the way for a virtual explosion of this technology in pharmacology. In 1993, scientists developed the first map of the human genome.[8]

The Human Genome Project

The term "genome" means the totality of genetic information found in an organism's DNA and/or ribonucleic acid (RNA).[5] The international endeavor known as the Human Genome Project (HGP) began in 1990. The project's goal was to use using new technology in automated DNA sequencing to map, or determine the DNA nucleotide sequence of, the human genome by 2005. The working draft of the human genome was announced at a White House ceremony in June 2000, published in *Nature* and *Science* in February 2001, and completed in 2003. The HGP also sequenced the genetic code of several other species including fruit flies, mice, and *Escherichia coli*. Although the genome of each member of a species is unique, the HGP sequenced multiple variations of each gene to find commonalities among species representatives. After publication of the HGP draft, scientists confirmed the ability to sequence an individual's DNA in 2007.[8]

Basic Concepts

In any nurse's practice, patients question the possible effect of genetics on their risk for a multitude of diseases and conditions. The etiology of a genetic disease is now understood to be a change in DNA structure that alters the expression of a particular gene. **Fig. 1** illustrates the location of a gene within a DNA segment. A genetic disease may be caused by a single gene change or by chromosomal abnormalities such as the duplication or deletion of a gene segment, or a change that occurs during cellular division. These genetic changes may be inherited from one or both parents, or may occur spontaneously as a "new mutation."[9]

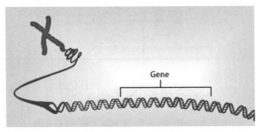

Fig. 1. Location of a gene within a DNA segment. (*Courtesy of* Greg R. Gaiker Jr, University of Tennessee, Knoxville, TN.)

Genograms

Mendel's experiments elucidated inheritance patterns that are still used in clinical practice when a genogram or pedigree, a pictorial display of an individual's family relationships and medical history, is created. Albeit simple, a genogram is still one of the most powerful tools available to health care providers. In 2004, Guttmacher and colleagues[10] asserted that the information gleaned from a careful, 3-generation family history can help practitioners discuss disease risk, prevention, and detection, and make best use of genetic tests as they become more widely available. Whereas some practitioners question the accuracy of patient-reported family histories, Guttmacher maintained that the accuracy of the genogram increases when families complete it together. In addition, completing the genogram together gives all participating family members access to more accurate health information. Online software programs to record and save family genograms are available to individuals and health care practitioners. One such widely used program is the Department of Health and Human Services' *My Family Health Portrait*, available at https://familyhistory.hhs.gov/fhh-web/home.action. The US Surgeon General declares every Thanksgiving Day to be "Family History Day," and encourages people to collect family history data while family members are gathered for the holiday. After filling the document with information, families can save it, add to it as additional information becomes available, and share it with other family members. **Fig. 2** provides an example of a 3-generation genogram. From this genogram it is possible to identify dominant patterns of genetic conditions as well as sex-linked traits and diseases. It is important to remember, however, that not all genetic mutations and diseases appear in a family genogram. Individuals and health care providers must always consider the possible development of new mutations.

All nurses should be skilled in gathering a family's historical information as well as diagramming and interpreting a family genogram. Nurses also can educate patients about genetic testing and help them make informed decisions about which tests to undergo for themselves or for their families. Although the genogram is an excellent visual assessment tool, genetic testing provides a more comprehensive picture of the molecular basis of disease.

GENOMICS APPLICATIONS

This section briefly examines several common genomic diagnostic applications (genotyping, inheritable disease screening, whole-genome sequencing, and gene expression), how genomics are being used to advance disease treatment (gene therapy and pharmacogenomics), and how such technology has created the demand for direct-to-consumer (DTC) genetic testing.

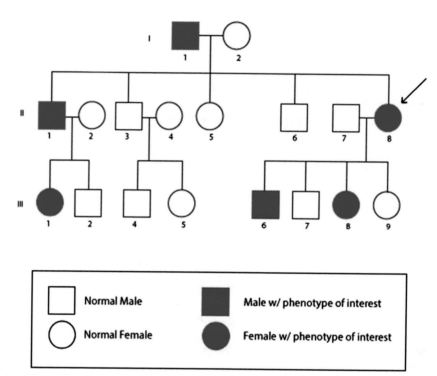

Fig. 2. Three-generation genogram. Open circles represent normal-appearing females, filled circles represent females with the phenotype of interest, open boxes represent normal-appearing males, and filled boxes represent males with the phenotype of interest. Each generation is labeled with a roman numeral and each person within that generation is labeled with an Arabic number. The arrow indicates the proband or the person providing the history. In this case, the proband was person number 8 in generation II, and her father and 2 children have the phenotype of interest. (*Courtesy of* Greg R. Gaiker Jr, University of Tennessee, Knoxville, TN.)

Genotyping

Genotyping explores the genetic makeup of the elements of life (ie, a cell, an organism, or an individual). It objectively examines diseases, syndromes, and conditions while emphasizing the phenotypic (or observable) similarities and differences at a biological, psychological, and environmental level. Genotyping single-nucleotide polymorphisms (SNPs) can show how diseases might be linked to a gene on a specific chromosome. SNP genotyping has determined that stroke risk is linked to gene variants on chromosomes 9p21.3,[11] 4q25,[12] and 16q22.[13] Type 2 diabetes and its sequelae have been associated with specific genetic mutations.[14–17] The occurrence of asthma has been linked to a gene variant on chromosome 5q.[18] Researchers also linked a single gene variant on chromosome 17 to several conditions including Alzheimer disease,[19,20] coronary artery disease,[21] hypertension,[22] and systemic lupus erythematosus.[23] While SNP genotyping can help the genetics of diseases become recognizable and possibly treatable, it lacks the specificity needed to determine the exact genes related to a specific disease. This limitation will decrease as genomic-driven technology facilitates more expansive genotyping (genome genotyping) and potential DNA profiling.

Compared with SNP genotyping, genome genotyping offers a more rigorous, efficient, and accessible application to examine diseases' biomolecular foundations and/or contributions. It also aids in the development of genotype databases, and is able to examine gene heterogeneity and uncover the presence of haplotypes (groups of alleles that are transmitted/inherited together) and environmental DNA influences. Genome genotyping techniques involve DNA sequencing, multilocus genotyping or sequencing, genome-wide association, and SNP tagging, which uses the information from SNP genotyping to link gene variants to several loci within and across chromosomes. Results from these techniques indicate that most diseases, syndromes, and conditions (eg, neurodegenerative diseases, depression, or attention deficit/hyperactivity disorder [ADHD]) involve several factors or causes.

Using comparative quantitative genotyping, 14 high-risk subtypes of the human papillomavirus have been associated with certain phenotypes.[24] This discovery may lead to potential treatment options for female infertility and cervical cancer.[25] Multilocus genotyping or sequencing enhances the detection of invasive and lethal pathogens, including *Listeria monocytogenes,*[26] *Bacillus anthracis,*[27] and *Campylobacter jejuni.*[28] Genome genotyping decreases the dependence on phenotypes, resulting in a more comprehensive and thorough examination of possible alleles (1 of 2 or more versions of a gene) associated with a disease.[29] This ability is evident in the success achieved by scientists in connecting the susceptibility for asthma in persons from India with the haplotypes of the ADRB2 gene on chromosome 5q.33.1,[30] and linking the risk of end-stage renal disease to type 2 diabetes in African Americans with the gene variant rs730947 of the GCK1 gene on chromosome 7.[31]

With genome genotyping, genes that have been poorly researched in the past are now being examined and connected to diseases such as Parkinson disease,[32] essential hypertension,[33] and peripheral arterial disease.[34] Larger and more diverse samples can be genotyped to gain a better understanding of gene variants' prevalence in populations with amplified DNA,[35] DNA pools,[36] tagged SNPs,[37] or tagged mitochondrial DNA.[38] Establishing common genetic variants helps create a genomic risk profile for ischemic stroke,[39] identify the susceptible alleles of rheumatoid arthritis,[40] describe the homozygosity of alleles related to early-onset Parkinson disease,[32] and match transplant donors with recipients via the genotyped human leukocyte antigen (HLA) gene.[41]

Genome genotyping strengthens the research on sporadically occurring diseases because genetic linkage, not the phenotypes manifested in a family, now determines the selection of possible candidate genes. This change allows for a more conclusive understanding of disease genetics. Candidate genes have been identified for diseases such as amyotrophic lateral sclerosis,[42] which has a 95% sporadic occurrence in the community.[43] The caveat for such genetic advances is their dependence on the prevalence of the known gene variants in the general population and published information.[44] Unfortunately, there is minimal information about the presence, occurrence, and linkage of SNPs within and across the chromosomes for ethnic-minority and vulnerable populations, which limits the construction and use of reference panels for SNPs, DNA pooling, or SNP tagging.[45] Caution must be exercised when genome genotyping these populations to avoid erroneous conclusions, biased interpretations, and incorrect application of results.[44]

Phenotype-driven SNP genotyping has emphasized the gene variants' role in disease onset and progression. The process also has served as a first step in understanding the utility of genetic information in health care professions. However, genomics has seen the evolution of SNP genotyping into genome genotyping, which increases the applicability of genetics as evidenced by the genetic research about inheritable diseases.

Inheritable Disease Screening

With the application of genomics, researchers can give the health care industry a more comprehensive understanding of genetic-driven inheritability and the potential to address diseases proactively, as seen with the global application of newborn screening. Genomics has helped expand newborn screening practice from the detection of a single metabolic disorder, phenylketonuria, to 30 to 40 disorders with 29 recommended core disorders.[46] Early screening allows clinical manifestation of these disorders to be better assessed, significantly reducing the risk of misdiagnosis or missed treatment during infancy.[46] However, care must be taken with the expanded newborn screening practices because of the increased risk of false-positive outcomes and inconclusive information about the "natural history" of some screened disorders.[46] Early, age-appropriate treatments have increased newborn survival rates for these diseases. As a result, federal guidelines recommend that the benefits and risks be considered before using newborn screening.[47]

Genomics can recognize and address other highly inheritable diseases. Although ADHD is often treated as a social disorder because of the social unrest resulting from its phenotypes, it actually has an inheritability of 80% to 90%.[48] This multifactorial disease is now better understood as a result of genome genotyping; its symptoms have been linked to variants in dopaminergic genes, serotonergic genes, and the synaptosomal-associated protein gene.[48] Several de novo and rare copy-number variations (CNV) have been linked to ADHD risk and the susceptibility of genes related to ADHD symptoms.[49] Gene variants on chromosome 6q25–6q27 have been used to explain ADHD's heritability level of 83%.[50] These same gene variants also have been used to associate the risk of schizophrenia with the phenotype of insufficient myelination.[51]

For inheritable diseases that may not be preventable at birth, genomics has promoted the discovery of treatment modalities such as genetic testing, early aggressive treatments, and ongoing management. By monitoring the genomic expression of gene mutations, the quality of life is enhanced for persons with cystic fibrosis (CF),[52] Tay-Sachs disease,[53] hemochromatosis,[54] and Down syndrome.[55] Genomics may contribute to the discovery of innovative screening methods for inheritable diseases, such as using maternal serum to screen for Down syndrome[55,56] and nasal/bronchial epithelium to screen for CF.[57] Even if screening is unable to conclusively identify the suspected gene variant, it provides a better understanding of disease heterogeneity and how the synergistic functioning of gene variants affects the phenotypes.[58,59] Such understanding can help pave the way for whole-genome sequencing.

Whole-Genome Sequencing

Whole-genome sequencing represents the future of genotyping. This detailed analysis of genomic elements offers a reliable and accurate examination of the DNA basepairs' variability, degree of loci association, level of activation, and conformation over time, along with the phenotypic reaction to environmental stimuli. Using a whole-genome shotgun resequencing approach, scientists were able to distinguish one bacterial strain from others by examining the gene variants to determine how these mutations contributed to the biological phenotypes indicating the strain.[60] This level of sequencing facilitates many processes, including the detection of SNPs, chromosomes' conformations or constitutions, aberrations from deletions and duplications, patterns or genomic waves, and the defining signals of CNVs, SNPs, and microsatellites across multiple loci,[61] that can yield a chromosome's genomic profile.[62,63] This work may make it feasible for researchers to chart the genes of a disease, associate the gene mutations within and across the genome, and predict the genes' influence on the expressed phenotype. By screening for a gene variant and predicting how it will manifest, whole-genome sequencing also may allow for proactive patient care. Through genomics, the process of whole-genome sequencing will facilitate population genotyping for a uniform and accurate examination of the diversity in human genetics.[64] The next step in advancing the process and application of whole-genome sequencing is understanding gene expression.

Gene Expression

Gene expression detects which genes are turned on and which are turned off. This process is necessary, as not all DNA is expressed in all tissues. Understanding the tightly regulated process of gene expression in normal human functioning provides important insights into disease states. In simple terms, gene expression refers to the complex process of DNA being transcribed to RNA and then being translated into a protein product. DNA contains many noncoded regions (introns) that are interspersed with regions that are coded for transcribed genes (exons). An intermediary messenger RNA (mRNA) undergoes splicing to remove introns so that the mRNA is composed of only the coded gene regions. The final protein product can be studied, although most researchers study mRNA transcripts. Because mRNA degrades more easily than DNA, it often is translated back into DNA (using reverse transcriptase) for easier handling. This translated form of DNA, known as cDNA, contains only the coded gene regions.[6]

DNA microarrays and the real-time, quantitative polymerase chain reaction allow for the study of gene expression. Microarray chips are ordered arrangements of DNA sequences or expressed sequence tags bound to a glass slide. Complementary DNA strands hybridize to these bound sequences and can be quantitatively detected with florescent tags. There are numerous platforms capable of interrogating thousands of genes simultaneously, and the technology continues to evolve. Beyond gene chips, glass beads can be tagged with DNA sequences to measure gene expression using flow cytometry–based approaches. More than 123,000 articles have been published on gene expression in the past 2 years. A few examples of discoveries based on such gene-expression studies are provided here.

Hypertension

Hypertension leads to changes in the vasculature and other potentially detrimental effects such as atherosclerosis, stroke, and renal disease. Anwar and colleagues[65] reviewed gene-expression changes caused by pressure-induced stretch injuries on the vascular walls in a variety of tissue types and cell cultures. Vascular wall stretching activates intracellular pathways and transcription factors that lead to the expression of genes that mediate cell growth and apoptosis, vasomotor and inflammatory response, and extracellular matrix metabolism. Continuous stretch results in upregulation of proinflammatory mediators through a nuclear factor κB–dependent pathway.[65] Understanding which genes are expressed, or not expressed, allows for better targeting of efforts to improve treatment strategies for the disease process being investigated.

Cancer

Cancer is a leading cause of morbidity and mortality, and has been the focus of intense research for decades. Expression profiling has helped to identify breast-tumor tissue of origin and classify breast cancer tumors more effectively than conventional histologic staining and immunohistochemistry estrogen and progesterone receptor staining.[66] Through expression studies, the Cancer Genome Atlas Network has identified

4 subtypes of breast cancer.[67] Expression profiles can be used to provide prognostic risk for relapse in early-stage breast cancer through signatures expressed in as few as 21 genes (Oncotype DX) or as many as 76 genes (Rotterdam signature).[66] Researchers have identified expression signatures with as few as 12 genes that can help predict the recurrence of colon cancer. The use of expression profiles is slowly changing the delivery of health care in the twenty-first century. Unfortunately, few expression studies have passed the rigorous testing needed for use in clinical practice (www.ClinicalTrial.gov), so most remain in the research arena. As more knowledge accumulates, more results will be translated into practice.

Treatment interventions

Several researchers have investigated changes in gene expression in response to treatment interventions. A well-known study by Ornish and colleagues[68] identified gene-expression changes in 501 genes (48 upregulated and 453 downregulated) among men undergoing intensive nutrition and lifestyle interventions. These findings highlighted areas where nursing interventions promoting health and lifestyle changes such as proper nutrition,[69] diet and exercise,[70] and smoking cessation,[71,72] can significantly influence gene expression. Furthermore, alternative health care approaches, such as acupuncture[73] and mind-body-spirit therapies,[74] also have been shown to result in changes in gene expression.

Epigenomics

Current understanding of gene regulation extends beyond DNA's nucleotide sequence and into the epigenetic changes (chemical and packaging modifications) that can affect gene transcription either positively or negatively.[75,76] Epigenomics is a rapidly growing field that provides insights into how the environment affects gene expression. An example is epigenetic studies on monozygotic twins. Older twin pairs have more epigenetic differences than do younger twin pairs. Researchers have attributed the differences primarily to unique environmental experiences by the twins over their lifetimes.[77] The extent to which the environment induces these changes and how epigenetics regulates gene expression is an emerging area of research.

Commonly investigated epigenetic biomarkers include DNA methylation, MicroRNAs, and posttranslational histone modifications. Epigenomics involves the study of neurodegenerative diseases, complex multifactorial diseases, rare diseases, and cancer.[78] The National Center for Biotechnology Information provides more information about the field and its common nomenclature at http://www.ncbi.nlm.nih.gov/epigenomics.

One epigenetic mechanism that warrants consideration is DNA methylation. The pattern of DNA methylation (hypermethylation or hypomethylation) plays an important role in many diseases. Common DNA methylation terms include Islands (CpG islands), Shores (methylated regions adjacent to the islands), Shelves (methylated regions beyond the shores), and Open Sea (other areas). CpG islands, highly conserved CpG-rich regions in DNA, have a crucial role in gene regulation.[79] Hypermethylation of cytosines within CpG islands works like an off-switch to silence transcription. Likewise, hypomethylation of normally methylated sites may promote transcription. The absence or presence of methylation can be detected through a process called bisulfate conversion followed by simple electrophoresis, or through a more rapid technique using DNA methylation microarrays. Recently, an array (Illumina's Infinium HumanMethylation450 BeadChip) capable of interrogating up to 450,000 CpG sites was validated using colorectal cancer and DNA methylation models.[80]

DNA is tightly packaged in chromosomes. **Fig. 3** shows how the DNA structure must be opened to reveal the familiar double-helix formation. Highly compact DNA is known as chromatin. For DNA to be processed, the DNA strands must be accessible to the "copying machinery" or transcription factors in the cell. Histones modification, which helps package and compact DNA, is another epigenetic mechanism that prevents or permits transcription-factor access to DNA for replication.

Epigenetic mechanisms have been used to investigate broad areas of functioning and disease, including neurobehavior, neurodevelopment, diabetes, obesity, cancer, and autoimmune, cardiovascular, Alzheimer, and infectious diseases, as well as how environmental signals induce DNA change.[81–83] These mechanisms deepen the understanding of gene regulation in disease and offer exciting new treatment possibilities.[84]

Gene Therapy

Although the concept of gene therapy has existed for more than 20 years, it has had limited practical success. Scientists first targeted inherited recessive disorders in

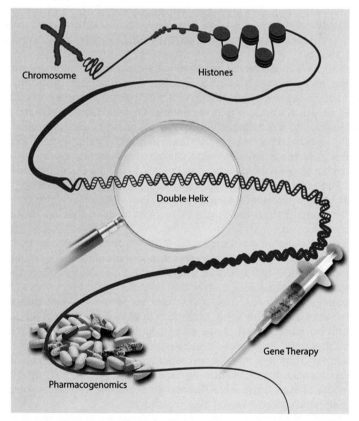

Fig. 3. DNA structure and treatment applications. DNA is tightly bound in the chromosome and wrapped around histones. Unpackaged DNA has the characteristic double-helix structure. The way individuals respond to drugs differs depending on their genetic code. These response variations are investigated through pharmacogenomics. Faulty DNA may be supplemented with normal DNA through gene therapy. (*Courtesy of* Greg R. Gaiker Jr, University of Tennessee, Knoxville, TN.)

hopes of transferring a normal gene copy to persons with a single defective gene.[85] Since that time the range of target diseases has increased, but serious immune dysfunction and deaths among some subjects, first occurring in 1999, halted some attempts and led researchers to proceed with caution.[86] According to a registry of publicly and privately funded research (www.ClinicalTrials.gov), there have been a huge number of gene-therapy studies, but only a handful have successfully reached the market.

The goal of gene therapy is to transfer normal genetic material via some type of vector to replace or augment the function of faulty genetic material. Traditionally, most vectors have been viral and have had high gene-delivery efficiency. The inability of these viral vectors to self-replicate limits the potential for unintended release. These replication-deficient viruses include the retrovirus, adenovirus, adeno-associated virus, and herpes simplex virus. Nonviral vectors are less immunogenic and have a flexible delivery size.[87] Of all the viral vectors, adenoviral vectors are the most studied. Lentiviral vectors are the most frequently studied retroviruses. These vectors are considered safe because they require several accessory viral proteins for infectivity, they can facilitate transfer through the nucleopore, and their replication is inhibited. Kamimura and colleagues[87] concluded that approximately 67% of trials used viral vectors and approximately 24% used nonviral vectors. Magnetic nanoparticles also have been proposed as a target for gene therapy, as they may allow imaging-monitored delivery.[88]

Researchers have made recent progress in therapies for CF, primary immunodeficiencies, the nervous system, ocular disease, and muscular dystrophy.[89–92] For example, it has been shown that the loss of the CF transmembrane conductase regulator (CFTR) adversely affects airway secretions. There is debate about the best therapy target to address this loss: surface epithelium or submucosal glands. More than 25 CF clinical trials have been completed using viral and nonviral vectors. Researchers have achieved success in a mouse model using an aerosolized, nonviral gene-transfer technique with a single-dose plasmid carrying the CFTR cDNA coupled with cationic lipid GL67. This technique is currently being tested in humans to determine if monthly dosing over 1 year improves CF lung disease.[92] Two viral vector weaknesses, immunogenicity and transient transgene expression, must be overcome before success can be established in clinical trials.

Primary immunodeficiencies include more than 300 genetic disorders that affect the immune system. The first to be treated was adenosine deaminase severe combined immunodeficiency (ADA-SCID). In this disorder, the faulty protein adenosine deaminase (ADA) allows toxic purine metabolites to build up in the thymus, negatively affecting lymphocyte function. There was early success using hematopoietic stem cell gammaretroviral gene therapy in patients with ADA-SCID as 29 of 40 participants (73%), combined from 3 small phase I/II clinical trials, no longer required enzyme replacement therapy.[91] Rivat and colleagues also summarized less successful gene therapy trials for 3 primary immunodeficiencies: X-linked severe combined immunodeficiency, chronic granulomatous disease, and Wiskott-Aldrich syndrome. The varying benefits of these trials were sometimes overshadowed by the development of T-cell acute lymphoblastic leukemia or myelodysplasia.

Despite the few successfully marketed gene therapies to date, the science continues to move forward as technology grows. Researchers face the dual challenges of the high cost of developing these therapies and the need to recruit and study large numbers of patients with sometimes rare genetic conditions. Success in developing and eventually implementing new gene therapies may depend in part on the market's ability to pay for therapies costing up to $300,000 per year or $1.6 million for a one-time injection.[93] In the meantime, the discovery of epigenetic mechanisms in gene regulation and investigations of new treatment strategies, such as histone deacetylases and methyl-donor–rich diets, are promising areas of research.[94]

Pharmacogenomics

Among genomic applications, pharmacogenomics holds the greatest promise to customize treatment based on an individual's unique drug response. The role of inherited genetic variation in drug response has been studied for more than half a century and research has mushroomed over the past decade, with more than 2500 related articles published in just the past 2 years.

The term pharmacogenomics was first coined in 1959 and first conceptualized in 1957.[95] In 1977, the pivotal discovery that cytochrome P450 oxidase in the liver controls debrisoquine and sparteine metabolism led to isolation of the responsible enzyme (CYP2D6). It is held that CYP2D6 is directly involved in one-fourth of all commonly used drugs. To date, researchers have identified more than 80 CYP2D6 enzyme variants and can make drug-response predictions based on a patient's genotype. However, these predictions are not based on individual pharmacokinetic measurements.[96] The enzyme superfamily cytochrome P450 (commonly called CYP) has several subfamilies. Researchers have identified 2 important 2C subfamilies, CPY2C19 and CYP2C9, as the cause of impaired mephenytoin metabolism and reduced clopidogrel metabolism, respectively. Racial variations in *CYP2C* gene metabolism also have been reported.[96]

Warfarin is one of the most commonly used anticoagulants (prescribed to 0.5%–1.5% of the population). One major problem with this drug's administration is the variation in interindividual dosages required to maintain the drug's therapeutic range (international normalized ratio 2.0–3.0) from less than 10 mg to more than 100 mg per week.[97] Strong evidence suggests that the starting dose of warfarin should be based on CYP2C9 and VKORC1 genotypes.[97,98] Candidate gene studies in the mid-1990s focused on the enzyme CPY2C9, which metabolizes warfarin. A person with the normal CPY2C9 genotype (*1/*1) metabolizes the drug much faster than a person with a severely impaired CPY2C9 genotype (*3/*3), with a striking half-life difference range of 30 to 37 hours and 92 to 203 hours, respectively. Much later, VKORC1 mutations were discovered that conferred sensitivity to warfarin.[98] In 2007, the Food and Drug Administration (FDA) modified the warfarin label to include optional dosing recommendations both with and without consideration of these genotypes. In general, persons with the CPY2C9 *3/*3 genotype should be started on a lower dose. The FDA now includes pharmacogenomic indications for drugs used to treat chronic hepatitis and CF.[99]

Researchers have identified another important application of pharmacogenomics in the area of human immunodeficiency virus (HIV) treatment. Individuals with allele variant T-cell 1 have an increased risk of hypersensitivity reaction to the anti-HIV drug abacavir. The presence of at least 1 HLA-B*57:01 allele is considered positive. It is estimated that up to 6% of patients will have an adverse, sometimes life-threatening, reaction; thus, screening is very important.[100]

Pharmacogenomics is the realization of personalized medicine: it uses a person's genetic information to guide individual treatment. An updated list of clinical pharmacogenomic implementation guidelines can be retrieved from http://www.pharmgkb.org/. As personalized medicine seeks to transform the care of patients with cardiovascular disease, cancer, and HIV, this is an exciting time for researchers and health care practitioners. Some have envisioned the future of personalized medicine to include access to a person's genetic profile in their electronic medical record (EMR) to guide treatment options. Hicks and colleagues[101] described methods of summarizing genetics variants in the EMR with interpretive consultation and actionable alerts. Clinical implementation has been challenged by a perceived lack of clinical utility, the need to develop and disseminate guidelines, and the need to increase insurance reimbursement for testing.[96] Meanwhile, data that may lead to additional discoveries among genes involved in drug metabolism and response continue to accumulate from genetic-association, gene-expression, proteomic, and metabolomic studies. Drug response is a complex trait. The study of functional genomics and network biology may provide important insights into this attribute.[102] In parallel with the mass of information waiting to be explored and applied, discerning consumers are pushing for provider utilization of such information through their increased use of DTC genetic testing.

Direct-to-Consumer Genetic Testing

Along with the rapid growth in genetics knowledge, there has been a dramatic increase in the number of companies offering a variety of genetic tests directly to consumers.[103–106] Most require the consumer to mail a simple saliva sample or cheek swab to the testing laboratory. Results usually are mailed to the consumer or offered via secure password-protected Web sites. Current offers range from personalized counseling about nutrition and exercise based on genetic information to direct testing for specific illnesses. These tests are usually genome-wide analyses that provide an estimate of one's risk for 1 or more, sometimes more than 100, diseases. Many of these kits are marketed directly to consumers by for-profit companies without requiring counseling with a health care professional before or after the test. Some kits do require a prescription.

Consumers may obtain results on tests for everything from ancestry and non–health-related traits, such as hair curl or sense of smell, to responses to drugs and risks for complex and life-threatening diseases. In addition to well-established genetic tests, there are options to participate in research on a broad range of areas including sexual orientation.[107] These tests measure susceptibility genes. Environmental and lifestyle factors are significant contributors to many of the tested conditions; this fact may or may not be clearly explained with the test results. In addition, some explanations of test results are easier to interpret than others.

Regulation of DTC testing is less specific than that for pharmaceuticals or medical equipment. In addition, reliability and validity data about most of the offered tests is not readily available to consumers. There are many potential positive outcomes of DTC genetic testing, such as motivation for lifestyle changes, relief about negative tests, and earlier diagnosis and treatment of conditions. However, the potential risks of false-negative results, increased anxiety, and unnecessary demand for health care must be considered. Several individuals and groups have called for industry-wide codes of practice and written informed consent for such testing.[103,104,106]

GENOMICS IN NURSING PRACTICE

Genetics/genomics should not be considered a specialty discipline, as it affects every point along the health to illness continuum. This fact makes advances in genetics/genomics relevant to all nurses regardless of educational preparation or practice setting. As part of the largest health care profession, nurses are in a key position to integrate the latest genetic/genomic technologies and information into their daily practice, whether at the bedside, in the classroom, or with policy makers. In 2010, Calzone and colleagues[108] published a white paper describing how nurses are transforming the United States health care system using genetics and genomics. This document highlighted the impact of genetics and genomics on nursing research, education, insurance/reimbursement, and policy. It also provided strategies and solutions for addressing current knowledge gaps. Although tremendous strides have been made to prepare nurses in the United States to be competent in genetics and genomics, several factors complicate these efforts: a critical shortage of nurses; scarce resources to meet the needs of educators, practitioners, and policy makers; increasing patient acuity; and exponential advances in the science of genetics/genomics.[108] The "omics" revolution—the exploration of large biological datasets—has revolutionized medicine and will continue to do so. However, the more important issue is resolving the challenging debate about how to apply information from large biological data sets to the care of individuals or groups of patients. As a profession, nursing lies at the crux of this debate.

Nursing Education

In the last 2 years, several authors have published comprehensive articles describing the importance of genomics in nursing education. Many of these were part of a 2-year series on genetics and genomics in the *Journal of Nursing Scholarship*.[109–114] In the United States, competencies published by consensus through the American Nurses Association (ANA) serve as benchmarks for curricular guidelines and outcome indicators for practicing registered nurses (RNs)[115] and nurses with graduate degrees.[116] Competencies for the practicing RNs center around 4 major areas: nursing assessment; identification; referral activities; and provision of education, care, and support.[115] Similarly, the 38 competencies specific to advanced practice nurses build on those for RNs and fall into the following categories: risk assessment and interpretation; genetic education, counseling, testing, and results interpretation; clinical management; ethical, legal, and social implications; professional role; leadership; and research.[116] The National Coalition for Health Professional Education in Genetics (NCHPEG) issued competencies for the interdisciplinary health care workforce.[117]

Nurses face many challenges in meeting the essentials presented in these documents. Studies have cited several factors that contribute to the lack of progress in including genetics/genomics in nursing education[109–111,118]:

- An underappreciation of the relevance of genetics/genomics to nursing practice
- The fact that competency expectations seem daunting
- A lack of nursing faculty prepared to teach genetics content
- A lack of licensure or relicensure competency requirements by state boards of nursing
- A lack of emphasis of genetics/genomics in certification exams
- Overcrowded curricula

A 2012 study of faculty readiness to integrate genomic content into curricula demonstrated that, while most faculty had positive feelings about the *2008 Essentials of Genetic and Genomic Nursing: Competencies Curricula Guidelines, and Outcome Indicators* (2008 Essentials),[115] the majority felt unprepared to teach genetics/genomic content, rating their genetics/genomics knowledge as low or very low. Most respondents failed to answer the question about their intentions to include genetics/genomics information in their course or curricular materials.[119]

Another investigation sought to determine the extent to which the 2008 Essentials had been implemented by nurse faculty and researchers attending the Council for Advancement of Nursing Science conference.[120] Although the sample size was small and biased toward faculty members and researchers, most respondents reported not having read the 2008 Essentials and that their institution was not meeting the competencies.[120]

Researchers have proposed strategies to help prepare faculty to integrate genomics into nursing education,[111,121] including offering content delivery models.[109] Williams and colleagues[111] described successful strategies that were used in the United States and United Kingdom to enhance faculty preparedness in genetics/genomics, including having faculty participate in a genetics/genomics faculty champion network, and receive doctoral, postdoctoral, and continuing education. Daack-Hirsch and colleagues[109] proposed models to integrate the genetics/genomics essentials into nursing curricula based on published literature and anecdotal experience. Suggested models include creating a curriculum thread or a stand-alone required or elective course. The investigators also discussed covering genetics/genomics content via simulation in the clinical practicum setting or through the dissemination of printed and technological resources.[117] Other teaching strategies, including the use of case studies, storytelling, online genomics resources, student self-assessment, guest lecturers, and genetic focus groups, have also been shown to be effective.[121] Shuster[122] proposed integrating the 2008 Essentials into a prenursing microbiology course. In another study, faculty were encouraged to refer to published resources for genomic education.[112]

Redefining and Strengthening Evidence-Based Nursing Practice

Rapid technological advances in whole-genome sequencing will cause an inevitable increase in the use of genomic information in clinical patient care. This shift will have a profound effect on disease prevention, screening, diagnosis, prognosis, treatment selection, and treatment efficacy. Several single-gene tests have already been incorporated into patient care, especially in oncology. For example, individuals identified to be at high risk based on personal and family history can choose to have genetic testing for hereditary breast ovarian cancer syndrome, Lynch syndrome, familial adenomatous polyposis, and others. The health care profession continues to face the challenge of translating rapidly advancing genomic technologies into clinical patient care. Furthermore, health practitioners must confront the possibly dramatic yet unknown impact that such genomic information will have on patients' psychosocial outcomes. In many ways, history is repeating itself. When single-gene tests were first introduced, there was little known about how to share the genetic information with patients and about how patients would then communicate disease risk to their family members. While these knowledge gaps are beginning to close, there is little time to "catch up" and investigate the impact genetic information will have on the health care providers who deliver it and the patients who receive it. At present, there is even a lack of evidence about how genetic information benefits patients. A recently published editorial addressed these issues and cited nurse faculty as being vital in the process of preparing future generations of nurses to take on these challenges.[113]

Interpreting and Delivering Genomic Information

In July 2011, the Institute of Medicine (IOM) hosted a workshop to explore the integration of large-scale genomic information into clinical practice.[123] The content highlighted the implications of the interpretation and delivery of genomic information, as well as health professional workforce development and ethical issues. One section of the report set forth 4 clinical vignettes to demonstrate how genomic information may be applied in the future. In one vignette about an older patient with asthma, genomic information was used to determine the specific condition subtype and identify pharmacogenomic treatment recommendations. In another vignette, a couple has each of their genomes tested for serious congenital disorders before conceiving a child. The report raised the important point that genomic information often provides more data than the clinician is able to address. Therefore, clinicians will need to learn how to filter the information for data that is applicable and usable. In essence, clinicians will need to integrate genomics in a way that does not necessarily change patient care, but improves it.[123] For this to happen, the health care industry will need to address several regulatory issues and develop an infrastructure capable of generating, storing, and interpreting genomic data. Before genomic data is given to a patient it must be determined to have both clinical and social utility, and be packaged in a format clinicians can interpret that also is sensitive to the privacy issues of health care data sharing, including the use of EMRs.[123]

Implications for Nursing Practice

Integrating genetic/genomics into the nursing care of patients imposes certain challenges. In 2012, Calzone and colleagues[114] published the results of a survey exploring these challenges using a Web-based, investigator-constructed, 43-item instrument. A convenience sample of practicing nurses was surveyed to assess their attitudes, practices, receptivity, confidence, and competency in integrating genomics into nursing practice. The findings revealed that, while acknowledging that genetic knowledge was an important aspect in the optimal care of patients, 81% of nurses rated their understanding of the genetics of common diseases as fair or poor, and reported feeling ill-prepared to care for the genomic aspects of their patients' diseases.

Investigators have described the use of genomic-focused nursing assessments as an important intersection of the nursing process and genomic competencies.[124] Some of genomic assessments regularly conducted by nurses include obtaining a family history and constructing/updating a 3-generation family genogram. Other emerging assessments include[124]:

- Asking patients about environmental factors that might influence gene expression
- Evaluating clinical data relating to genomic conditions
- Asking patients if they desire to know more about the genetics of a certain condition
- Discussing preventive measures for genomic conditions
- Providing genetic referrals, if indicated

Further emphasis has been placed on nurses becoming proficient in applying biomarkers for certain specialties (eg, oncology),[125] and using pharmacogenomics and nutrigenomics to care for patients with chronic illnesses.[126]

Pestka and colleagues[124] published the findings of a study exploring nurses' perceived benefits, barriers, and educational recommendations for using family genograms in the clinical setting. The study used a qualitative design with focus groups. In general, nurses cited the benefits of the use of family genograms in the clinical setting as being the positive outcomes for patients and families, and strong support for the tool in primary care. Nurse respondents also emphasized that the genogram format should be electronic and easy to access/complete in a short amount of time. Barriers cited were the time-consuming nature of constructing a genogram and a lack of knowledge and confidence in constructing a genogram. Although nurses generally supported the use of genograms in clinical practice, they placed the biggest emphasis on obtaining more evidence for the defined patient benefits of using the tool.[124]

Ethical, Legal, and Social Issues

Expanding the understanding of genetics comes with many related ethical, legal, and social issues (ELSI). The HGP stimulated the hope that genetic aberrations causing physical and mental illnesses and disabilities could soon be identified, treated, and possibly prevented by gene manipulation or genetic sequencing. This hope must be tempered with the risk of genetic differences being used to foster ethnic stereotypes or stigmatize groups by race or other characteristics. The practice of eugenics—the attempt to rid society of negatively perceived physical, social, and intellectual characteristics believed to be caused by defective genes—resulted in such atrocities as forced sterilization and the genocide of millions in Nazi Germany.[127] Clearly, the enthusiasm for scientific advances and the possibilities of eliminating diseases should be balanced with the perils of stigmatizing and discriminating against any group or individual.

When the HGP began in 1990, those involved recognized the imperative to address the legal, ethical, and social issues related to this new understanding of genetics and an individual's genetic information. For this reason, the National Human Genome Research Institute (NHGRI) established the Ethical Legal and Social Implications Research Program just as the HGP commenced. This program established 4 research priorities[128,129]:

1. *Genomic research*, focusing on issues of design and conduct of genomic research
2. *Genomic health care*, focusing on the effect of genetic information on the provision of health care
3. *Broader social issues*, including how the understanding of health, disease, and individual responsibility may be affected by genomics research
4. *Legal, regulatory, and public policy issues*, focusing on the effect this research will have on current and future policies and regulations

The program also provided funding for research and educational programming related to these priorities.

In 2008, The US Congress passed, and President George W. Bush signed into law, the Genetic Information Nondiscrimination Act of 2008 (GINA) (P.L. 110-233, 122 Stat.881), which prohibits discrimination in health coverage and employment based on genetic information. While some state laws offer even more protection against discrimination, GINA requires that all states must comply, at a minimum, with the Act's provisions that prohibit requiring genetic information from a person or family member or using such information in decisions about health coverage, rates, or identification of preexisting conditions. These protections do not extend to noncivilians such as US Military personnel and veterans.[130] For this Act, genetic information includes genetic testing and family history data, as well as any request for or receipt of genetic counseling. The Act does not offer the same protections concerning life, disability, or long-term care insurance, or require coverage for any genetic testing. Companies with fewer than 15 employees are exempt, and health insurers may use genetic test results in making payment determinations for health care claims.[129,131] Whereas GINA prohibits discrimination based on results from a genetic test for disease risk, it is silent about other tests or consultations such as mental health counseling or blood tests associated with increased disease risk. Nurses should keep apprised of GINA specifics and changes so as to provide clear and accurate information to patients and their families.

Several additional ethical issues were addressed during the 2011 IOM workshop. Attendees discussed the importance of health care providers disclosing genomic information to patients in person rather than through a written report or phone call. One of the complicating issues in delivering genomic information is that it takes hours for providers to cover all of the clinically significant gene variants.[123] In an already rushed health care system, keeping the disclosure strictly within the clinician-patient relationship may not be feasible. Furthermore, practitioners must consider how receiving so much detailed information will affect a patient's anxiety levels about future health concerns. Certainly, privacy issues with electronic medical/health records and patient access to genomic tests/personalized medicine data must also be critically evaluated.[123] Other issues identified during the 2011 ELSI Congress included the blurring of boundaries between research and treatment, the uncertainty surrounding the incomplete nature of genomic information, and the debate between scientific and nonscientific stakeholders in determining the priorities for biomedical research.[132]

The use of genetics/genomics in patient care likely will expand and complicate existing concerns about equity of and access to health care. In other words, will all individuals have access to genetic/genomic tests? Many such questions remain, especially given the pending implementation of the 2010 Patient Protection and Affordable Care Act (ACA).[133] In fact, the entire 905-page ACA document used the word genomics only once. It is also unclear whether the ACA and GINA will work in parallel or at cross purposes. The ethical debate about "duty to warn" (ie, whether a health care provider should notify patient's family members about the risk for genetic health problems) also will persist with the use of genomics.[134] Providers need to remain mindful of the balance between caring for the patient, or proband, and the impact the patient's genetic/genomic information will have on other family members.

While the ACA requires insurance to cover clinician counseling about genetic testing for *BRCA* mutations for women at higher risk for breast cancer, it does not cover the actual testing itself. Preventive services for those at higher risk of cancer arising from their family history are covered. The law prohibits insurance companies from using genetic information or newborn screening results to determine rates (http://www.healthcare.gov/law/).

Health care providers must understand and consider these issues in patient care, in every setting. Understanding the science of genetics is critical for nurse clinicians, scientists, and educators. No less critical is understanding the legal and ethical issues that this knowledge creates.

SUMMARY

Nurses should realize that the presence of high-risk genotypes is not always associated with future disease, particularly in complex diseases involving multiple genes. There are still many unknowns about the complexity of the human genetic code, such as how genes interact with one another and the environment to manifest differential expressions of disease and health. Although there is not a genetic test for every disease, the ability to determine disease risk will continue to advance with genomics. While there is ample room for progress in the area of gene therapy, scientists have been successful in harnessing genetics knowledge to target optimal drug therapy based on an individual's genotypes. As health care consumers become more knowledgable and continue to engage the marketplace to determine their genetic risks and phamacogenomic profiles, the health care industry must work to keep up. Technological advances in genetics have created ethical and legal dilemmas, which likely will become more complicated as more advances are achieved. Nurse clinicians, scientists, and educators in the twenty-first century will be challenged to remain informed of the issues, become proficient in genetic competencies, and provide the best available evidenced-based care to patients.

ACKNOWLEDGMENTS

The authors are grateful to Dr Sandra Thomas and Ms Laurie Wyatt for their editorial reviews and critiques, and to Mr Greg R. Gaiker Jr for creating the illustrations used in this article.

REFERENCES

1. Lorentz CP, Wieben ED, Tefferi A, et al. Primer on medical genomics part I: history of genetics and sequencing of the human genome. Mayo Clin Proc 2002; 77(8):773–82.
2. Mikail CN. Public health genomics: the essentials. San Francisco (CA): Jossey-Bass; 2008.
3. Beery T, Workman M. Genetics and genomics in nursing and health care. Philadelphia: FA Davis; 2012.
4. Nickla H, Klung WS, Cummings MR. Essentials of genetics student handbook & solutions manual. 5th edition. Upper Saddle River (NJ): Pearson Prentice Hall; 2004.
5. Hartl DL. Essential genetics: a genomics perspective. Sudbury (MA): Jones and Barlett; 2012.
6. Hartl DL, Jones EW. Genetics: analysis of genes and genomes. 6th edition. Sudbury (MA): Jones and Barlett; 2005.
7. McPhee SJ, Hammer GD. Pathophysiology of disease: an introduction to clinical medicine. New York: McGraw Hill; 2010.
8. Tobias ES, Conner M, Ferguson-Smith M. Essential medical genetics. 6th edition. Hoboken (NJ): Wiley Blackwell; 2011.
9. Barsh G. Genetic disease. In: McPhee SJ, Hammer GD, editors. Pathophysiology of disease: an introduction to clinical medicine. New York: McGraw Hill; 2010. p. 2–29.
10. Guttmacher AE, Collins FS, Carmona RH. The family history—more important than ever. N Engl J Med 2004;351(22):2333–6.
11. Anderson CD, Biffi A, Rost NS, et al. Chromosome 9p21 in ischemic stroke: population structure and meta-analysis. Stroke 2010;41(6):1123–31.
12. Lemmens R, Buysschaert I, Geelen V, et al. The association of the 4q25 susceptibility variant for atrial fibrillation with stroke is limited to stroke of cardioembolic etiology. Stroke 2010;41(9):1850–7.
13. Gudbjartsson DF, Holm H, Gretarsdottir S, et al. A sequence variant in ZFHX3 on 16q22 associates with atrial fibrillation and ischemic stroke. Nat Genet 2009; 41(8):876–8.
14. Froguel P, Vaxillaire M, Sun F, et al. Close linkage of glucokinase locus on chromosome 7p to early-onset non-insulin-dependent diabetes mellitus. Nature 1992;356(6365):162–4.
15. Garay-Sevilla ME, Nava LE, Malacara JM, et al. Advanced glycosylation end products (AGEs), insulin-like growth factor-1 (IGF-1) and IGF-binding protein-3 (IGFBP-3) in patients with type 2 diabetes mellitus. Diabetes Metab Res Rev 2000;16(2):106–13.
16. Laakso M, Malkki M, Kekalainen P, et al. Glucokinase gene variants in subjects with late-onset NIDDM and impaired glucose tolerance. Diabetes Care 1995; 18(3):398–400.

17. Vozarova B, Fernandez-Real JM, Knowler WC, et al. The interleukin-6 (-174) G/C promoter polymorphism is associated with type-2 diabetes mellitus in Native Americans and Caucasians. Hum Genet 2003;112(4):409–13.
18. Thomas NS, Holgate ST. Candidate locus approach for studying the genetics of asthma and atopy. Monaldi Arch Chest Dis 1997;52(3):296–302.
19. Elkins JS, Douglas VC, Johnston SC. Alzheimer disease risk and genetic variation in ACE: a meta-analysis. Neurology 2004;62(3):363–8.
20. Skeehan K, Heaney C, Cook-Deegan R. Impact of gene patents and licensing practices on access to genetic testing for Alzheimer disease. Genet Med 2010;12(Suppl 4):S71–82.
21. Vargas-Alarcon G, Zamora J, Sanchez-Garcia S, et al. Angiotensin-I-converting enzyme (ACE) insertion/deletion polymorphism in Mexican patients with coronary artery disease. Association with the disease but not with lipid levels. Exp Mol Pathol 2006;81(2):131–5.
22. Bouzekri N, Zhu X, Jiang Y, et al. Angiotensin I-converting enzyme polymorphisms, ACE level and blood pressure among Nigerians, Jamaicans and African-Americans. Eur J Hum Genet 2004;12(6):460–8.
23. Uhm WS, Lee HS, Chung YH, et al. Angiotensin-converting enzyme gene polymorphism and vascular manifestations in Korean patients with SLE. Lupus 2002;11(4):227–33.
24. Tadokoro K, Akutsu Y, Tanaka K, et al. Comparative quantitative analysis of 14 types of human papillomavirus by real-time polymerase chain reaction monitoring Invader reaction (Q-Invader assay). Diagn Microbiol Infect Dis 2010;66(1):58–64.
25. Burd EM. Human papillomavirus and cervical cancer. Clin Microbiol Rev 2003;16(1):1–17.
26. Ward TJ, Ducey TF, Usgaard T, et al. Multilocus genotyping assays for single nucleotide polymorphism-based subtyping of *Listeria monocytogenes* isolates. Appl Environ Microbiol 2008;74(24):7629–42.
27. Rasko DA, Worsham PL, Abshire TG, et al. *Bacillus anthracis* comparative genome analysis in support of the Amerithrax investigation. Proc Natl Acad Sci U S A 2011;108(12):5027–32.
28. Taboada EN, Ross SL, Mutschall SK, et al. Development and validation of a comparative genomic fingerprinting method for high-resolution genotyping of *Campylobacter jejuni*. J Clin Microbiol 2012;50(3):788–97.
29. Gleen K, Du ZQ, Eisenmann JC, et al. An alternative method for genotyping of the ACE I/D polymorphism. Mol Biol Rep 2009;36:1305–10.
30. Bhatnagar P, Gupta S, Guleria R, et al. beta2-Adrenergic receptor polymorphisms and asthma in the North Indian population. Pharmacogenomics 2005;6(7):713–9.
31. Leak TS, Langefeld CD, Keene KL, et al. Chromosome 7p linkage and association study for diabetes related traits and type 2 diabetes in an African-American population enriched for nephropathy. BMC Med Genet 2010;11:22.
32. Simon-Sanchez J, Kilarski LL, Nalls MA, et al. Cooperative genome-wide analysis shows increased homozygosity in early onset Parkinson's disease. PLoS One 2012;7(3):e28787.
33. McBride MW, Graham D, Delles C, et al. Functional genomics in hypertension. Curr Opin Nephrol Hypertens 2006;15(2):145–51.
34. Murabito JM, White CC, Kavousi M, et al. Association between chromosome 9p21 variants and the ankle-brachial index identified by a meta-analysis of 21 genome-wide association studies. Circ Cardiovasc Genet 2012;5(1):100–12.

35. Berthier-Schaad Y, Kao WH, Coresh J, et al. Reliability of high-throughput gen-otyping of whole genome amplified DNA in SNP genotyping studies. Electro-phoresis 2007;28(16):2812–7.
36. Macgregor S, Zhao ZZ, Henders A, et al. Highly cost-efficient genome-wide as-sociation studies using DNA pools and dense SNP arrays. Nucleic Acids Res 2008;36(6):e35.
37. Wiltshire S, de Bakker PI, Daly MJ. The value of gene-based selection of tag SNPs in genome-wide association studies. Eur J Hum Genet 2006;14(11): 1209–14.
38. Sigurdsson S, Hedman M, Sistonen P, et al. A microarray system for genotyping 150 single nucleotide polymorphisms in the coding region of human mitochon-drial DNA. Genomics 2006;87(4):534–42.
39. Meschia JF. Ischaemic stroke: one or several complex genetic disorders? Lancet Neurol 2003;2(8):459.
40. Steer S, Abkevich V, Gutin A, et al. Genomic DNA pooling for whole-genome association scans in complex disease: empirical demonstration of efficacy in rheumatoid arthritis. Genes Immun 2007;8(1):57–68.
41. Bentley G, Higuchi R, Hoglund B, et al. High-resolution, high-throughput HLA gen-otyping by next-generation sequencing. Tissue Antigens 2009;74(5):393–403.
42. Schymick JC, Scholz SW, Fung HC, et al. Genome-wide genotyping in amyotro-phic lateral sclerosis and neurologically normal controls: first stage analysis and public release of data. Lancet Neurol 2007;6(4):322–8.
43. Piedmont and Valle d'Aosta Register for Amyotrophic Lateral Sclerosis (PARALS). Incidence of ALS in Italy: evidence for a uniform frequency in West-ern countries. Neurology 2001;56(2):239–44.
44. Wilkening S, Chen B, Bermejo JL, et al. Is there still a need for candidate gene approaches in the era of genome-wide association studies? Genomics 2009; 93(5):415–9.
45. Chanda P, Yuhki N, Li M, et al. Comprehensive evaluation of imputation perfor-mance in African Americans. J Hum Genet 2012;57(7):411–21.
46. Levy HL. Newborn screening conditions: what we know, what we do not know, and how we will know it. Genet Med 2010;12(Suppl 12):S213–4.
47. Deluca J, Zanni KL, Bonhomme N, et al. Implications of newborn screening for nurses. J Nurs Scholarsh 2013;45(1):25–33.
48. Thapar A, O'Donovan M, Owen MJ. The genetics of attention deficit hyperactiv-ity disorder. Hum Mol Genet 2005;14(Spec No 2):R275–82.
49. Lionel AC, Crosbie J, Barbosa N, et al. Rare copy number variation discovery and cross-disorder comparisons identify risk genes for ADHD. Sci Transl Med 2011;3(95):95ra75.
50. Cannon TD, Kaprio J, Lonnqvist J, et al. The genetic epidemiology of schizo-phrenia in a Finnish twin cohort. A population-based modeling study. Arch Gen Psychiatry 1998;55(1):67–74.
51. Aberg K, Saetre P, Lindholm E, et al. Human QKI, a new candidate gene for schizophrenia involved in myelination. Am J Med Genet B Neuropsychiatr Genet 2006;141B(1):84–90.
52. Chandrasekharan S, Heaney C, James T, et al. Impact of gene patents and licensing practices on access to genetic testing for cystic fibrosis. Genet Med 2010;12(Suppl 4):S194–211.
53. Colaianni A, Chandrasekharan S, Cook-Deegan R. Impact of gene patents and licensing practices on access to genetic testing and carrier screening for Tay-Sachs and Canavan disease. Genet Med 2010;12(Suppl 4):S5–14.

54. Chandrasekharan S, Pitlick E, Heaney C, et al. Impact of gene patents and licensing practices on access to genetic testing for hereditary hemochromatosis. Genet Med 2010;12(4 Suppl):S155–70.
55. Kang Y, Dong X, Zhou Q, et al. Identification of novel candidate maternal serum protein markers for Down syndrome by integrated proteomic and bioinformatic analysis. Prenat Diagn 2012;32(3):284–92.
56. Papageorgiou EA, Karagrigoriou A, Tsaliki E, et al. Fetal-specific DNA methylation ratio permits noninvasive prenatal diagnosis of trisomy 21. Nat Med 2011;17(4):510–3.
57. Ogilvie V, Passmore M, Hyndman L, et al. Differential global gene expression in cystic fibrosis nasal and bronchial epithelium. Genomics 2011;98(5):327–36.
58. Pyeritz RE. Evaluation of the adolescent or adult with some features of Marfan syndrome. Genet Med 2012;14(1):171–7.
59. Vylet'al P, Kublova M, Kalbacova M, et al. Alterations of uromodulin biology: a common denominator of the genetically heterogeneous FJHN/MCKD syndrome. Kidney Int 2006;70(6):1155–69.
60. Srivatsan A, Han Y, Peng J, et al. High-precision, whole-genome sequencing of laboratory strains facilitates genetic studies. PLoS Genet 2008;4(8):e1000139.
61. Diskin SJ, Li M, Hou C, et al. Adjustment of genomic waves in signal intensities from whole-genome SNP genotyping platforms. Nucleic Acids Res 2008;36(19):e126.
62. Peiffer DA, Le JM, Steemers FJ, et al. High-resolution genomic profiling of chromosomal aberrations using Infinium whole-genome genotyping. Genome Res 2006;16(9):1136–48.
63. Xing J, Watkins WS, Zhang Y, et al. High fidelity of whole-genome amplified DNA on high-density single nucleotide polymorphism arrays. Genomics 2008;92(6):452–6.
64. Xing J, Watkins WS, Shlien A, et al. Toward a more uniform sampling of human genetic diversity: a survey of worldwide populations by high-density genotyping. Genomics 2010;96(4):199–210.
65. Anwar MA, Shalhoub J, Lim CS, et al. The effect of pressure-induced mechanical stretch on vascular wall differential gene expression. J Vasc Res 2012;49(6):463–78.
66. McDermott U, Downing JR, Stratton MR. Genomics and the continuum of cancer care. N Engl J Med 2011;364(4):340–50.
67. Cancer Genome Atlas Network. Comprehensive molecular portraits of human breast tumors. Nature 2012;490(7418):61–70.
68. Ornish D, Magbanua MJ, Weidner G, et al. Changes in prostate gene expression in men undergoing an intensive nutrition and lifestyle intervention. Proc Natl Acad Sci U S A 2008;105(24):8369–74.
69. Kaput J, Rodriguez RL. Nutritional genomics: the next frontier in the postgenomic era. Physiol Genomics 2004;16(2):166–77.
70. Campbell KL, Foster-Schubert KE, Makar KW, et al. Gene expression changes in adipose tissue with diet- and/or exercise-induced weight loss. Cancer Prev Res (Phila) 2013;6(3):217–31.
71. Morozumi T, Kubota T, Sugita N, et al. Alterations of gene expression in human neutrophils induced by smoking cessation. J Clin Periodontol 2004;31(12):1110–6.
72. Zhang X, Lenburg ME, Spira A. Comparison of nasal epithelial smoking-induced gene expression on Affymetrix Exon 1.0 and Gene 1.0 ST arrays. ScientificWorldJournal 2013;2013:951416.

73. Shiue HS, Lee YS, Tsai CN, et al. Gene expression profile of patients with phadiatop-positive and -negative allergic rhinitis treated with acupuncture. J Altern Complement Med 2010;16(1):59–68.
74. Rossi EL. Psychosocial genomics: gene expression, neurogenesis, and human experience in mind-body medicine. Adv Mind Body Med 2002;18(2):22–30.
75. Conley YP, Biesecker LG, Gonsalves S, et al. Current and emerging technology approaches in genomics. J Nurs Scholarsh 2013;45(1):5–14.
76. Mazzio EA, Soliman KF. Basic concepts of epigenetics: impact of environmental signals on gene expression. Epigenetics 2012;7(2):119–30.
77. Talens RP, Christensen K, Putter H, et al. Epigenetic variation during the adult lifespan: cross-sectional and longitudinal data on monozygotic twin pairs. Aging Cell 2012;11(4):694–703.
78. Garcia-Gimenez JL, Sanchis-Gomar F, Lippi G, et al. Epigenetic biomarkers: a new perspective in laboratory diagnostics. Clin Chim Acta 2012;413(19–20):1576–82.
79. Singh H. Teeing up transcription on CpG islands. Cell 2009;138(1):14–6.
80. Sandoval J, Heyn H, Moran S, et al. Validation of a DNA methylation microarray for 450,000 CpG sites in the human genome. Epigenetics 2011;6(6):692–702.
81. Dawson MA, Kouzarides T, Huntly BJ. Targeting epigenetic readers in cancer. N Engl J Med 2012;367(7):647–57.
82. Hardison RC. Genome-wide epigenetic data facilitate understanding of disease susceptibility association studies. J Biol Chem 2012;287(37):30932–40.
83. Tollefsbos T. Epigenetics in human disease. Oxford (United Kingdom): Elsevier; 2012.
84. Jakovcevski M, Akbarian S. Epigenetic mechanisms in neurological disease. Nat Med 2012;18(8):1194–204.
85. Vachani A, Moon E, Wakeam E, et al. Gene therapy for lung neoplasms. Clin Chest Med 2011;32(4):865–85.
86. Evans CH, Ghivizzani SC, Robbins PD. Arthritis gene therapy's first death. Arthritis Res Ther 2008;10(3):110.
87. Kamimura K, Suda T, Zhang G, et al. Advances in gene delivery systems. Pharmaceut Med 2011;25(5):293–306.
88. Li C, Li L, Keates AC. Targeting cancer gene therapy with magnetic nanoparticles. Oncotarget 2012;3(4):365–70.
89. Bowers WJ, Breakefield XO, Sena-Esteves M. Genetic therapy for the nervous system. Hum Mol Genet 2011;20(R1):R28–41.
90. Goyenvalle A, Seto JT, Davies KE, et al. Therapeutic approaches to muscular dystrophy. Hum Mol Genet 2011;20(R1):R69–78.
91. Rivat C, Santilli G, Gaspar HB, et al. Gene therapy for primary immunodeficiencies. Hum Gene Ther 2012;23(7):668–75.
92. Sinn PL, Anthony RM, McCray PB Jr. Genetic therapies for cystic fibrosis lung disease. Hum Mol Genet 2011;20(R1):R79–86.
93. Whalen J. Gene-therapy approval marks major milestone. Wall St J 2012. Available at: http://online.wsj.com/article/SB10001424052970203707604578095091940871524.html. Accessed March 22, 2013.
94. Day JJ, Sweatt JD. Epigenetic treatments for cognitive impairments. Neuropsychopharmacology 2012;37(1):247–60.
95. Vessell ES. Drug therapy, pharmacogenetics. N Engl J Med 1972;287(18):904–9.
96. Scott SA. Personalizing medicine with clinical pharmacogenetics. Genet Med 2011;13(12):987–95.

97. Eriksson N, Wadelius M. Prediction of warfarin dose: why, when and how? Pharmacogenomics 2012;13(4):429–40.
98. Carlquist JF, Anderson JL. Using pharmacogenetics in real time to guide warfarin initiation: a clinician update. Circulation 2011;124(23):2554–9.
99. Auffray C, Caulfield T, Khoury MJ, et al. 2012 highlights in translational 'omics. Genome Med 2013;5(1):10.
100. Martin MA, Klein TE, Dong BJ, et al. Clinical pharmacogenetics implementation consortium guidelines for HLA-B genotype and abacavir dosing. Clin Pharmacol Ther 2012;91(4):734–8.
101. Hicks JK, Crews KR, Hoffman JM, et al. A clinician-driven automated system for integration of pharmacogenetic interpretations into an electronic medical record. Clin Pharmacol Ther 2012;92(5):563–6.
102. Kasarskis A, Yang X, Schadt E. Integrative genomics strategies to elucidate the complexity of drug response. Pharmacogenomics 2011;12(12):1695–715.
103. Bunnik EM, Janssens AC, Schermer MH. Informed consent in direct-to-consumer personal genome testing: the outline of a model between specific and generic consent. Bioethics 2012. [Epub ahead of print].
104. Janssens AC, Gwinn M, Bradley LA, et al. A critical appraisal of the scientific basis of commercial genomic profiles used to assess health risks and personalize health interventions. Am J Hum Genet 2008;82(3):593–9.
105. Myers MF. Health care providers and direct-to-consumer access and advertising of genetic testing in the United States. Genome Med 2011;3(12):81.
106. European Academies Science Advisory Council. Direct-to-consumer genetic testing for health-related purposes in the European Union. 2012. Available at: http://www.easac.eu/home/reports-and-statements/detail-view/article/direct-to-co.html. Accessed January 12, 2013.
107. Anderson-Minshall D. Can Your Genes Explain Sexual Orientation? The Advocate 2012;2. Available at: http://www.advocate.com/print-issue/current-issue/2012/10/30/can-your-genes-explain-sexual-orientation. Accessed March 22, 2013.
108. Calzone KA, Cashion A, Feetham S, et al. Nurses transforming health care using genetics and genomics. Nurs Outlook 2010;58(1):26–35.
109. Daack-Hirsch S, Dieter C, Quinn Griffin MT. Integrating genomics into undergraduate nursing education. J Nurs Scholarsh 2011;43(3):223–30.
110. Kirk M, Calzone K, Arimori N, et al. Genetics-genomics competencies and nursing regulation. J Nurs Scholarsh 2011;43(2):107–16.
111. Williams JK, Prows CA, Conley YP, et al. Strategies to prepare faculty to integrate genomics into nursing education programs. J Nurs Scholarsh 2011;43(3):231–8.
112. Tonkin E, Calzone K, Jenkins J, et al. Genomic education resources for nursing faculty. J Nurs Scholarsh 2011;43(4):330–40.
113. Jenkins J, Bednash G, Malone B. Bridging the gap between genomics discoveries and clinical care: nurse faculty are key. J Nurs Scholarsh 2011;43(1):1–2.
114. Calzone KA, Jenkins J, Yates J, et al. Survey of nursing integration of genomics into nursing practice. J Nurs Scholarsh 2012;44(4):428–36.
115. Consensus Panel on Genetic/Genomic Nurse Competencies. Essentials of genetic and genomic nursing: competencies curricula guidelines, and outcome indicators. 2nd edition. Silver Spring (MD): American Nurses Association; 2009.
116. Greco K, Tinley S, Seibert D. Essential genetic and genomic competencies for nurses with graduate degrees. 2nd edition. Silver Spring (MD): American Nurses Association and International Society of Nurses in Genetics; 2012.

117. National Coalition for Health Professional Education in Genetics. Core competencies in genetics for health professionals. 3rd edition. 2007. Available at: http://www.nchpeg.org/index.php?option=com_content&view=article&id=237&Itemid=84. Accessed February 1, 2013.

118. Calzone KA, Jenkins J. Genomics education in nursing in the United States. Annu Rev Nurs Res 2011;29:151–72.

119. Jenkins JF, Calzone KA. Are nursing faculty ready to integrate genomic content into curricula? Nurse Educ 2012;37(1):25–9.

120. Thompson HJ, Brooks MV. Genetics and genomics in nursing: evaluating Essentials implementation. Nurse Educ Today 2011;31(6):623–7.

121. Garcia S, Greco K, Loescher L. Teaching strategies to incorporate genomics education into academic nursing curricula. J Nurs Educ 2011;50(11):612–9.

122. Shuster M. Can genetics and genomics nursing competencies be successfully taught in a prenursing microbiology course? CBE Life Sci Educ 2011;10(2): 216–21.

123. Institute of Medicine. Integrating large-scale genomic information into clinical practice: workshop summary. Washington, DC: The National Academies Press; 2011.

124. Pestka EL, Meiers SJ, Shah LL, et al. Nurses' perceived benefits, barriers, and educational recommendations for using family pedigrees in clinical practice. J Contin Educ Nurs 2012;43(11):509–17.

125. Richmond ES, Dunn D. Biomarkers: an overview for oncology nurses. Semin Oncol Nurs 2012;28(2):87–92.

126. Beery TA, Smith CR. Genetics/genomics advances to influence care for patients with chronic disease. Rehabil Nurs 2011;36(2):54–9, 88.

127. Saunders M. The human genome project: an historical perspective for social workers. Soc Work Public Health 2011;26(4):336–48.

128. Roberts L, Davenport RJ, Pennisi E, et al. A history of the Human Genome Project. Science 2001;291(5507):1195.

129. National Human Genome Research Institute. Genetic Information Nondiscrimination Act (GINA) of 2008. 2012. Available at: http://www.genome.gov/24519851. Accessed February 9, 2013.

130. Badzek L, Henaghan M, Turner M, et al. Ethical, legal, and social issues in the translation of genomics into health care. J Nurs Scholarsh 2013;45(1):15–24.

131. McGuire AL, Majumder MA. Two cheers for GINA? Genome Med 2009;1(1):6.

132. Henderson GE, Juengst ET, King NM, et al. What research ethics should learn from genomics and society research: lessons from the ELSI Congress of 2011. J Law Med Ethics 2012;40(4):1008–24.

133. Patient Protection and Affordable Care Act (2010). H.R. 3590. U.S 111th Congress. Available at: http://www.gpo.gov/fdsys/pkg/PLAW-111publ148/pdf/PLAW-111publ148.pdf. Accessed September 27, 2013.

134. Offit K. Personalized medicine: new genomics, old lessons. Hum Genet 2011; 130(1):3–14.

Nursing Genomics
Its Role in Health Trajectory

Pei-Ying Chuang, PhD, MSN, RN[a],*, Ching Hsiu Hsieh, EdPhD, RN[b],
Bashira Addullah Charles, PhD, RN[c]

KEYWORDS

- Human genomics • Nursing science • Essential competencies • Clinical practice
- Bioscience skills

KEY POINTS

- Genomics refers to understanding all the genes in the human genome, including how the genes interact with each other and with environmental, psychosocial-behavior, and cultural factors.
- New strategies in nursing genomics science provide enhanced care and promote healthier outcomes through academic preparation, clinical practice, and research.
- Health care providers recognize the aspects of translational medicine from bench science to bedside on overall health so as to provide more effective concepts/benefits from a genomics perspective in personalized medicine.
- Future direction should reach out to global professional entities in nursing leadership and research collaboration.

INTRODUCTION

The World Health Organization (WHO) has successfully recognized the potential that genomic science and advanced biotechnologies have for achieving public health goals.[1] As a result, the Human Genome Project (HGP) has, for the past decade, celebrated its remarkable discoveries of 1800 disease genes and 2000 genetic tests for human health.[2] The HGP not only accomplishes the whole genome sequence of the individual, but it also has at least 350 biotechnology-based products in current clinical trials to analyze and understand the enormous amount of bioinformatics data. The human genome is the complete set of human genetic information, including how the

Disclosures: No financial conflict of interest.
[a] School of Nursing, University of Texas Health Science Center at Houston, 6901 Bertner Avenue, Room 613, Houston, TX 77030, USA; [b] Department of Nursing, Chang Gung University of Science and Technology, No.2 Chia-Pu West Road, Putzu City, ChiaYi County 61363, Taiwan, Republic of China; [c] Center Research Genomics & Global Health, National Human Genome Research Institute, National Institutes of Health, BG12A Room 4047, 12 South Drive, Bethesda, MD 20814, USA
* Corresponding author.
E-mail address: peiyingc@yahoo.com

genes interact with each other.[3,4] Conversely, genetics, a discipline of molecular biology, focuses more on the study of individual genes and the genes' impact on heredity.[5,6] To date, human genomics has had a huge effect on the caregiver's ability to assess individual health risks, whether those risks are inherited or result from environmental, psychosocial, or cultural interaction. Because of this, personalized medicine in the twenty-first century has embraced a health care approach that incorporates both the prevention and treatment of diseases. At the same time, some scientists and health care providers deal with more complex ethical, legal, and social implications (ELSI) relevant to human genomics.

The Ethics Committee for the Human Genome Organization (HUGO, 1995)[7] has proposed 6 ethical principles regarding "Ethical Issues in International Collaborative Research on the Human Genome" from the HGP and the Human Genome Diversity Project (HGDP): (1) competence on training planning, pilot and field testing, and quality control; (2) communication when dealing with socially and culturally sensitive topics; (3) research studies that acknowledge and include consultation needs, consent decisions, choices made, and collaboration benefits; (4) confidentiality code with the purpose of controlling access; (5) review of conflict of interest; and (6) continual review for the implementation.[7–9] These principles respect the client and protect the client's health information. In 2005, the General Conference of the United Nations Educational Scientific and Cultural Organization (UNESCO) approved the Universal Declaration on Bioethics and Human Rights.[10] The Declaration does not diminish human dignity to the individual's genetic characters, but it instead respects each person's uniqueness and common bond with other humans. The Genetic Information Non-Discrimination Act (GINA), signed by President George W. Bush on May 21, 2008, reflects the realization that the need to understand ELSI issues has risen due to personal genetic information against discrimination based on health insurance and employment issues.[11] Therefore, WHO's Human Genetics (HGN) prioritizes 4 genomic areas (genetic testing and screening, genetic patents, genetic databanks, and pharmacogenomics), based on the ELSI goals.[12] All health care providers in all professional fields need to learn about and be aware of these goals.

The American Nurses Association (ANA) endorses the *Code of Ethics for Nurses* (2001),[13] Canadian nurses embrace the *Code of Ethics for Registered Nurses*,[14] and UK nurses use the *Standards of Conduct Performance and Ethics of Nurses and Midwives*[15]; all of these codes emphasize the ideals and morals of the nursing profession. Nurses, regardless of their academic preparation, clinical specialty, and research experience, play a central role in applying human genomics to the health trajectory so as to improve patient outcomes. This review article summarizes nursing genomics in health trajectory on (1) essential nursing competencies in fundamental molecular biology/pathophysiology, ELSI, Web site resources, and training opportunities into nursing licensure requirements and institutional/academic accreditation; (2) evidence-based classification of genomic tests/biomarkers and family health history in adults, women/children, and public health in clinical practice; and (3) updated and innovative technology resources to better analyze hands-on bench science skills and bioinformatics through nursing programs in the United States and improved comprehensive expertise in the laboratory.

NURSING GENOMIC/GENETIC ACADEMIC PREPARATION: FROM CLASSROOMS TO CREATIVE LEARNING ENVIRONMENTS

The National Coalition for Health Professional Education in Genetics (NCHPEG), National Human Genome Research Institute, American Medical Association, American

Nurses Association, more than 50 interdisciplinary professional organizations, and consumers, volunteers, government agencies, private industries, managed care organizations, and genetics professional leaders have published genomic competencies for all health professional.[16] All health professionals believe that integrating genomics education into their profession is fundamental. Recently, more than 49 professional nursing organizations and experts successfully developed the Essential Nursing Competencies and Curricula Guidelines for Genetics and Genomics.[16,17] The purpose of this standard document is to define essential competencies and to incorporate ELSIs into nursing education and practice for all registered nurses (RNs). In addition, a Consensus Panel in 2011 established the American Association of Colleges of Nursing's (AACN) Essential Master's Education in Nursing.[18] Seven categories address 38 competencies, including risk assessment and interpretation; genetic education, counseling, testing, and result interpretation; clinical management and ELSI; professional roles and leadership; and research. Professional responsibility and professional practice domains, which are the main themes, each deals with specific areas of knowledge and clinical performance indicators.

However, fewer than one-third of all baccalaureate nursing programs in the United States include a genomics content in the curricula.[19–24] In 2010, US Human Service[25] reported that more than 40% of RNs who worked as faculty in their principal nursing position were between the ages of 50 and 59, and more than 19% of RNs whose principal position was as faculty were 60 years or older. These findings brought attention to the lack of progress of nursing genomic education for both students and faculty. Furthermore, Jenkins and Calzone[26] reviewed the transtheoretical model core construct guide in a genetic/genomic curriculum based on the nursing faculty point of view (n = 156). One point 5% (n = 2) of the respondents identified that they were in the precontemplation stage with no intent to adopt any curriculum course change related to genetic/genomics. Thirty-five percent (n = 55) of the faculty was in the contemplation stage, suggesting that it would adopt curriculum changes within the next 6 months; 4% (n = 6) had plans to make changes within the next 30 days within the preparation stage. Only 9% (n = 14) already reported curriculum changes for less than 6 months within the action stage. Hence, pursuing genomic knowledge in a nursing program faces many challenges: (1) limited comprehension of genetic/genomic relevancy to practice; (2) insufficient knowledge to understand emerging literature; (3) faculty inadequately prepared to teach content; (4) long, complex process involving existing genetic/genomic competencies; (5) rapid changes in the field that make it difficult to remain current; and (6) no regulations requiring integration of genetics/genomics.[20,23,27,28]

Shuster[29] reported that the genetics/genomics competencies course emerged as an initial method for teaching nursing students. Nursing students were required to take 3 courses—Biology 219 and public health microbiology with a 3-credit lecture and 2-credit laboratory based on the American Society for Microbiology and Genetics and Genomics instruction—over 3 semesters; nurses also received precontent and postcontent knowledge (3 themes) and attitudinal assessments (open-ended questionnaire). Overall, postknowledge scores revealed a significant improvement ($P<.001$) within the 3 semesters; a significant gain of knowledge occurred in microbiology and the biologic basis of diversity with the technology of genetics/genomics, but the courses did not yield significant difference. Enhancing biologic/microbiology courses might explain this trend in genetics/genomics learning. Garcia and colleagues[16] highlighted teaching strategies for genomic education by using 2 conceptual frameworks: Learning Engagement Model[30] and Diffusion of Innovation Theory by Roger and Floyd.[31] Moreover, Internet-based tools, such as WebQuest, Second

Lie, wikis, clickers, bulletin board, blogs, and up-to-date platforms, also address the area of genetics/genomics.

The New Mexico State University[16] provides biologic/microbiological courses for nursing students that focus on the biologic basis of genetic diversity (genotype, phenotype, alleles, mutations, horizontal transfer in bacteria, and genetic drift and shift in viruses), implications of genetic diversity in the context of natural selection, and technological aspects of assessing genetic diversity and making genetic-based identifications (polymorphism chain reaction-PCR genotyping, gel electrophoresis genotyping, and sequencing).[29] Hamilton[32] addressed physiologic and molecular processes as a foundation form of basic genetics/genomics clinical practice. Nursing competencies have the responsibility of incorporating genetics as follows: genetics at the molecular level (DNA transcription, RNA translation protein, type of mutations); genetics behind human diversity (polymorphisms and small gene changes that impact diversity); types of genetic disorders (single vs complex genes); interactions between the environment and genetic expression; genetic testing; and prevention and treatment of genetic diseases. These factors create a wide range of learning environments for all nurses. **Table 1** provides formal and informal Internet genetic/genomic learning resources, which are categorized according to the special needs associated with education, clinical practice, and research purposes.

Recently, 50 US schools of nursing reputed to have exemplary nursing programs have engaged in informal phone interviews. Despite the high standard of these schools, only 30 schools have incorporated genetics/genomics contents into their baccalaureate science of nursing (BSN), master's (n = 25) programs, and doctoral degree (n = 17) studies (**Table 2**). In these schools/institutes, 11 have their own wet biologic laboratory settings in nursing departments, whereas 26 have access to multiple discipline laboratories. Currently, 24 school of nursing programs in the United States have established their own molecular biologic laboratories that provide settings for the analysis of human genome studies. This pilot data will serve as a foundation for a continuing investigation of all genetic/genomic curriculums in nursing programs and as a way to follow up with current databases in the United States.

NURSING GENOMIC/GENETIC CLINICAL PRACTICE: GENERAL CARE TO SPECIALTY COMPONENTS PROVIDED

The United States has 3,063,163 licensed RNs who have earned a hospital-based diploma (20.4%), an associate's degree (45.4%), or a bachelor's or other advanced degree (34.2%).[25] Nearly 85% of nurse practitioners (NPs) reported that they held a master's degree and 3.9% reported holding a doctorate degree. Approximately 35% of NPs are 45 years old or younger.

The Genetic Nursing Credentialing Commission (GNCC),[33] which offers 2 special genetic nurses certification opportunities, works closely with the International Society of Nurses in Genetics (ISONG) and the National Human Genome Research Institute. Fifteen genetic clinical nurses (GCN) in 10 states throughout the United States are RNs who have completed a bachelor's degree and obtained credentials from the Genetic Nursing Credentialing Commission, which includes 50 genetic cases in the preceding 5 years, 4 written case studies reflecting ISONG standards, and 45 contact hours of genetic content within 3 calendar years of application. The job duties of the nurses involve taking detailed medical histories, assessing for the presence of genetic and nongenetic risk factors of disease, and managing patients. The genetic health care needs include the following: creating patient care plans; teaching patients about their conditions; administering treatments and medications; interpreting laboratory

Table 1	
Genetic/genomic Web site resources	
Name	**Web site**
Education	
Ask a Geneticist	http://www.thetech.org/genetics/index.php
Bank of stories	http://www.tellingstories.nhs.uk
Centers for Disease Control and Prevention, Genomics, & Health Weekly E-mail Update	http://www.cdc.gov/genomics/update/about.htm
Clinical Children's Hospital Genetics Education Program for Nurses (United States)	http://www.cincinnatichildren.org/edu/clincal/gpnf/default.htm
Credible Genetics (ATCG) Resource Network, Trust It or Trash It	http://www.trustortrash.org
Dolan DNA Learning Center Cold Spring Harbor Laboratory	http://www.dnalc.org
Eurogene-Learning Portal for Genetic Medicine	http://137.204.230.143/eugeu
Eurogene Project	http://eurogene.eu
GeneReviews	http://www.genetests.org
Genetics—a topic area within Scitable by Nature Education	http://www.nature/com/scitable/topic/genetics-5
Genetics Education Supporting Education in Genetics and Genomics for Health	http://www.geneticseducation.nhs.uk
Genetics/Genomics Competency Center for Education [G2C2]	http://www.g-2-c-2.org
Genetic Science Learning Center	http://learn.genetics.urah.edu
Gene Sense	http://www.genesense.org/uk/
Genetic Tools Web Site	http://staff.washington.edu/sbtrini/index/shtml
Global genetic-genomic community [G3C]	www.g-3-c.org
National Cancer Institute—Targeted Therapies Tutorials	http://www.caner.gov/cancertopics/understandingcaner/targetedtherapies
Murdoch Children's Research Institute—Genetics Education & Health Research Group (Australia)	http://111.mcri.edu.au/pages/research/education/default.asp
National Center for Case Study Teaching in Science	http://Ublib.buffalo.edu/libraries/projects/cases/ubcase.htm
National Coalition for Health Professional Education in Genetics	http://nchpeg.org
National Human Genome Research Institute (NHGRI)	http://www.nihi.gov
National Health Services National Genetics Education and Development Center (United Kingdom)	http://www.geneticseducation.nhs.uk/about-us/resources.aspx
Public Health Genetics Foundation (PHG; United Kingdom)	http://www.phgfoundation.rog/pages/edu_resources.htm

(continued on next page)

Table 1 *(continued)*	
Name	**Web site**
Online Mendelian Inheritance in Man (OMIM)	http://www.omim.org
The PharmGenEd Program	http://pharmacogenomics.ucsd.edu
Wellcome Trust Sanger Institute (United Kingdom)	http://yourgenome.org
Your Genes, Your Health	http://www.ygyh.org
Culture	
Genetic counseling cultural competence toolkit	www.geneticcounselingtoolkit.com/efault.htm
Clinical practice	
Cancer Genome Atlas	http://cancergenome.nih.gov
Catalog of published Genome-Wide Association Studies	http://www.genome.gov/gwastudies
Chromatin Structure and Function	http://www.chromatin.us
ClinSeq; A large-Scale Medical Sequencing Clinical Research Pilot Study	http://www.genome.gov/20519355
Collecting Family history	http://ghr.nlm.niih.gov
Database for DNA Methylation and Environmental Epigenetic Effects	http://www.methdb.de
Database of Genotypes and Phenotypes (dpGap)	http://www.ncbi.nlm.nih.gov/gap
Database of Noncoding RNAs	http://www.noncode.org
Epigenomic Datasets	http://www.ncbi.nlm.nih.gov/epigenomics
Epigenomics Fact Sheet	http://www.genome.gov/27532724
Evaluation of genomics applications in practice and prevention	www.egappreviews.org
GeneBank	http://www.ncbi.nlm.nih.gov/genbanck
Gene Expression Omnibus	http://www.ncbi.nlm.nih.gov/geo
Genetic Home Reference (GHR)	http://ghr.nlm.nih.gov/
Genetics and your Practice	http://www.marchofdimes.com/gyponline/index.bms
Genetic clinic simulation	http://lml.dartmouth.edu/education/cme/genetics/
Genetic Education	http://www.geneticseducation.nhs.uk/
Genetics in Clinical Practice: A team approach	http://lml.dartmouth.edu/education/cme/genetics
Genetic/Genomic Competency Center for Education [G2C2]	
Gene tests	www.ncbi.nlm.nih/gov/sites/genetests
Genetic Test Registry (GTR)	http://www.ncbi.nlm.nih.gov/gtr
Histone Database	http://reserach.nhgri.nih.gov/histones
Human Epigenome Project	http://www.epigenome.org
Human Gene Mutation Database (HGMD)	http://www.hgmd.cf.ac.uk/ac/index/php

(continued on next page)

Table 1 (*continued*)	
Name	**Web site**
Human Genome resources	http://www.ncbi.nlm.nih.gov/genome/guide/human/
International Cancer Consortium	http://www.icgc.org
International Human Epigenome Consortium	http://ihec-epigenomes.org/index.html
Locus-Specific Mutation Databases (HGVS/LSMD)	http://www.hgvs.org/dblist/glsdb.html
My Family Health Portrait	http://familyhistory.hhs.gov/fhhweb/home.action
National Organization for Rare Diseases (NORD)	http://rarediseases.org/
Online Mendelian Inheritance in Man (OMIM)	http://www.ncbi.nlm.nih.gov/Omim/
Orphanet	http://www.orpha.net/consor/cgi-bin/index.php
Pharmacogenomics	http://wwww.ornl.gov/sci/techresorces/human_genome/medicine/pharma.shtml
Rare Genetic Diseases in Children (RGDC)	http://mcrcr2.med.nyu.edu/murphp01/homenew.htm
Talking Glossary of Genetic Terms	http://www.genome.gov/glossary
Telling stories	http://www.tellingstories.nhs.uk
Power analysis	
Quanto	http://hydra.usc.edu/gxe/
Bio-informatics databases	
Gene Ontology	http://www.geneontology.org/
Database of SNP (dbSNP)	http://www.ncbi.nlm.nih.gov/projects/SNP
HapMap Project	http://mhapmap.ncbi.nlm.nih.gov/
Genomic Structural Variation (dbVar)	http://www.ncbi.nlm.nih.gov/dbvar
Trust Sanger Institute	http://www.sanger.ac.uk/humgen/cnv
Real-Time PCR Allele Discrimination	http://www.roche-applied–science.com http://allele-specific fluorescence intensity signals
Technology	
Real-time PCR allelic discrimination	http://www.appliedbiosystems.com http://www.roche-applied-science.com
Genotyping assay	http://www.sequenom.com http://www.illumia.com
Candidate copy number variations	http://appliedbiosystems.com
Center for Inherited Disease Research (CIDR)	http://www.cidr.jhmi.edu/requirements/applications.html
Database of Genotypes	http://www.ncbi.nlm.nih.gov/entrez/query.fcgi?db=gap

Table 2
Schools of nursing with genetic/genomic curriculum and bio-laboratory in United States

School of Nursing	Genetics/Genomics Curriculum			Biologic Laboratory
	BSN	MS	Doctoral	
Arizona State University Phoenix, AZ	$Y_{courses}$	$Y_{clinical\ track}$	$Y_{clinical\ track}$	Access to other discipline laboratories
Boston College Chestnut Hill, MA	N	$Y_{courses}$	N	
Case Western Reserve University Cleveland, OH	$Y_{courses}$	$Y_{courses}$	$Y_{courses}$	Center of Excellence: Building End-of-Life Science through Positive Human Strengths and Traits (BEST) Center (Oncology/Genetics) Access to other discipline laboratories
Columbia University New York, NY	$Y_{courses}$	$Y_{courses}$	$Y_{courses}$	Access to Interdisciplinary Research to Reduce Antimicrobial Resistance (CIPAR)
Duke University	$Y_{courses}$	Y_{option}	Y_{option}	Center for Interdisciplinary Salivary Bioscience Research Access to other discipline laboratories
Emory University Atlanta, GA	$Y_{courses}$	$Y_{courses}$	N_{option}	Access to other discipline laboratories
Frontier School of Midwifery and Family Nursing Hyden, KY	N	N	N	
Georgetown University Washington, DC	$Y_{courses}$	$Y_{courses}$	N	Access to other discipline laboratories
George Washington University Washington, DC	N	Y	N	Access to other discipline laboratories
Georgia Regents University Augusta, GA	$Y_{courses}$	$Y_{courses}$	$Y_{courses}$	Access to other discipline laboratories
Indiana University-Purdue University Indianapolis, IN	N	N	N	Access to other discipline laboratories
Johns Hopkins Baltimore, MD	$Y_{courses}$	Y_{option}	Y_{option}	Center for Interdisciplinary Salivary Bioscience Research Access to other discipline laboratories

University				
Marquette University Milwaukee, WI	N	N	N	
New York University New York, NY	$Y_{courses}$	$Y_{courses}$	Y_{DNP}	NYU Cancer Institute, NYU Bluestone Center for Clinical Research, Comprehensive Center on Brain Aging, and Clinical Translational Science Institute
Ohio State University Columbus, OH	$Y_{courses}$	N	N	College of Nursing Research Laboratory
Oregon Health and Science University Portland, OR	$Y_{courses}$	Y_{option}	Y_{option}	Access to other discipline laboratories
Pennsylvania State University University Park, PA	$Y_{courses}$	Y	N	Access to other discipline laboratories
Rush University Chicago, IL	N	Y	N	Access to other discipline laboratories
University of Alabama Birmingham, AL	$Y_{courses}$	N	N	Access to other discipline laboratories
University of Arizona Tucson, AZ	$Y_{courses}$	$Y_{courses}$	N	Biochemical/Biologic laboratories
University of Arkansas of Medical Sciences Little Rock, AR	N	N	N	
University of California-Los Angeles Las Angeles, CA	$Y_{courses}$	$Y_{courses}$		
University of California-San Francisco San Francisco, CA	$Y_{courses}$	$Y_{courses}$	Y_{option}	UCSF Clinical and Translational Science Institute (CTSI) Access to other discipline laboratories
University of Colorado Denver, CO	$Y_{courses}$	Y_{option}	Y_{option}	Access to other discipline laboratories
University of Florida Gainsville, FL	$Y_{courses}$	$Y_{courses}$	N	Health Professions, Nursing, and Pharmacy (HPNP)
University of Kansas Kansas City, KS	$Y_{courses}$	$Y_{courses}$	N	Access to other discipline laboratories
University of Kentucky Lexington, KY	N	N	N	

(continued on next page)

Table 2
(continued)

| School of Nursing | Genetics/Genomics Curriculum | | | Biologic Laboratory |
	BSN	MS	Doctoral	
University of Illinois Chicago, IL	N$_{??}$	N	N	Access to other discipline laboratories
University of Iowa Iowa City, IA	Y$_{courses}$	N	Y$_{courses}$	Access to other discipline laboratories
University of Maryland Baltimore, MD	Y$_{courses}$	Y$_{courses}$	Y$_{courses}$	
University of Michigan-Ann Arbor Ann Arbor, MI	N	N	N	Access to other discipline laboratories
University of Minnesota-Twin Cities Minneapolis, MN	N	N	N	
University of Nebraska Medical Center-Omaha, NE	Y$_{courses}$	N	N	Access to other discipline laboratories
University of North Carolina-Chapel Hill Chapel Hill, NC	Y$_{option}$	N	N	Biobehavioral laboratory
University of Pennsylvania Philadelphia, PA	Y$_{courses}$	Y$_{courses}$	Y$_{option}$	Laboratory of Innovative and Translating Nursing Research
University of Pittsburgh Pittsburgh, PA	Y$_{courses}$	N	N	Targeted Research and Academic Training Program for Nurses in Genomics Access to other discipline laboratories
University of Rochester Rochester, NY	Y$_{courses}$	N	N	Access to other discipline laboratories

Institution				Laboratories
University of Tennessee Health Sciences Center Memphis, TN	$Y_{courses}$	N	N	Access to other discipline laboratories
University of Texas-Austin Austin, TX	$Y_{courses}$	$Y_{courses}$	$Y_{courses}$	Biobehavioral Laboratory
University of Texas-Dallas	Y	Y	Y	Genomics Translational Research Laboratory
University of Texas Health Science Center at Houston	$Y_{courses}$	N	N	Center for Nursing Research Biologic Laboratory Services
University of Utah Salt Lake City, UT	N	N	N	Access to other discipline laboratories
University of Virginia Charlottesville, VA	N	$Y_{courses}$	N	Access to other discipline laboratories
University of Washington Seattle, WA	N	N	N	Biobehavioral Nursing & Health Systems (BNHS)
University of Wisconsin-Madison Madison, WI	N	Y_{option}	Y_{option}	
University of Wisconsin-Milwaukee Milwaukee, WI	N	N	N	Biobehavioral Research Lab
Vanderbilt University Nashville, TN				
Virginia Commonwealth University	N	N	N	Center for Biobehavioral Clinical Research
Wayne State University East Lansing, MI	$Y_{courses}$	$Y_{courses}$	Y_{DNP}	Access to other discipline laboratories
Yale University New Haven, CT	N	Y_{option}	Y_{option}	Access to other discipline laboratories

Abbreviations: $Y_{courses}$, Yes- Incorporated into courses; Y_{DNP}, Yes-Doctoral nurse practitioner program; Y_{option}, Yes-Incorporate into courses (optional).

data; coordinating care needs with other health care professionals; and assisting families so they can better cope with their circumstances. Fifty-five advanced practice nurses in genetics (APNG) in 28 states throughout the United States are RNs with a master's degree; these nurses have accumulated 300 hours of genetic practicum experience, completed 50 cases within 5 years of application, written 4 genetic case studies, and provided evidence of professional achievement by providing health care to patients afflicted by genetic conditions. They receive referrals from other health care providers, perform detailed assessments, construct pedigrees, develop plans of care, diagnose medical conditions, prescribe treatments, and provide genetic counseling. They often assume roles of leadership in their professional communities by conducting research, writing articles to educate health care professionals and the public, and coordinating community health resources.

Clinical researchers have launched a new era in medicine by assuming a significant role in detecting the biologic basis of disease and discovering more effective ways to diagnose, treat, and prevent illness. Health promotion, disease prevention, acute care, and palliative and end-of-life care have altered the perspective of the transitional health trajectory across the individual's life span. Nurses remain actively committed to engaging in genomics in clinical practice by assessing family pedigree, interpreting risk factors, offering counseling on genetic testing, and providing education.[34] Nurses also conduct ELSI communication with patients and families, all of whom span a wide spectrum of populations, related to informed consent, confidentiality, and personal genomic information.

The qualitative study of Pestka and colleagues[35] identified that 79% of female nurse participants (n = 19) felt confident to use the electronic family pedigrees tool in a primary or critical care setting after they had used the family history practice. The data indicate the importance of the nurses feeling comfortable when taking personal information from patients and family members and when dealing with emotional issues and discussion. In addition, electronic family pedigree, which will be recognized as a part of patient records, will play an essential role in determining prognosis and optional treatments in advance. Calzone and colleagues[36] used an online nursing genomics integration survey on a 239-convenience sample of RNs employed at the National Institutes of Health. The Diffusion of Innovation Theory and family history assessments were examined according to the domains of attitudes and receptivity, confidence, competency and knowledge, social system, and decision and adoption. Seventy-one percent (n = 170) of the respondents considered genetics/genomics as very important to the nursing practice; however, 81% (n = 191) rated poor or fair on their genetics/genomics knowledge of common diseases. Thirty-four percent (n = 81) of the respondents had known about or read the Essential Nursing Competencies; and 24% (n = 57) felt very or somewhat confident in assessing a patient's genetic susceptibility. Most reported only a fair (56%; n = 133) knowledge of genetics/genomics, whereas 60% (n = 143) stated they had never had a course in genetics/genomics. A similar result emerged from Crane and colleagues' study,[37] which used an online survey based on genetic activities in clinical practice to determine the effect of personal confidence in carrying out the genetic activities in 612 American College of Nurse-Midwives. Although nurses recognized that they must incorporate genetics/genomics care into their profession, they did not routinely use genetics/genomics when taking a family history. In conclusion, these nurses have demonstrated their knowledge of clinical advanced practice and have indicated that ELSI should play an essential role in clinical settings.

In general, newborn screening (NBS) can identify serious metabolic, hormonal, blood, or hearing disorders and/or genetic conditions; although the screening procedure is not always diagnostic, it can suggest early treatment approaches or appropriate referrals.[38–40] Screening protocols, which vary among states, regions, and countries, are based on each particular condition. Professional nurses can use their knowledge of NBS procedures, policies, and implications to make sure the parents of the young patients receive accurate information (eg, purpose, meaning, risks, advantages, and rights of enrollment depending on the locale, specimen collection, and retention) before testing. Professional nurses can oversee follow-up results and interpret outcomes related to the NBS. Furthermore, some technologies, such as electrospray-ionization tandem mass spectrometry of amino acids,[41] quantitative amino acid high-performance liquid chromatography (HPLC) analysis,[42] enzyme-linked immunosorbent assay (ELISA),[43] and genotype,[44] have proven to be beneficial to NB testing results.

There are several types of genetic disorders in children. Some are hereditary; parents with a genetic disorder or family history of genetic disorders make it more likely that one or more of their children will also have a genetic disorder. Most common genetic diseases are related to chromosomal abnormalities, single gene defects, multifactorial problems, and teratogenic problems.[45] A genetic disorder in the family history (occurring with another child, one parent, or the fetus) again increases the risk of a chromosomal abnormality in the child. The National Human Genome Research Institute (NHGRI)[46] reported that about 30% to 40% of children with special needs do not have an exact diagnosis; therefore, undiagnosed conditions in children often create challenges for both the children and their families. For instance, the Centers for Disease Control and Prevention's (CDC's) Autism and Developmental Disabilities Monitoring Network (ADDM)[47] identified approximately 1 in 88 children with an autism spectrum disorder (ASD) in 2013. This ASD occurs 5 times more frequently in boys than in girls (1:252); about 1 in 6 children in the United States had a developmental disability between 2006 and 2008. The risk factors associated with autism include the following: identical twins (36%–95%); parents who have a child with an ASD (2%–18%); children with autism associated with genetic or chromosomal conditions with Down syndrome, fragile X syndrome, and tuberous sclerosis (10%); children born to older parents (62%); or children with a low birth weight. In summary, family pedigree may help health care providers to determine the risks for certain health problems; in addition, the parents' genetic contribution can indicate any possible genetic inheritance patterns. Medical management and ethical and legal resources depend on the sensitive time during the entire clinical evaluation period and how much information the parents are seeking or are prepared to receive. Because nurses are often the first health care providers, they play an important role in initiating the process.

For 12 years, the National Institutes of Health (NIH)-funded Women's Genome Health Study (WGHS) has followed common major health events (myocardial infarction, stroke, cancer, diabetes, osteoporosis, venous-thromboembolism, cognitive decline, and age-related visual disorders, such as macular degeneration and cataracts) in the genome-wide data of 65,169 American women, 45 years or older.[48] This study has found that dietary, behavioral, and traditional exposure affected the gene-environment and gene-gene interactions as they relate to incident disease states. Although only 12% of women in the general population develop breast cancer, 60% of these breast cancers are associated with an inherited mutation; a similar association exists between ovarian cancer and an inherited mutation (15%–50% of women found a harmful BRACA1 or BRCA2 mutation).[49] For women's health, BRCA1 and BRACA2 are still the only earliest significant detection biomarkers of hereditary breast and ovarian cancers to this point, according to the National Cancer

Institute.[41,50] For this reason, the health care profession offers women BRACA genetic testing and strongly recommends professional consultations. On the other hand, the Prostate Cancer Foundation, with the economic support of $480 million, has established 1500 prostate cancer research programs at 200 universities in 20 countries over 15 years. However, the US Preventive Services Task Force recently announced that the prostate-specific antigen (PSA) test for men's health is not as beneficial as previously believed,[51–54] although the PSA test may prevent a biopsy procedure, which can be both harmful and unnecessary. In recent years, reproductive genetic testing has become a controversial issue, motivating both the government and institutions to examine the value of such testing and the potential medical benefits of such testing, including treating infertility.[55] To make wise decisions about medical experiments, researchers must consider what most benefits the people who will be affected. Although some individuals focus on finding ways to increase the number of family members, others deal with the repercussions of a dramatically increased life expectancy in wealthier populations due to better public health, nutrition, and medicine.

According to the Administration on Aging from the Department of Health and Human Services, 12.9% of the population in the United States in 2009 was age 65 or older (29.6 million). It is estimated that by 2030, the older population will reach 72.1 million, an increase of 19%.[56] Both the Hartford Geriatric Nursing Initiative and the Building Academic Geriatric Nursing Capacity lead the way in training the next generation of nurses to effectively deal with America's aging population.[57] Eighty percent of people 65 and older have at least one chronic illness, such as heart disease, diabetes, or arthritis.[58] These complex diseases are linked with multiple genomic risks and environmental factors, which have a wide range of traits and a large number of effects in the human genome. In addition, late-onset genomic diseases, such as neuropsychiatric diseases (dementia, and Parkinson, Alzheimer, and Huntington disease), and chronic complex diseases (diabetes, heart disease), require a great deal of genomic innovation.[59]

Overall, cancer, which is a genomic disease, creates complex conditions that transcend all ages. The higher mortality and morbidity risk of cancer makes it a top research priority for embarking on an intensive genomic analysis. Cancer and other common and rare diseases have implications for the nursing profession, specifically because the profession deals with such diverse areas as pediatrics, obstetrics/gynecology health, adult health care, and geriatrics. Although environmental factors often cause primary cancers (90%–95%), genomics also plays a role in cancer; as a result, cancer genomics in clinical practice investigates the relationship between genetic variation and cancer progression.[60] Detecting a biologic marker (biomarker) provides an objective characteristic that serves as an indicator of a normal biologic process, pathogenic process, or response to pharmacologic therapeutic intervention.[61,62] The classification scheme of biomarkers includes the following: (1) type 0 biomarkers measure the natural history of a disease correlated over time with known clinical indicators; (2) type I biomarkers are associated with the effectiveness of pharmacologic agents; and (3) type II biomarkers or surrogate end point biomarkers are intended to substitute for a clinical end point. The Division of Cancer Prevention at the National Cancer Institute[63] established the early detection research network with biomarker development as a formal process to guide researchers in general clinical studies.

An oncology clinical practice makes the integration of biomarkers into symptoms management a priority: how to refine the conceptualization of the symptom phenotype; how to develop valid and reliable measures of the symptom phenotype; and how to define sensitive and specific biomarkers. Biomarkers of cancer risk can be considered as follows: (1) low penetrance (relative risk ≥ 1.0 to <1.5); (2) moderate penetrance (relative risk ≥ 1.5 to ≤ 5.0); and (3) high penetrance (relative risk ≥ 5.0).[62] The following cancer risk assessment (CRA)[64,65] benefits those individuals who have a potential risk from a genomics perspective: (1) earlier age of cancer onset; (2) the same type of cancer in 2 or more close relatives in the same lineage; (3) 2 or more primary cancers in the same person; (4) constellation of cancer's characteristic of a hereditary syndrome; (5) male breast, ovarian, or medullary thyroid cancer at any age; (6) breast cancer in woman of Jewish ancestry; and (7) a previously identified cancer-associated mutation in the family. Likewise, the American Society of Clinical Oncology[66] wrote the following guidelines concerning when to consider a genetic test: (1) family or individual history consistent with an inherited cancer syndrome; (2) genetic test results that can be interpreted; (3) results of genetic test to guide further medical management; and (4) the individual is a legal adult (18 years of age or older), or the individual had cancer risks in childhood and associated changes in medical management. Moreover, the CDC[67,68] has also developed a guideline for assessing genetic tests: the ACCE model that has analytic validity (A), clinical validity (C), clinical utility (C), and ethical, legal, and social implications (E). This model has been used worldwide to evaluate genetic tests and to contribute to the identification of gaps between genetic test results and standard policy decision making. In conclusion, nurses, who focus on identifying ways to improve the quality of health care and of life for older adults across care settings, highlight the interpersonal interaction in this population's health outcomes and interventions, and reduce the caregiver burden experienced by involved family members.

NURSING GENOMIC/GENETIC BIOSCIENCE SKILLS: BENCH EVIDENCE TO BEDSIDE PRACTICE

Future genomics research must recognize comprehensive major themes in the fields of biology, health, and society that emphasize cytogenetics, genomics, epigenetics, and proteomics analyses. Research must focus on significant single-gene disorders, complex multiple genes, and sequencing exome/noncoding regions so as to identify the structure and function that cause human disease, develop molecular diagnostic tests that can detect a predisposition to disease within individuals, and guide pharmacologic treatment in an efficient manner while minimizing drug-associated side effects.[59] Therefore, researchers need to gain an understanding of how high-throughput biochemistry molecular technologies manage a number of genome data scale views; how bioinformatics has accurate interpretations in the analysis resources; and how to determine which categories of biologic methods and experimental skills will best detect target biomolecule materials. A new long-term mission of the 1000 Genomes Project for human genomic studies involves merging data from 2 databases in Europe and the United States.[69] To achieve this goal requires that the databases have uniform quality control, that all resources for publication needs are immediately released, and that different populations offer their unique perspectives of biologic interpretations. With scientific nurses taking the lead in the genomic era, translational nursing research application is necessary to bring the bench evidence into bedside care. According to the National Institute of Nursing Research (NINR),[70] the nursing genomic science strategic plan includes 5 areas: (1) promoting good health and preventing disease through risk assessment; (2) making decisions that support communication; (3) advancing the quality of life by focusing on family, symptom, and self-management; (4) implementing innovations in technology/informatics development and environmental interaction; and (5) creating training opportunities and cross-cutting themes, especially leadership in health disparities, cost, policy, and public education.

This year, the *Journal of Nursing Scholarship Genomic Nursing Webinar* Series invited nursing experts and authors of articles published in the *Journal of Nursing Scholarship* 2013 *Genomic Special Issue* to the NHGRI[71] of NIH. These scholars, who represented a vast range of research fields, spoke on a diversity of topics related to the genomic application in health care across the individual's life span. **Table 3** gives a summary of what nursing experts, those in ISONG and those currently involved in active research, recommend in terms of genetics/genomics studies. Because nurses play a pivotal role in helping patients go through their medical treatment/intervention, nurses need to enhance their professional knowledge, practical skills, and research so as to be effective givers of care. By becoming the practitioners of beside-centered health care, nurses will expand evidence-based research by applying bench data to clinical practice. Moreover, according to an active NINR research funding report in 2013, 5 individual fellowship F awards (F31, n = 4) have been awarded to the Oregon Health and Science University, University of California–San Francisco, University of Pittsburgh, and University of Tennessee Health Science Center; one postdoctoral fellow award (F32) was given to the Brigham and Women's Hospital; and one recipient of K99 NIH Pathway to Independent award was given to the University of Pittsburgh. Two institutes (Virginia Commonwealth University and Duke University) have benefits to the R00 awards and 9 institutes have also received RO1 awards (University of Pittsburgh, University of Maryland–Baltimore, University of Tennessee Health Science Center, and Virginia Commonwealth University). Three senior investigators have received intramural project award at the National Institute of Nursing Research (NINR) (**Table 4**). There is no doubt in nursing that nurse education, clinical practitioner, and nursing faculty researchers have been accomplished in many ways.

The Human Genome

The genome is made up of 46 chromosomes that reside in the nucleus (22 pairs of autosomes and 1 pair of sex chromosomes: XX in females and XY in males), as well as a small, circular DNA molecule within the mitochondria. Interestingly, humans are 99.9% identical at the DNA level. There are estimated to be 3 billion base pairs (bp) in the human genome, of which only about 1.5% are used to code for the estimated 22,000 genes. In addition, about 3.5% of the genome is highly conserved but lies in noncoding regions.[72–74]

DNA is made up of long sequences of double-stranded nitrogenous bases (A, adenine; T, thymine; C, cytosine; and G, guanine) that direct the synthesis of single-stranded RNA molecules, containing the bases A, C, G, and uracil (U), which in turn direct the synthesis of proteins.[72–74] In regions of coding DNA, the process of transcription from DNA to RNA involves splicing (ie, the DNA is copied and exons are joined together but introns are removed), which yields a mature messenger RNA (mRNA). Translation refers to the process of protein synthesis from an mRNA template. However, more than 98% of the human genome consists of noncoding DNA (eg, transfer RNA, ribosomal RNA, and regulatory RNA), which are associated with activities such as the regulation of gene expression, organization of chromosomal architecture, and the control of epigenetic inheritance.[72–75] There can also be genetic variations, called single nucleotide polymorphisms (SNPs), that exist between individuals (about 10–20 million SNPs or 1 in 1000 bp).[76,77] Most known SNPs have an allele frequency in the general population that is greater than 1% and do not cause any change in the protein sequence or function. However, if SNPs are rare and lead to a

Table 3
Genetic/genomic experts in education, research, clinical practice, consulting, policy, and technology

Name	University/Institute	Special Clinical Field
Ethical/legal and social issues		
Laurie Badsek, LLM, JD, MS, RN, FAAN	Professor, West Virginia University School of Nursing; Director, Center for Ethics and Human Rights at the American Nurses Association	Ethical, legal, policy
Kathy Sparbel, PhD, FNP-BC	University of Illinois at Chicago	Clinical decision making
Jacqueline M. Hale, RN, MSN, APNC, AOCN, APNG	Open Society Foundations	Central Asia and South Caucasus, energy, and human rights issues
Maggie Kirk, PhD, FRCN, BSc Hons, RGN	Professor, University of Glamorgan, UK	Education, policy
Emma Tonkin, PhD, BSc Hons	Faculty, University of Glamorgan, UK	Education, policy
Oncology		
Alice Kerber, MS	Saint Joseph's Hospital in Atlanta	Oncology
Ellen Giarelli, EdD, RN, MS, CRNP	Associate Professor, Drexel University	Psychosocial oncology
Lauri A. Linder, PhD, APRN, CPON	Assistant Professor; University of Utah	Teen cancer
Rebekah Hamilton, PhD, RN	Associate Professor, Rush University	Oncology
Erika Santos, PhD, MS, RN	International Center for Research and Teaching in Brazil	Colorectal cancer/Oncology
Deborah MacDonald, PhD, MS, APNG	Assistant Professor and Cancer Risk Counselor at City of Hope	Oncology
Kathleen Calzone; PhD, RN, APNG, FAAN	Senior Nurse Specialist (research), NCI, Center for Cancer Research/Genetics Branch, NIH	Oncology
Jean Jenkins; PhD, RN, FAAN	Staff, Genomic Healthcare Branch, NHGRI, NIH	Oncology
Newborn screening		
Jane DeLuca, PhD, CRNP, APNG, MS, BS	Assistant Professor, University of Rochester School of Nursing	Newborn screening
Childhood disorders		
Cynthia Prows, MSN, CNS, FAAN	Genetics Clinical Nurse Specialist, Cincinnati Children's Hospital	Education
Martha Turner, PhD, RN	RN Assistant Director, American Nurses Association	Ethical and legal approach

(continued on next page)

Table 3
(continued)

Name	University/Institute	Special Clinical Field
Cynthia Prows, MSN, RN, APNG, FAAN	Cincinnati Children's Hospital	Children with genetic disorders
Catherine Rice, PhD	Behavioral Scientist, National Center on Birth Defects and Developmental Disabilities at the Centers for Disease Control and Prevention	Autism spectrum disorders
Adult		
Shu-Fan Wung; PhD, CNRN, RN, FAAN	Associate Professor, University of Arizona	Cardiovascular genomics
Matthew J. Gallek; PhD, CNRN, RN	Assistant Professor, University of Arizona	Stroke
Kathleen T. Hickey; PhD, RN	Assistant Professor, Columbia University	Sudden cardiac death
Nicole Zangrilli Hoc; PhD, RN	Assistant Professor, University of Pittsburgh	Traumatic brain and spinal cord injuries
Sheila Alexander; PhD, RN	Assistant Professor, University of Pittsburgh	Traumatic brain and stroke
Debra Schutte, PhD, RN	Associate Professor, Michigan State University College of Nursing	Neuropsychiatric disorders (AZ; Huntington)
Norah Johnson, PhD, RN, CPNP	Faculty, Marquette University College of Nursing	Autism spectrum disorder
Jacquelyn Y. Taylor; PhD, PNP-BC	Associate Professor, Yale University	Racial/ethnic and gender difference in cardiovascular disease
Aldi T. Kraja, Dsc, PhD	Associate Professor, Washington University at St. Louis	Metabolic syndrome
Ann Cashion, PhD, RN, FAAN	Scientific Director, NINR, NIH	Metabolic syndrome
Maria Adamaian, ACNP, PhD	Doctoral student; Seton Hall University in South Orange New Jersey	Acute care
Lynnette Howington, DNP, RNC, WHNP-BC	Texas Christian University	Critical care
Marsha Tadje, APRN, AOCN	Assistant Professor; University of Utah	Sleep in elderly cancer
Sandra Founds, CNM, FNP, PhD, RN	Associate Professor, University of Pittsburgh	Education; midwifery

Counseling/education		
Audrey Tluczek, PhD, RN	Associate Professor, University of Wisconsin-Madison	Counseling psychology
Mindy Tinkle; PhD, RN, WHNP-BC	Scientific Review Officer, NINR, NIH	Education
Cathy Y. Read, PhD, RN	Associate Dean, Boston College	Education
Susan Gennaro, DSN, RN, FAAN	Dean and Professor, Boston College	Education; perinatal
Technology		
Mary Beth Steck, PhDc, APRN, BC	Doctoral student; University of Pittsburgh	Technology
Nick Nicol, PhD, FCN	Professor of Human Genetics, Universal College of Learning in New Zealand	Education; genetics
Heather Skirton, PhD, RGN, RGC, QMW	Nurse Researcher (CNS), University of Plymouth (UK)	Genetics researcher
Alexis Bakos, PhD, MPH, RN, C	Chief of the Diversity Training Branch, Center to Reduce Cancer Health Disparities at the National Cancer Institute in Maryland	Management; education
Ellen Giarelli, EdD, RN, MS, CRNP	Associate Professor, Division of Graduate Nursing at Drexel University College of Nursing and Health Professions	Education
Diane Seibert, PhD, ARNP, FAAN,	Uniformed Services University of Health Sciences	Skin disorders
Erika Monteiro Santos; PhD, MS, RN	Researcher, Center for Research and Teaching and National Institute of Oncogenomics, Sao Paulo, Brazil	Oncology genomics
Deborah Tamura, MS, RN	Research APN, National Cancer Institute Dermatology Branch	Skin disorders/oncology genetics

Table 4
Active Health Research Funding Focused on Human Genetics/Genomic Studies at National Institute of Nursing Research at the National Institutes of Health

Research Project	University/Institute	Research Field
F31	Oregon Health and Science University	Association of poststroke fatigue trajectories with cytokine polymorphisms
F31	University of California-San Francisco	Identification of genetic markers associated with attention fatigue
F31	University of Pittsburgh	Genomic of the vascular endothelial growth factor pathway in neonatal respiratory distress syndrome
F31	University of Tennessee Health SCI Center	Dopaminergic genetic contributions to obesity in kidney transplant recipients
F32	Brigham and Women's Hospital	A translational study of the caveolin-1 gene and human cardio metabolic disease
K99	University of Pittsburgh at Pittsburgh	Transcriptomics in traumatic brain injury: relationship to brain oxygenation
R00	Virginia Commonwealth University	Exhaled biomarkers of pulmonary infection in the critically ill
R00	Duke University	Expanding evidence of genetic contributions to survivorship in coronary artery disease
R01	University of Pittsburgh	Determining genetic and biomarker predictors of delayed cerebral ischemia and long term outcomes after
R01	University of Pittsburgh at Pittsburgh	Genomic variability and symptomatology after traumatic brain injury
R01	University of Pittsburgh at Pittsburgh	Epigenomics of patient outcomes after aneurysmal subarachnoid hemorrhage
R01	University of Maryland Baltimore	Epigenetic modifications of *BDNF* and *TRKB* genes underlie pain plasticity
R01	University of Maryland Baltimore	Spinal mechanisms underlying spinal cord injury-induced pain: implications for targeted therapy
R01	University of Maryland Baltimore	Center for the genomics of pain
R01	University of Arkansas for Medical Sciences	Interactions among depressive symptoms and genetic influences on cardiac outcomes
R01	University of Tennessee Health Science Center	Genetics, environment, and weight gain posttransplantation
R01	Virginia Commonwealth University	Epigenetics and psychoneurologic symptoms in women with breast cancer
ZIA	National Institute of Nursing Research	Molecular-genetic mechanisms underlying effects of anti-inflammatory/analgesic drugs
ZIA	National Institute of Nursing Research	Genomic approaches for elucidating novel targets for pain and symptom management
ZIA	National Institute of Nursing Research	Investigating molecular-genetic correlates of fatigue

disease, they are typically referred to as mutations. These fundamental biologic principles are the basis of some advanced technologies that allow us to study genetic networks and protein pathways.

The Genome Revolution in Biotechnology

Following the discovery of the structure of DNA in 1953[78] by James D. Watson and Francis Crick, in 1977 Frederick Sanger[79] played a major role in the development of a standard procedure for DNA sequencing. This eventually led to the establishment of comprehensive genome sequencing projects. The 3 classical components of genome analysis are DNA sequencing (such as shotgun and high-throughput, also known as next-generation sequencing [NGS]), the assembly of that sequence to create a representation of the original chromosome (using expressed sequence tags and bacterial artificial chromosomes), and the annotation and analysis of that representation with respect to its biologic information.[80,81] The Human Genome Project[80,82] (2003) and the International HapMap Project[83] (2005) are dedicated to undertaking sequencing of the human genome for use by researchers worldwide. However, other avenues of research are also under study. The following sections discuss the areas of genomics, cytogenetics, epigenetics, and proteomics (**Table 5**).

Genomics/Genetics

In the early efforts of genomics, developing advanced DNA sequencing techniques was critical. These have included NGS (also known as whole genome sequencing [WGE]), genome-wide association studies (GWAS), whole exon sequencing (WES), and single nucleotide variants (SNVs, or SNPs).[75,84] NGS captures information from the entire human genome; most NGS studies are associated with large sample sizes and diagnostic studies (case-control). In contrast, WES is a more cost-efficient approach that concentrates on the protein-coding regions of genes (exons), which make up only 1% of the genome, but carry 85% of disease-causing or pathogenic variants. Both WGS and WES have had a significant effect on our understanding of the pathogenesis of both common and rare human diseases. The base-position error rate in NGS sequencing is approximately 0.5% to 2.0%.[85] Thus, a significant rate of false-positives can result from a combination of errors and irregularities arising from the many steps and processes involved in NGS, and so these data need to be interpreted with a great deal of caution.[75,84] SNVs or SNPs can be used to indicate relationships in a family tree by selecting polymorphisms through the genome and using linkage analysis. Gene expression profiling focuses on detecting the expression of mRNA in specific tissues/cells of interest over time. For example, after the onset of a cerebral ischemia, the brain tissue may highly express mRNA for specific apoptosis signaling factors.

Other, newer methods of cost-effective high-throughput sequencing include nanopore technology at Harvard University, Illumina from Oxford Nanopore Technologies, the SOLiD System from Applied Biosystems, and SMART sequencing from Pacific Biosciences.[86]

Cytogenetics/Cytogenomics

Cytogenetics/cytogenomics refers to the study of the structure and function of the cell, particularly the chromosomes.[87] The 23 pairs of chromosomes in humans are made up of both DNA and protein. A centromere is located near the middle of each chromosome. It divides the chromosome into a short arm (p) and a long arm (q) and is also involved in chromosome movement. Telomeres are located at the ends of the p and q arms; these deter the degradation of DNA during chromosome replication

Table 5
Genetics/genomics technologies

Domain	Cytogenetics/Cytogenomics	Genetics/Genomics	Epigenetics/Epigenomics	Proteomics

Methods	**Chromosome Analyses**
	Karyotyping
	• Chromosome Banding
	  ○ G banding
	  ○ R banding
	  ○ C banding
	  ○ T banding
	  ○ Nucleolar Organizing region (NOR) stains
	• Fluorescent *in situ* Hybridization (FISH)
	• Comparative Genomic Hybridization (CGH)
		Genome-Wide Association Studies (GWAS)
		• Affymetric Genome-Wide Single Nucleotide Polymorphism (SNP) Array
		• Illumina Omi Microarray
		Candidate Gene and Polymorphism Selection
		• Polymorphisms
		  ○ Single Nucleotide Polymorphisms (SNPs)
		  ○ Repeat Polymorphisms (short tandem repeat; STR)
		  ○ Insertion/Deletion Polymorphisms (INDELs)
		  Real-time PCR allelic discrimination
		  ○ Copy number of variants (CNVs)
		TaqMan Copy Number Assays
		Fluorescence in situ Hybridization (FISH)
			Histone Modification
			Whole-Genome Analysis
			• Chromatin Immunoprecipitation (ChIP) and DNA microarray (ChIP-Chip)
			Candidate Gene Analysis
			• Single Gene ChIP
			• Mass Spectrometry (MS)
			DNA Methylation
			Whole-Genome Analysis
			• Affinity-based Immunoprecipitation(MeDIP) and microarray (MeDIP-Chip) and Infinium plateform
			• Candidate Genes Analysis
			  ○ HELP
			  ○ Pyrosequencing
			  ○ Single gene ChIP
			  ○ Mass Spectrometry (MS)
			Bisulfite-Conversion Based Methylation
			Whole-Genome
				Protein Isolation with Immunoassays
				• ELISA (Enzyme Linked Immunosorbent Assay)
				• MS (Mass Spectrometry)
				• SISCAPA(Stable Isotope Standard Capture with Anti-Peptide Antibodies)
				Identifying Proteins that are Post-Transnationally Modified
				• Two-dimensional gel electrophoresis
				• SDS-PAGE with shotgun proteomics
				• Antibody methods
				  ○ Enzyme-linked Immunosorbent assay (ELISA)
				  ○ Western Blot (WB)
				  ○ Immunohistochemistry (IHC)
				Protein-protein interactions
				• Two-hybrid analysis
				• Protein microarray

- Genotype:
  - Polymerase chain reaction-restriction fragment length polymorphism (PCR-RFLP)
  - Real-time PCR allelic discrimination (TaqMan)
  - iPLEX Gold-SNP Genotyping Assay
  - GoldenGate Genotyping Assay: (larger)
  - Mass Spectrometry (MS) Bead Chip
  - Infinium HumanMethylation450K

4.2 Candidate Gene
  - EpiTyper

1.3 Bisulphite-based sequencing (BS-seq)

Affinity Based Methylation

5.1 Whole-genome microarray
  - Methylation DNA immune precipitation-chromatin immune precipitation (MeDIP-chip) + PCR

Restriction Endonuclease-Based Methylation

As methylation mapping method

For both whole-genome and candidate genes

Next-Generation Sequencing for histone modification and methylation (ChIP-seq)

- Immunoaffinity chromatography
- MS

and are associated with aging.[87] Each chromosome has unique patterns and characteristics that chromosome 1 is the largest whereas chromosome 21 is the smallest.

During mitosis and meiosis, chromosomes play vital roles in genetic diversity. The 2 most common types of chromosomal abnormalities are constitutional abnormalities and somatic (or acquired) abnormalities. A constitutional abnormality begins in early development (resulting in abnormal chromosome numbers in the sperm or eggs) and is therefore present in all cells of the body. Somatic chromosomal abnormalities are present in only certain cells or tissues, causing mosaicism.[74,87,88] These chromosomal abnormalities are visible during metaphase or interphase of the cell cycle, which is the basis for cytogenetic technologies. Some of the current, routine clinical applications of cytogenetics are karyotyping, fluorescent in situ hybridization (FISH), comparative genomic hybridization (CGH), and chromosomal microarray analysis (CMA).[74,87,88] These methods have all been advantageous to medical diagnostics.

Karyotyping identifies chromosome abnormalities using staining techniques (G, R, C, and nuclear organizing region stains), which produce unique banding patterns on each chromosome.[87,89] Cells can be prepared from bone marrow, blood, amniotic fluid, cord blood, and tissue. A mitotic inhibitor (such as colchicine) is added to disrupt the mitotic spindle, leading to an increased yield of mitotic cells for analysis. A hypotonic solution is then used to swell the cells for better viewing on slide preparations under a microscope. Normally, the lighter regions are GC rich, whereas darker regions are AT rich.

FISH detects the presence or absence of specific DNA sequences using fluorescent probes for specific chromosomal regions.[74,90,91] FISH can also be used to detect the expression of specific RNA targets. Comparative genomic hybridization (CGH) is a molecular method for determining copy number variations (CNVs) within the DNA, usually between 2 sources (for instance normal tissue as a reference sample versus abnormal tissue as a test sample).[74,92] The CGH approach can be performed using either the whole genome or using specific chromosomal target regions. Different-colored fluorescent signals can distinguish the length of a chromosome in specific regions between 2 sources; a higher intensity of color in the sample group represents a gain of material in a specific region while a higher intensity of color the reference sample indicates loss of material in that region. A neutral color indicates no difference between 2 sample sources.

Epigenetics/Epigenomics

Epigenetics is the study of heritable changes in gene expression without changes to the DNA sequence itself, and usually involves chemical modifications of the bases or proteins bound with the DNA.[93] Two mechanisms of epigenetic/epigenomic modification include histone modifications and DNA methylation.[75,84,94]

Histone modification regulates transcription, DNA repair,[95] DNA replication,[96] alternative splicing, and chromosome condensation.[97] Positively charged histone proteins (the core histones are H21, H2B, H3, and H4) are associated with negatively charged DNA in the chromatin.[97,98] The disruption of the contact between nucleosomes and the recruitment of chromatin remolding ATPases are key histone modifications that affect gene expression. Histone modifications can include chromatin remodeling, the positions of nucleosomes, and histone-modifying enzymes, and there is no single histone modification that can completely predict the chromatin state or DNA activity.[97]

DNA methylation is an important process that allows particular gene expression patterns to become stably transmitted to daughter cells. The most common form of DNA methylation often involves regions containing copies of the dinucleotide CpG (called CpG islands), which is a common target for cytosine methylation.[84] A CpG island is defined as a region in which at least 50% of bases are G and C. About 60% of human gene promoters are associated with CpG islands.[99] DNA methylation can inhibit gene expression by various mechanisms, including inhibiting transcription via DNA binding proteins.[100] Hypermethylation of DNA triggers the suppression of gene transcription and causes gene silencing; in contrast, hypomethylation leads to gene activation/expression.

Whole-genome histone modification assays include chromatin immunoprecipitation (ChIP), ChIP with a DNA microarray (ChIP-Chip), and next-generation sequencing (ChIP-Seq).[98,100] ChIP captures the position of modifications in the genome, whereas ChIP-Chip identifies areas of transcriptional activation or repression associated with certain histone modifications in specific regions. In addition, single gene ChIP and mass spectrometry (MS) can quantify the changes in specific histone modifications. Recently, high-throughput technologies, including serial analysis of gene expression (ChIP-SAGE) and paired-end ditag sequencing (ChIP-PET) have also been developed.[84,98] ChIP-Seq uses the same mechanisms as ChIP for both global and local histone modifications.

Other DNA methylation technologies include bisulfite conversion-based, affinity-based, and restriction endonuclease-based technologies. Bisulfite conversion-based technologies rely on the chemical conversion of unmethylated cytosine residues into uracil,[84] such as the Infinium Human Methylation 450K Bead Chip (whole-genome), which contains most common human DNA methylations, as well as EpiTyper for quantitative analysis. Methylated DNA immunoprecipitation (MeDIP) and MeDIP with a microarray (MeDIP-Chip) and quantitative polymerase chain reaction (PCR) is an affinity-based method that combines enzyme recognition and CpG sites to identify methylated regions on the genome.[84] The restriction landmark genome scanning method identifies methylated DNA via methylation sensitive enzymes.[101] Chip-Seq provides DNA sequencing for both histone modifications and DNA methylations.

Proteomics

Large-scale proteomics is devoted to understanding protein structure and function, which underlies our understanding of the metabolic pathways of cells.[102] The aim of proteomics experiments is to identify significantly different levels of proteins across samples. However, proteomics studies have some limitations due to the complexity of gene expression. First, the level of protein expressed in specific tissues/cells can vary based on the efficiency of protein degradation.[101–103] Also, although some proteins may still be active, they may be abnormal because of genetic alternations. Second, protein networks (protein-DNA or protein-protein interactions) may exhibit enhanced functions in the presence of some proteins, but may also inhibit other activities at the same time. Overall, the amount of protein produced differs from cell to cell and at different times. Although noncoding RNAs are not involved in protein transcription, they can affect the interaction between transcription and translation. Typically, microRNAs (miRNAs) are small portions of noncoding RNA that downregulate gene expression causing gene silencing.[104] Therefore, gene silencing via miRNAs can be a powerful tool for apoptosis and cell proliferation analysis. In medicine, epigenomics have applied to congenital genetic diseases and oncology therapies.

In the current environment of rapidly advancing technologies, methods for proteomics studies now also include immunoassays (ELISA, MS,[105,106] and sodium dodecyl sulfate polyacrylamide gel electrophoresis [SDS-PAGE], which identify proteins that are post-translationally modified),[107] as well as methods to study protein-protein interactions (2 hybrid analyses, protein microarrays, immunoaffinity chromatography, and MS). Fluorescence 2-dimensional differential gel electrophoresis[108] has also been widely used in protein research to identify quantitative changes across samples, with statistically valid results. The major goal of proteomics profiling is to investigate how gene and protein function can be associated with disease.

Many training opportunities are available for nursing professionals. The Summer Genetic Institute (SGI),[109] which the NINR sponsors, offers 6 weeks of intense lectures and laboratory skills training at NIH's main campus in Bethesda, MD. The SGI program started in 2000; Drs Roland Nardone, Patricia Grady, and Francine Nichols are the course directors. Most students were doctoral/post-doctoral nursing scholars, nursing faculty, or advanced clinical practitioners. Participants from more than 15 universities/institutes enrolled each year. By 2013, 233 students had completed this course, and more than 130 peer-reviewed publications have come from SGI participants; in addition, 47 SGI graduates have received federal funding for the research proposals they developed during the SGI. The SGI gives participants an opportunity to increase their knowledge in (1) using the molecular genetics methods in bio-behavioral research in a laboratory setting; (2) analyzing strategies used for genomic-based therapies and describing trends in molecular therapeutics; (3) identifying the strengths, weaknesses, and applications of genetic test; and (4) examining the ethical and legal issues related to genetic testing and genetic counseling and their implications for practice and research. SGI limits its applicants to either American citizens or permanent residents; it allows only a certain number of participants per term.

Second, the Junior Scientist Laboratory Training program (6 graduate credits), sponsored by the BioTract Program at NIH,[110] takes place at the main campus in Bethesda. The goal is to provide a quality training program that bridges the gap between the levels of laboratory skills biology graduates have acquired and the proficiency level these graduates need to be productive in a research laboratory setting. Ideal candidates need to be post baccalaureates, recent college graduates, fourth-year biology majors, or other science students who want to strengthen their laboratory skill set. Finally, the Cincinnati Children's Hospital[111] provides 2 specific programs for either nursing educators (18-week Web-based Genetics Institute course) or practitioners (5 weeks applying genomics in nursing practice and an independent self-paced module online). These courses stipulate that the educators, clinicians, and researchers already have a sophisticated knowledge of genetics/genomics. The courses are available for American citizens, permanent residents, and foreign scholars training online.

In conclusion, it is essential for nurses to have genetic knowledge, clinical practice, and research skills. Professional nurses need to be familiar with genetic terminology and principles, as well as with clinical genetic tests and technology application with molecular biology skills in laboratory evidence/work. More research will identify which areas still need to be explored. An understanding of genomics by nurses will have implications on the well-being of the global community. **Box 1** provides more textbook information related to genomics/genetics.

FUTURE DIRECTION

The practice of genomics to personalized medicine is a groundbreaking one. Personalized medicine focuses on the individual's genes, proteins, and environment to prevent, diagnose, and treat disease; it also provides information about genome changes in cancer, nature heritability, genomic technology application, and education

Box 1
Textbooks resources

1. Alberts B, Johnson A, Lewis J, et al. Molecular Biology of the Cell. 5th edition. New York: Garland Science; 2008.

2. Brooker RJ. Genetics: Analysis Principle. New York: McGraw-Hill, Inc; 2011.

3. Current Protocols in Immunology. (2013). Wiley Online Library. Online ISBN: 9780471142737. DOI: 10.1002/0471142735. http://onlinelibrary.wiley.com/book/10.1002/0471142735.

4. Current Protocols in Human Genetics. (2013). Wiley Online Library. Online ISBN: 9780471142904 DOI: 10.1002/0471142905. http://onlinelibrary.wiley.com/book/10.1002/0471142905.

5. Current Protocols in Mice Biology. (2013). Wiley Online Library. Online ISBN: 9780470942390 DOI: 10.1002/9780470942390. http://onlinelibrary.wiley.com/book/10.1002/9780470942390.

6. Current Protocols in Protein Science. (2013). Wiley Online Library. Online ISBN: 9780471140863 DOI: 10.1002/0471140864. http://onlinelibrary.wiley.com/book/10.1002/0471140864.

7. Cooper GM, Hausman RE. The Cell: A Molecular Approach. 5th edition. Sunderland (MA): Sinauer Associates, Inc; 2009.

8. Monsen RB. Genetics and Ethics in Health Care: New Questions in the age of genomic health (2008). ISBN: 9781558102637; PUB# 9781558102637.

9. Haydon J. Genetics in Practice: A clinical approach for healthcare practitioner (2008). Print ISBN: 9781861564641; Online ISBN: 9780470697726.

10. Skirton H, Patch C. Genetics for the health sciences: a handbook for clinical healthcare (2009). UK: Scion Publishing Ltd. ISBN 10: 1904842704; ISBN 13: 9781904842705.

11. Hartl DL, Jones EW. Genetics: Analysis of Genes and Genomes. 6th edition. Jones and Bartlett Publishers, Inc; 2005.

12. Huether SE, McCance KL, Rote B. Understand Pathophysiology. 5th edition. (MO): Elsevier; 2010.

13. McCance KL, Huether SE, Brashers VL, et al. Pathophysiology: The Biologic Basis for Disease in Adults and Children. 6th edition. (MO): Mosby Elsevier; 2010.

14. Krebs JE, Goldstein ES, Kilpatrick ST. Lewin's Genes X. Jones and Bartlett Publishers, LLC; 2011.

15. Miller OJ, Therman E. Human Chromosomes. 4th edition. New York: Springer-Verlag Inc; 2010.

16. Petrucci RH, Hardwood WS, Herring FG, et al. General Biochemistry: Principles and Modern Applications. 9th edition. Upper Saddle River (NJ): Prentice-Hall, Inc; 2006.

17. Strachan T, Read A. Human Molecular Genetics. 4th edition. Garland Science, Taylor & Francis Group, LLC; 2011.

for better health care. Managing numerous amounts of genome data is a major health care responsibility because it leads to a better understanding of the entire human genomic map and the association between the genetic map and disease. As genome sequence data sets continue to grow, new computational tools with compression algorithms will efficiently store the findings. Researchers will then have the obligation to understand how the data sets work and how to use and improve error-corrected results.

Kirk and colleagues[112] used a questionnaire survey for global nursing professional leaders/organizations on genomics/genetics competencies in nursing curricula and regulatory standards. More than 10 countries (Brazil, Israel, Italy, Japan, Netherlands, Oman, Pakistan, South Africa, United Kingdom, and United States) have responded to this survey. The questionnaire results showed that the nursing curriculum has demonstrated significant achievements and offers future strategies that include the participation of government and other policy-making organizations. The results of this study showed that genetics/genomics components are still neither fully developed in nursing education nor fully incorporated as a standard for registration and licensure. The 2012 NINR Roundtable (NNRR)[113–115] recognized the vision and innovation of nursing research in the following areas: (1) creating challenges and opportunities for symptom research at the interface of technology, informatics, and engineering; (2) prioritizing research questions related to the use of technology in symptom management; (3) accelerating research translation into evidence-based practice; and (4) implementing best practice for training clinicians and scientists. Nursing genomics presents professional roles in health trajectory and enables nurses to implement their mission through education preparation, advance clinical practice experience, and bring bench evidence to bedside care research. The 2005 Global Health Conference of the International Council of Nurses[116] adopted a human genomics perspective as its target mission and implemented links to guidelines, best practices, publications, benchmarking tools, and education. In the future, genomic nurses will bridge the activities among educators, clinical leaders, and research collaborators to improve global health.

REFERENCES

1. World Health Organization. The Initiative on Genomics & Public Health. 2013. Available at: http://www.who.int/rpc/igph-projects/en/. Accessed May 5, 2013.
2. National Human Genome Research Institutes (NHGRI). Human Genome Project. 2010. Available at: http://report.nih.gov/nihfactsheets/ViewFactSheet.aspx?csid=45. Accessed May 5, 2013.
3. National Human Genome Research Institute (NHGRI). Education-Talking Glossary. 2013. Available at: http://www.genome.gov/Glossary/index.cfm?id=532. Accessed May 5, 2013.
4. Genomics and World Health. Report of the advisory committee on health research. Geneva (Switzerland): World Health Organization; 2002. 2004. Available at: http://apps.who.int/gb/ebwha/pdf_files/WHA57/A57_R13-en.pdf. Accessed May 5, 2013.
5. Huether SE, McCance KL, Rote B. Understand pathophysiology. 5th edition. (MO): Elsevier; 2010.
6. McCance KL, Huether SE, Brashers VL, et al. Pathophysiology: the biologic basis for disease in adults and children. 6th edition. (MO): Mosby Elsevier; 2010.
7. Knoppers BM, Hirtle M, Lormeau S. Ethical issues in international collaborative research on the human genome: the HGP and the HGDP. Genomics 1996;34:272–82.
8. Human Genome Project Information. Ethical, Legal, and Social Issues. 2011. Available at: http://www.ornl.gov/sci/techresources/Human_Genome/elsi/elsi.shtml. Accessed May 20, 2013.
9. Badzek L, Henaghan M, Turner M, et al. Ethical, legal, and social issues in the translation of genomics into health care. J Nurs Scholarship 2013;45(1):15–24.

10. UNESCO. Universal Declaration on Bioethics and Human Rights. United National Educational, Scientific and Cultural Organization. Division of Ethics of Science and Technology Social and Human Science Sector. Paris, France. January, 2006. Available at: http://www.unesco.org/shs/ethics. Accessed May 20, 2013.

11. President Bush Signs H.R. 493, the Genetic Information Nondiscrimination Act of 2008. Office of the Press Secretary. 2008. Available at: http://georgewbushwhitehouse.archives.gov/news/releases/2008/05/20080521-7.html. Accessed May 20, 2013.

12. World Health Organization. HGN activities in ELSI of human genomics. 2013. Available at: http://www.who.int/genomics/elsi/elsiatwho/en/index.html. Accessed May 5, 2013.

13. Nursing World-code of Ethics. Code of ethics for nurses with interpretive statements. The American Nurses Association, Inc; 2001. Available at: http://nursingworld.org/MainMenuCategories/EthicsStandards/CodeofEthicsforNurses/Code-of-Ethics.pdf. Accessed May 20, 2013.

14. Centennial Edition. Canadian Nurses Association. The Code of Ethics for Registered Nurses. Ottawa, ON. 2008. Available at: http://www2.cna-aiic.ca/cna/documents/pdf/publications/Code_of_Ethics_2008_e.pdf. Accessed May 20, 2013.

15. Nursing & Midwifery Council. The Code: Standards of Conduct, Performance and Ethics for Nurses and Midwives. London, UK. 2007. Available at: http://www.nmc-uk.org/Documents/Standards/nmcTheCodeStandardsofConductPerformanceAndEthicsForNursesAndMidwives_LargePrintVersion.PDF. Accessed May 20, 2013.

16. Garcia SP, Greco KE, Loescher LJ. Teaching strategies to incorporate genomics education into academic nursing curricula. J Nurs Educ 2011;50(11):612–9.

17. American Nurses Association. Consensus panel on genetic/genomic nursing competencies. Essentials of genetic and genomic nursing: competencies, curricula guidelines, and outcome indicators. 2nd edition. Silver Spring (MD): 2009.

18. Calzone KA, Jenkins J, Prows CA, et al. Establishing the outcome indicators for the essential nursing competencies and curricula guidelines for genetics and genomics. J Prof Nurs 2011;27(3):179–91.

19. Greco KE, Tinley S, Seibert D. Development of the essential genetic and genomic competencies for nurses with graduate degrees. Annu Rev Nurs Res 2011;29:173–90.

20. Calzone KA, Jenkins J. Genomics education in nursing in the United States. Annu Rev Nurs Res 2011;29:151–72.

21. Daack-Hirsch S, Dieter C, Quinn Griffin MT. Integrating genomics into undergraduate nursing education. J Nurs Scholarsh 2011;43(3):223–30.

22. Pestka E, Lim SH, Png HH. Education outcomes related to including genomics activities in nursing practice in Singapore. Int J Nurs Pract 2010;16(3):282–8.

23. Prows CA, Glass M, Nicol MJ, et al. Genomics in nursing education. J Nurs Scholarsh 2005;37(3):196–202.

24. Jenkins J, Calzone K. Establishing the essential nursing competencies for genetics and genomics. J Nurs Scholarsh 2007;39:10–6.

25. U.S. Department of Health and Human Services Health Resources and Services Administration (HRSA). 2010. The registered nurse population: findings from the 2008 National Sample Survey of Registered Nurses. Available at: http://bhpr.hrsa.gov/healthworkforce/rnsurveys/rnsurveyfinal.pdf. Accessed May 20, 2013.

26. Jenkins JF, Calzone KA. Are nursing faculty ready to integrate genomics content into curricula? Nurse Educ 2012;37(1):25–9.

27. Burke S, Kirk M. Genetics education in the nursing profession: literature review. J Adv Nurs 2006;54(2):228–37.

28. Calzone KA, Cashion A, Feetham S, et al. Nurses transforming health care using genetics and genomics. Nurs Outlook 2010;58(1):26–35.

29. Shuster M. Can genetics and genomics nursing competencies be successfully taught in a prenursing microbiology course? CBE Life Sci Educ 2011;10(2): 216–21.

30. Guthrie JT, McRae A, Coddington CS, et al. Impacts of comprehensive reading instruction on diverse outcomes of low- and high-achieving readers. J Learn Disabil 2009;42(3):195–214. http://dx.doi.org/10.1177/0022219408331039.

31. Roger EM, Floyd SF. Communication of innovations—a cross-cultural approach. New York: The Free Press; 1971.

32. Hamilton R. Nursing advocacy in a postgenomic age. Nurs Clin North Am 2009; 44(4):435–46.

33. Genetic Nursing Credentialing Commission (GNCC). Advanced Practice (APNG) and Genetics Nurse (GCN) credential. 2013. Available at: http://www.geneticnurse.org/. Accessed May 5, 2013.

34. American Association of Colleges of Nursing. The essentials of Baccalaureate education for professional nursing practice. 2008. Washington, DC. Available at: http://www.aacn.nche.edu/education-resources/baccessentials08.pdf.

35. Pestka EL, Meiers SJ, Shah LL, et al. Nurses' perceived benefits, barriers, and educational recommendations for using family pedigrees in clinical practice. J Contin Educ Nurs 2012;43(11):509–17.

36. Calzone KA, Jenkins J, Yates J, et al. Survey of nursing integration of genomics into nursing practice. J Nurs Scholarsh 2012;44(4):428–36.

37. Crane MJ, Quinn Griffin MT, Andrews CM, et al. The level of importance of level of confidence that midwives in the United States attach to using genetics in practice. J Midwifery Womens Health 2012;57(2):114–9.

38. Kaye CI, Accurso F, La Franchi S, et al, Committee on Genetics. Newborn screening fact sheets. Pediatrics 2006;118(3):e934–63.

39. Lloyd-Puryea MA, Tonniges T, van Dyck PC, et al. American Academy of Pediatrics Newborn Screening Task Force recommendations: how far have we come? Pediatrics 2006;117(5 Pt 2):S194–211.

40. National Institutes of Health. Patient Education-Medline Plus: Newborn screen. U.S. National Library of Medicine. Available at: http://www.nlm.nih.gov/medlineplus/tutorials/newbornscreening/htm/_no_50_no_0.htm. Accessed May 5, 2013.

41. National Cancer Institute. BRCA1 and BRCA2: Cancer risk and genetic testing. 2013. Available at: http://www.cancer.gov/cancertopics/factsheet/Risk/BRCA. Accessed May 29, 2009.

42. National Cancer Institute. PDQ® Cancer information summary. Genetics of breast and ovarian cancer (PDQ®)-Health Professional. Date last modified 04/24/2009. Available at: http://www.cancer.gov/cancertopics/pdq/genetics/breast-and-ovarian/healthprofessional. Accessed May 15, 2013.

43. Vatanavicharn N, Ratanarak P, Liammongkolkul S, et al. Amino acid disorders detected by quantitative amino acid HPLC analysis in Thailand: an eight-year experience. Clin Chim Acta 2012;413(13–14):1141–4.

44. Wang C, Zhang W, Song F, et al. A simple method for the analysis by MS/MS of underivatized amino acids on dry blood spots from newborn screening. Amino Acids 2012;42(5):1889–95.

45. Adachi M, Soneda A, Asakura Y, et al. Mass screening of newborns for congenital hypothyroidism of central origin by free thyroxine measurement of blood samples on filter paper. Eur J Endocrinol 2012;166(5):829–38.

46. The Children's Hospital of Philadelphia. Types of genetic disease. 2013. Available at: http://www.chop.edu/healthinfo/types-of-genetic-diseases.html. Accessed May 5, 2013.

47. National Human Genome Research Institute (NHGRI). Learning about an undiagnosed condition in a child. 2011. Available at: http://www.genome.gov/17515951. Accessed May 5, 2013.

48. Centers for Disease Control and Prevention. Autism spectrum disorders (ASDs): data and statistics. 2013. Available at: http://www.cdc.gov/ncbddd/autism/data.html. Accessed May 5, 2013.

49. Ridker PM, Chasman DI, Zee RY, et al, Women's Genome Health Study Working Group. Rationale, design, and methodology of the Women's Genome Health Study: a genome-wide association study of more than 25,000 initially healthy American women. Clin Chem 2008;54(2):249–55.

50. National Cancer Institute. SEER Cancer Statistics Review, 1975–2005. 2009. Available at: http://seer.cancer.gov/csr/1975_2005/index.html. Accessed on April 20, 2013.

51. Hayes J, Barry MJ. Preventing prostate cancer overdiagnosis from becoming overtreatment. Oncology (Williston Park) 2011;25(6):468, 471, 478.

52. Hugosson J, Carlsson S, Aus G, et al. Mortality results from the Goteborg randomised population-based prostate-cancer screening trial. Lancet Oncol 2010; 11(8):725–32.

53. Shteynshlyuger A, Andriol GL. Cost-effectiveness of prostate specific antigen screening in the United States: extrapolating from the European study of screening for prostate cancer. J Urol 2011;185(3):828–32.

54. Tosoian JJ, Trock BJ, Landis P, et al. Active surveillance program for prostate cancer: an update of the Johns Hopkins experience. J Clin Oncol 2011;16:2185–90.

55. The National Human Genomics Research Institutes (NHGRI). National Institutes of Health Workshop Statement on Reproductive Genetic Testing: impact on women. 2012. Available at: http://www.genome.gov/10001753. Accessed May 30, 2013.

56: The Department of Health & Human Services. The Administration on Aging: aging statistics. 2013. Available at: http://www.aoa.gov/Aging_Statistics/. Accessed May 5, 2013.

57. Grady PA. Advancing the health of our aging population: a lead role for nursing science. Nurs Outlook 2011;59(4):207–9.

58. Wan He, Sengupta M, Velkoff VA. US Census Bureau, current population reports, p23–209, 65+ in the United States: 2005, U.S. Washington, DC; Government Printing Office. 2011. Available at: http://www.census.gov/prod/2006pubs/p23-209.pdf. 2005. Accessed May 5, 2013.

59. Korf BR, Rehm HL. New approaches to molecular diagnosis. JAMA 2013; 309(14):1511–21.

60. Anand P, Kunnumakkara AB, Sundaram C, et al. Cancer is a preventable disease that requires major lifestyle changes. Pharm Res 2008;25(9):2097–116.

61. Biomarkers Definitions Working, Group. Biomarkers and surrogate endpoints: preferred definitions and conceptual framework. Clin Pharmacol Ther 2001; 69(3):89–95.

62. Heckman-Stoddard BM. Oncology biomarkers: discovery, validation, and clinical use. Semin Oncol Nurs 2012;28(2):93–8.

63. National Cancer Institute (NCI). Early detection research network. 2013. Available at: http://edrn.jpl.nasa.gov/standards/wiki/index.php/Main_Page. Accessed May 30, 2013.

64. Lindor NM, McMaster ML, Lindor CJ. Concise handbook of familiar cancer susceptibility syndromes. 2nd edition. J Natl Cancer Inst Monogr 2008;38: 1–93.

65. Weitzel JN, Blazer KR, Macdonald DJ, et al. Genetics, genomics and cancer risk assessment: state of the art and future directions in the era of personalized medicine. CA Cancer J Clin 2011;61:327–59.

66. Robson ME, Storm CD, Weitzel J. American Society of Clinical Oncology policy statement update: genetic and genomic testing for cancer susceptibility. J Clin Oncol 2010;28:893–901.

67. Centers for Disease Control and Prevention (CDC). Genomic testing: ACCE model process for evaluating genetic tests. 2013. Available at: http://www.cdc.gov/genomics/gtesting/ACCE/. Accessed on May 5, 2013.

68. Burke W, Zimmern R. Moving beyond ACCE: an expanded framework for genetic test evaluation. A paper for the United Kingdom Genetic Testing Registry, PHG Foundation. 2007.

69. Clarke L, Zheng-Bradley X, Smith R, et al, 1000 Genomes Project Consortium. The 1000 Genomes Project: data management and community access. Nat Methods 2012;9(5):459–62.

70. Grady PA. Creating a healthier tomorrow through research, practice, and policy. Nurs Outlook 2010;58(5):268–71.

71. National Human Genome Research Institute (NHGRI). Journal of Nursing Scholarship Genomic Nursing Webinar Series. 2013. National Institutes of Health. Available at: http://www.genome.gov/27552312#al-2. Accessed May 20, 2013.

72. Brooker RJ. Genetics: analysis principle. New York: McGraw-Hill, Inc; 2011.

73. Cooper GM, Hausman RE. The cell: a molecular approach. 5th edition. Sunderland (MA): Sinauer Associates, Inc; 2009.

74. Strachan T, Read A. Human molecular genetics. 4th edition. Garland Science Publishing. New York: Wiley-Liss; 2011. ISBN: 978-0815341499.

75. Baumgartel K, Zelazny J, Timcheck T, et al. Molecular genomic research design. Annu Rev Nurs Res 2011;29:1–26.

76. Kurnat-Thoma EL. Genetics and genomics: the scientific drives of personalized medicine. Annu Rev Nurs Res 2011;29:27–54.

77. Nagele P. Perioperative genomics. Best Pract Res Clin Anaesthesiol 2011;25(4): 549–55.

78. Watson JD, Crick FH. Molecular structure of nucleic acids: a structure for deoxyribose nucleic acid. Nature 1953;171:737.

79. Sanger F. Determination of nucleotide sequences in DNA. Biosci Rep 2004; 24(4–5):237–53.

80. Collins FS, Patrinos A, Jordan E, et al. New goals for the U.S. Human Genome Project: 1998-2003. Science 1998;282(5389):682–9.

81. Venter JC. A part of the human genome sequence. Science 2003;299(5610): 1183–4.

82. DeLisi C. The human genome project. Am Sci 1988;76:488.

83. International HapMap Project. 2013. Available at: http://hapmap.ncbi.nlm.nih.gov/. Accessed May 5, 2013.

84. Conley YP, Biesecker LG, Gonsalves S, et al. Current and emerging technology approaches in genomics. J Nurs Scholarsh 2013;45(1):5–14.

85. Su Z, Ning B, Fnag H, et al. Next-generation sequencing and its applications in molecular diagnostics. Expert Rev Mol Diagn 2011;11(3):333–43.
86. Zhang J, Chiodini R, Badr A, et al. The impact of next-generation sequencing on genomics. J Genet Genomics 2011;38:95–109.
87. Miller OJ, Therman E. Human chromosomes. 4th edition. Springer-Verlag New York Inc; 2010. ISBN: 0-387-95046-X.
88. Hartl DL, Jones EW. Genetics: analysis of genes and genomes. 6th edition. Jones and Bartlett Publishers, Inc; 2005.
89. Barch MJ. Clinical cytogenetics: the act cytogenetics laboratory manual. New York: Raven Press, Inc; 1991.
90. Kurz CM, Moosdijk SV, Thielecke H, et al. Towards a cellular multi-parameter analysis platform: fluorescence in situ hybridization (FISH) on microhole-array chips. Conf Proc IEEE Eng Med Biol Soc 2011;2011:8408–11.
91. Amann R, Fuchs BM. Single-cell identification in microbial communities by improved fluorescence in situ hybridization techniques. Nat Rev Microbiol 2008;6(5):339–48.
92. Weiss MM, Hermsen MA, Meijer GA, et al. Comparative genomic hybridisation. Mol Pathol 1999;52(5):243–51.
93. Bird A. Perceptions of epigenetics. Nature 2007;447(7143):396–8.
94. Robertson KD, Wolffe AP. DNA methylation in health and disease. Nat Rev Genet 2000;1(1):11–9.
95. Huertas D, Sendra R, Munoz P. Chromatin dynamics coupled to DNA repair. Epigenetics 2009;4(1):31–42.
96. Luco RF, Pan Q, Tominaga K, et al. Regulation of alternative splicing by histone modifications. Science 2010;327(5968):996–1000.
97. Kouzarides T. Chromatin modifications and their function. Cell 2007;128(4):693–705.
98. Barski A, Cuddapah S, Cui K, et al. High-resolution profiling of histone methylations in the human genome. Cell 2007;129(4):823–37.
99. Portela A, Esteller M. Epigenetic modifications and human disease. Nat Biotechnol 2010;28(10):1057–68.
100. Kouzarides T. SnapShot: histone-modifying enzymes. Cell 2007;128(4):802.
101. Laird PW. Principles and challenges of genome-wide DNA methylation analysis. Nat Rev Genet 2010;11:191–203.
102. Dhingra V, Gupta M, Andacht T, et al. New frontiers in proteomics research: a perspective. Int J Pharm 2005;299(1–2):1–18.
103. Rogers S, Girolami M, Kolch W, et al. Investigating the correspondence between transcriptomic and proteomic expression profiles using coupled cluster models. Bioinformatics 2008;24(24):2894–900.
104. Chen K, Rajewsky N. The evolution of gene regulation by transcription factors and microRNAs. Nat Rev Genet 2007;8(2):93–103.
105. Klopfleisch R, Klose P, Weise C, et al. Proteome of metastatic canine mammary carcinomas: similarities to and differences from human breast cancer. J Proteome Res 2010;9(12):6380–91.
106. Gupta N, Tanner S, Jaitly N, et al. Whole proteome analysis of post-translational modifications: applications of mass-spectrometry for proteogenomic annotation. Genome Res 2007;17(9):1362–77.
107. Rath A, Glibowicka M, Nadeau VG, et al. Detergent binding explains anomalous SDS-PAGE migration of membrane proteins. Proc Natl Acad Sci U S A 2009;106(6):1760–5.
108. Tonge R, Shaw J, Middleton B, et al. Validation and development of fluorescence two-dimensional differential gel electrophoresis proteomics technology. Proteomics 2001;1(3):377–96.

109. National Institute of Nursing Research (NINR). Summer Genetics Institute (SGI). 2013. Available at: https://www.ninr.nih.gov/training/trainingopportunitiesintramural/summergeneticsinstitute. Accessed May 5, 2013.

110. Bio-Trac: Junior Scientist training program. National Institutes of Health. 2013. Available at: http://www.biotrac.com/pages/Tracs/Trac_Junior_Scientist_Training_Program.html. Accessed May 5, 2013.

111. Cincinnati Children's Hospital. Genetics education program for nurses. 2013. Available at: http://www.cincinnatichildrens.org/education/clinical/nursing/genetics/default/. Accessed May 5, 2013.

112. Kirk M, Calzone K, Arimori N, et al. Genetics-genomics competencies and nursing regulation. J Nurs Scholarsh 2011;43(2):107–16.

113. Genomic Nursing State of the Science Advisory Panel, Calzone KA, Jenkins J, Bakos AD. A blueprint for genomic nursing science. J Nurs Scholarsh 2013; 45(1):96–104.

114. Grady PA. The National Institute of Nursing Research: delivering on the promise. Appl Nurs Res 2012;25(4):229–30.

115. Grady PA. Vision and Innovation: the National Nursing Research Roundtable. Heart Lung 2012;41(4):319–20.

116. International Council of Nurses (ICN). Global health workforce alliance. 2010. Available at: http://www.who.int/workforcealliance/members_partners/member_list/icn/en/index.html. Accessed May 15, 2013.

How Advances in Genomics are Changing Patient Care

Elizabeth K. Bancroft, RN, PhD

KEYWORDS

• Genetics • Genomics • Nursing • Practice implications

KEY POINTS

- The understanding and application of genetic/genomic information is changing health care practice, and is becoming an integral part of routine health assessment and a standard component of a multidisciplinary approach to the diagnosis and treatment of disease.
- Primary care practitioners and nurses in particular will be at the forefront of using and interpreting genetic test results for the prevention and treatment of common chronic diseases, with only the more complicated cases referred to a genetics specialist.
- Keeping knowledge current in this rapidly advancing field is a challenge for all health professionals.
- Nurses are in a unique position to assist with the integration of genetics into everyday practice.
- The major challenge for professional leaders is in ensuring that nurses are satisfied they have adequate training and support in learning about genetics, which historically has been poorly covered in the nursing curricula.

INTRODUCTION

The integration of genetics and genomics into mainstream health care has been highlighted as a major change in practice that will affect the delivery of health care at all levels.[1–4] The complete sequencing of the Human Genome Project (HGP) in 2003 has led to a new direction, in particular to the understanding of common diseases. Thus treatments for both rare and common diseases are now better understood based on the genetic information available. Genetic conditions have historically been

Funding: E.K. Bancroft is funded by Cancer Research UK (Professor Eeles' Programme Grant, reference C5047/A15007). Funding is provided by the National Institute of Health Research to the Biomedical Research Center at The Royal Marsden NHS Foundation Trust and The Institute of Cancer Research.
Conflict of Interest: No conflict of interest has been declared by the author.
The Oncogenetics Team, The Royal Marsden NHS Foundation Trust and The Institute of Cancer Research, Downs Road, Sutton, Surrey SM2 5PT, UK
E-mail address: elizabeth.bancroft@rmh.nhs.uk

managed within specialist genetics centers; however, genetic and genomic information is slowly being integrated into the management of nearly all common diseases.

Understanding of the genetic/genomic basis of disease has risen exponentially since the completion of the HGP, and the use of the knowledge generated by this initiative has the potential to help identify individuals at most risk of certain diseases.[5-8] Such understanding will enable screening and prevention measures to be targeted at those who need it most, and improve diagnostics and treatments. This approach to health care is often referred to as "personalized medicine." However, most nurses have received minimal genetics education, so this change in practice may seem daunting.

Nurses in all roles, such as primary care, at the patient's bedside, and in tertiary specialties, have an important role in promoting health to ultimately prevent or reduce the burden of disease and to educate patients.[9] Nurses are particularly well placed, having close relationships with both patients and their families, to identify when a disease may have an inherited component. This more informal setting can often lead to discussions about the health of other family members rather than being mentioned during an often time-pressured medical consultation.

The aim of this article is to provide an overview of how genetics/genomics has the potential to improve health care within many different clinical scenarios, and in particular to highlight the key issues for nurses working across a variety of roles. First, definitions of personalized medicine, genetics, and genomics are provided to explain their importance in health care today. Second, a brief overview of traditional genetics services is presented, explaining why rare genetic conditions will continue to be managed within a specialist service. Third, the ways in which increased knowledge of genetics/genomics is being integrated into mainstream practice for all common diseases are described, for example, influencing choices of screening and therapeutics. Finally, how this knowledge has the potential to benefit both the individual patient and populations as a whole is discussed, highlighting the key issues and challenges for health care providers and, in particular, for nurses. The objective is to point out to nurses from every specialty why they will need a basic understanding of genetics to deliver optimal care to their patients.

PERSONALIZED MEDICINE

Personalized medicine describes the use of specific information about individuals to decide which interventions will best treat their disease, or prevent them from developing a disease. To some extent health care professionals have always practiced personalized medicine, using information about a person's lifestyle, family history, and environment to inform management decisions.[8] However, more recently the phrase personalized medicine has more commonly been applied to the use of genetic/genomic information in health care. Much of the variation in disease susceptibility and response to drugs is believed to be genetically determined, and there is an increasing expectation that the understanding of this will personalize the delivery of medicine.[8]

GENETICS AND GENOMICS

Every cell in the human body contains a nucleus, within which DNA is stored. DNA contains the 20,000 genes that make up the human genome. 'Genetics' and 'Genomics' are terms that are often used interchangeably. The World Health Organization refers to genetics as the study of heredity, and genomics as the study of genes and their function. The main difference is that whereas genetics examines the function and composition of a single gene, genomics incorporates all genes and their interrelationships so as to understand their combined effect on growth and development.[10]

A person's characteristics are determined by the interactions of these 20,000 genes, together with a host of external factors. These complex interactions determine that although genetic factors are important in the development of all diseases, no single genetic variant is predictive of when or whether a person will develop a disease, or of its severity[11,12] (There are some exceptions; for example, very rare genetic conditions such as Huntington's disease. If someone has a mutation in the Huntington's disease gene, they will definitely develop the disease at some point in their lifetime if they reach adulthood). An individual gene may make a contribution to disease, but on its own is insufficient to cause the disease. Instead, the disease will manifest in the presence of other factors (genetic and/or environmental). It is widely accepted that the development of the vast majority of common diseases is due to the action of multiple genes, termed polygenic (multiple gene) inheritance, rather than being due to the presence of a mutation in a single gene.[13,14]

There are two important definitions to understand when considering genetic mutations: *germline* and *somatic*. Mutations to genes that are acquired during a person's lifetime, which cannot be inherited, are termed somatic mutations. Mutations in genes that a person is born with, and which are found in the DNA of every cell in the body (except the gametes), are known as germline mutations. Germline mutations can also be found in some of the ova and sperm, therefore these mutations can be passed on to future generations.

SPECIALIST CLINICAL GENETICS SERVICE

Clinical genetics is a medical specialty that provides the diagnosis and management of genetic conditions. Genetic counseling and genetic testing can be offered to individuals and families with, or at risk of, conditions that may have a genetic basis; for example, chromosomal abnormalities such as Down syndrome, single gene disorders such as Huntington's disease or cystic fibrosis, and birth defects such as a cleft palate or neural tube defects. Families with hereditary cancer are also managed by clinical genetics services.

Management of Hereditary Cancer

Cancer is very common, affecting approximately 1 in 3 people in their lifetime, and is known to have a hereditary component in some families. Dominantly inherited germline mutations in genes with a predisposition to cancer account for an estimated 5% to 10% of all cases of cancer.[15] It is possible, however, that even more cases may have a genetic component, as some genetic variants are very common and, although each has a small effect, in combination the risks can be substantial. Patients with a strong family history of cancer can be referred to a clinical genetics service for a risk assessment and to consider genetic testing where applicable.

As cancer is common, it can be difficult to know what constitutes a family history of concern. The main indications are:

- The same type of cancer affecting more than one close relative
- Young onset (eg, younger than 40–50 years for breast cancer, younger than 50 years for bowel cancer)
- If one person has been affected by more than one type of cancer
- Close family members affected by cancer in successive generations (eg, mother and daughter, father and son)

- The occurrence of more than one rare type of cancer in a family (eg, sarcoma and brain tumor)
- Ethnicity: some populations are known to have a higher risk (eg, people with Ashkenazi Jewish ancestry have a higher risk of carrying a mutation in *BRCA1/2*)

If a family meets any of these criteria, they may benefit from a referral to a specialist genetics service for assessment. The majority of testing currently undertaken for hereditary cancer is for the breast/ovarian cancer-predisposition genes *BRCA1* and *BRCA2*, or the mismatch repair genes (*MLH1, MSH2, MSH6, PMS2*) that confer a predisposition to colorectal and gynecologic cancers. With both of these conditions, the penetrance (the chance a disease will occur as a result of the presence of a mutation in one of these genes) is very high, up to 70% to 80% in most cases.[16–18] An individual identified with a mutation therefore has a high chance of developing cancer in the future, and the benefit of knowing this information is that regular screening can be offered from a younger age and that preventive options, such as surgery, can be considered.

THE FUTURE OF GENETICS AND GENOMICS: INTEGRATION INTO EVERYDAY PRACTICE

As already described, for very high-risk individuals with rare genetic conditions caused by a mutation in a single gene, management within a specialist genetics service is the optimal care. However, since the completion of the HGP it is now understood that a large proportion of variation, in both disease susceptibility and response to drugs, may be genetically determined.

Multiple genetic changes, or genetic variants, have been identified as being associated with the development of all common diseases. Each of these genetic changes individually only slightly affects the risk of being affected by a disease, and they are commonly seen in the general population. The development of tests that detect the presence of multiple variants would enable people to be stratified into different risk categories, from which screening and prevention methods could be offered accordingly.[19,20]

Although more information is needed to fully understand the role of genetic variants, it is anticipated that in the not too distant future, a person's entire genetic code will be a part of their electronic medical record. Therefore it is likely that genetic information will become integrated into routine health assessments, particularly within primary care.[1,7,19,21–23] This shift in health care will change nursing practice over the next decade. Genomics will become a significant feature of health care and nursing practice, and primary care providers will be at the forefront of using and interpreting genetic test results in relation to the prevention and treatment of common chronic diseases (more complicated cases and rare genetic conditions will continue to be referred to a genetics specialist). This routine integration will move genetics away from being a specialty and to become a standard part of the care pathway.

Nurses within primary, secondary, and tertiary care are ideally placed to provide information and support to patients receiving information based on their genetic risk.[9] Equality of access is an important issue, and nurses could play a central role in ensuring that all patient groups have equal access to such information. Health professionals will need adequate training not only in genetic science, but also in communicating genetic information to the public in a language they can understand.

Knowledge about the genetic basis of disease could be beneficial for delivering health care for the following reasons. First, it identifies individuals at higher risk of disease such as cancer, and enables screening to be targeted at the people who need it most.[24–26] Such targeting offers both personal and economic benefits as screening enables earlier detection of disease, thus decreasing morbidity and mortality. Second, the knowledge about how genes work will help to develop preventive strategies that may help an individual to reduce the risk of developing a disease. Third, this knowledge will inform potential therapeutic targets and drug dosages in the treatment of disease.[1,4,19,27,28] All of these aspects have the potential to benefit public health, and each are now discussed in more detail with clinical examples.

Using Genetics to Target Screening for Those Who Need it Most

Using genetic markers as an indication of a person's risk of disease has an advantage over other screening tools, because markers are always present and do not change over time or with a clinical condition.[29]

At present, population cancer screening programs, for example, for bowel, breast, and cervical cancer, use age to determine when screening should start, and everyone in a population is treated as being at risk once they reach the age specified. There is growing interest in using genetic information to help stratify people into different risk categories to stagger screening age based on a person's individual risk. A person's risk can be calculated using both age and genetic risk. The benefit of this method is that it would reduce the number of people undergoing screening whilst most cancers that would have been identified through an age-based screening program would still be detected.[19,24,25] As controversy exists around screening, reducing the number of people offered screening has the potential to reduce some of the potential harms.[24,30] For example, false-positive results can be very stressful for the person receiving them, and lead to unnecessary diagnostic tests. Reducing the number of people undergoing further investigations therefore has benefits for both the individual and the health service.[26] Personalizing screening in this way also has the potential to reduce the harms associated with overdiagnosis and overtreatment, which have been identified as particular issues in screening for breast and prostate cancer.[31,32]

Many questions need to be answered before such an approach could become integrated into practice for cancer screening; for example, whether genetic markers are able to distinguish between a predisposition to develop life-threatening rather than indolent cancer, and whether genetic testing would be acceptable to both the public and health professionals. In addition, lifestyle factors may affect risk; for example, the risk of breast cancer has been linked to obesity, lack of physical exercise, alcohol consumption, use of oral contraceptives, and hormone replacement therapy.[15] If screening is to be targeted at those most at risk, lifestyle factors will also need to be included in risk algorithms.

Using Genetics to Inform Prevention Strategies

The knowledge that one is more genetically susceptible to a disease offers the individual the opportunity to personally manage one's health and take any necessary precautions. For example, someone known to have a higher susceptibility to heart disease can reduce their risk by eating a healthy diet, increasing physical activity, reducing alcohol intake, and not smoking. Personalized education and prevention strategies can be developed to help patients at higher genetic risk to use such lifestyle alterations to help modify their risk, ultimately aiming to reduce the burden of disease. It is hypothesized that personal knowledge that one is at increased genetic risk may be a powerful motivator to adopt lifestyle changes to decrease such risk, although more research is needed in this area.[11,33–35]

Other examples of methods to prevent disease can be seen in the high-risk setting for women who carry a mutation in one of the high-risk breast cancer genes, *BRCA1* or *BRCA2*. Women who are known to carry a mutation in one of these genes can be referred to a breast surgeon to consider having a prophylactic mastectomy to remove their breast tissue, which has been demonstrated to significantly reduce the risk of breast cancer.[36] Alternatively, for those at high risk of breast cancer, studies have shown that taking tamoxifen or raloxifene, which are selective estrogen receptor modulators, for a period of 5 years can reduce the risk of breast cancer in postmenopausal women by 50%.[37,38] These two powerful examples show how knowledge of being at a high risk of a disease can have an impact on clinical decision making about the use of prevention strategies. As more is learned about the genetic basis of disease, clinicians will be able to identify many more people at increased risk of various diseases, and health delivery will increasingly focus on screening and prevention.

Targeting Drugs on an Individual Basis

The third area where the impact of genetic information is apparent is in the choice of specific drugs that is informed by genetic status; often referred to as pharmacogenomics. It is well documented that different people have very different responses to drugs, and this presents a serious clinical problem. It is known that approximately one-third of drugs prescribed have no clinical benefit for the person they are prescribed for.[26] In addition, adverse drug reactions are documented to be responsible for 1 in 15 hospital admissions in the United Kingdom, and affect more than 2 million people per year in the United States.[26,39] Many factors (eg, age, weight, and sex) can affect a response to a drug, but a substantial proportion of variation (estimated to be between 20% and 95%) is thought to be genetic.[26] There is therefore huge potential for genetics to be used to help predict an individual's response to drug treatments, thus enabling clinicians to increase the efficacy of drugs prescribed and avoid adverse drug reactions. Two examples of how genetics can help to improve the treatments targeted at specific individuals are presented.

Warfarin dosage

Warfarin has a narrow therapeutic index; however, it has a wide inter-individual variability in the dosage required for a therapeutic effect. If too much is prescribed, the patient is at risk of excess bleeding; if too little is administered, the patient is at risk of clot formation. Treatment with warfarin is common and effective, but requires regular monitoring to ensure the patient is receiving the correct dosage, which can be expensive for the health care system and time consuming for patients.[40]

Two genetic variants have been identified that affect the metabolism of warfarin: CYP2C9 and VKOR.

- CYP2C9 is a liver enzyme responsible for metabolizing foreign chemicals and drugs, including warfarin. Variations in the gene encoding this enzyme result in different metabolic abilities of the enzyme.[40,41]
- Warfarin induces anticoagulation by inhibiting vitamin K epoxide reductase (VKOR), which is an enzyme involved in the recycling of vitamin K, an essential cofactor for clotting factors. Genetic variants in the gene encoding VKOR therefore affect a person's clotting rates.[40]

The Food and Drug Administration (FDA) have acknowledged the role of these genetic variants in individual response to warfarin dosages and have relabeled warfarin, stating that a lower initiation dose should be prescribed for those with genetic variations in CYP2C9 and VKOR enzymes. The use of this individualized genetic information can therefore be used to determine the optimal dosage of warfarin, resulting in less need for close monitoring and a reduction in side effects. Other factors also affect the response to warfarin, including age, gender, and weight, therefore these must also be taken into consideration by the prescriber.[42]

Herceptin and breast cancer

The use of trastuzumab (Herceptin) in the treatment of breast cancer is an example of how somatic genetic information can help to inform the optimal treatment for an individual. Approximately one-quarter of patients with breast cancer have tumors that overexpress the human epidermal receptor type 2 (*HER2*) gene. This overexpression results in high concentrations of the HER2 receptor in these cells, causing growth and progression of cancer cells. Breast tumors are tested for their HER2 status at diagnosis and, before the development of drugs such as trastuzumab, the prognosis for women with HER2-positive tumors was poor.

Herceptin is a monoclonal antibody that binds to the HER2 receptor, blocking the receptor to reduce its ability to accelerate division and development of cancer cells.[43–45] Therefore, it is prescribed only for the subset of women whose tumors express the HER2 receptor, and is an example of how understanding personalized genetic information about a tumor is already used to inform cancer treatment.

These two examples show how individual genetic variation can be used to optimize and personalize the treatments of patients. This area of medicine is developing rapidly, and nurses will need to have an understanding of why certain treatments may work for some patients, but not for others with seemingly very similar diseases. Patients themselves will question why they are advised to take certain medications, and explaining how complex genetic factors inform the decision-making process may prove to be a challenge.

CHALLENGES TO THE INTEGRATION OF GENETICS INTO ROUTINE CLINICAL PRACTICE

As already discussed, the advances in understanding the genetic basis of disease have huge potential to improve health care for the individual and to help truly personalize patient care. However, there are several challenges to routinely integrating genetics into mainstream practice in an effective way.

A note of caution in using genetic/genomic information to inform health care is that it should always be considered within the context of a patient's lifestyle and the family history of a disease. Making an assessment based on all of the information available will give the patient a more accurate understanding of his or her risk of disease. For example, if a person does not have a high genetic risk of heart disease but is overweight, inactive, smokes cigarettes, and has a high-fat diet, the genetic information would not be used in isolation to advise them that their risk of heart disease is low. Instead the patient would be counseled on lifestyle, highlighting the increased risk of heart disease based on these lifestyle factors alone.

Use and Interpretation of Genetic Information

Genetic information is perceived as being different to other types of personal and medical data, and this has been termed "genetic exceptionalism."[28,46] This difference is due to genetics being seen as family information, as our genetic makeup is shared with our immediate and wider family members and, as such, can give an indication about the likely genetic makeup of a close relative. People have no control over their genetic makeup, yet genetic information has the potential to predict future disease in people with no symptoms or any idea that they are at increased risk.[26,47] There is potential for anxiety in people identified to be at a higher risk of disease, and this could be a burden in terms of uncertainty about the future.[27] Difficult decisions will need to be made in regard of compliance with screening programs and preventive measures, despite being unable to predict if or when the disease will present.

Provision of Information

If a genetic risk assessment is to become a routine part of health care, the information provided to patients and their families will need careful consideration. There will be the need to counsel people about the benefits and limitations of genetic information, and for this information to be meaningful for them.[48,49] There is a common misconception that genetic information is extremely accurate,[50] but disease is the result of complex interactions between both genetic and environmental factors. It is the role of health care professionals to assist with the interpretation of individuals' risk of disease based on their family history and other risk factors alongside any genetic testing results that may be available. Nurses could play a key role in the provision of information and counseling, support, and follow-up of people undergoing such testing, and in assisting in the interpretation of test results,[51] and it is important that they fully understand the implications of any test results being used to inform a patient's care.

Accessing Genetic Information

Personalized medicine using genetic information has received much attention, both in the media and from health care providers, which has led to the rapid proliferation of Web-based companies offering genetic testing direct to the consumer (DTC) without the need to go through a medical practitioner[28,52] (eg, see Refs.[53–55]). The FDA does not oversee DTC genetic tests, and companies therefore do not need to provide evidence of the validity of the test results. Moreover, there is variability across the United States with regard to restrictions placed on these Web sites. Concern has been voiced by health professionals, regulators, policy advisors, and ethicists about this provision of genetic information outside the clinical context, for tests that are not yet considered to be clinically useful. For people accessing such tests without adequate information on their limitations, there is potential for negative consequences such as increased anxiety when a result indicates a higher risk of disease.[28,56]

Ethical Issues and the Right Not to Know

If a person's entire genetic code becomes part of his or her electronic medical record, the ability to test for a person's predisposition to multiple diseases will become commonplace.[57] Such testing will present particular challenges in terms of gaining consent from patients, as there may be information that people would prefer not to know. For example, people may prefer not to find out that they carry a mutation in a gene that predisposes them to Alzheimer's disease. When asked hypothetically, many people state that they want all information available, but this is when they are not aware of what all the information could be and what it might imply.[58] How health care professionals manage and communicate this information promises to be a considerable challenge.

Inherited disorders can be distinguished from other illnesses by the implications they carry for other blood relatives, and a person who is identified to have a genetic predisposition to a disease may then be faced with the choice of informing other family members. The impact of disease status may have untold repercussions on close relatives. Family dynamics and communication processes, notions of self-identity, culture, and the relationship with health services may all be affected. Family dynamics are often complex, with issues such as divorce, adoption, bereavement, geographic distance, and family rifts causing potential communication barriers.[59–61]

There is concern, particularly for younger people, that being identified as having a genetic predisposition to certain diseases may lead to future discrimination when seeking insurance and employment.[62,63] In the United States the Genetic Information Nondiscrimination Act, passed in 2008, is designed to prohibit the use of genetic information in health insurance and employment. In the United Kingdom, the Association of British Insurers has a moratorium until 2017 preventing the use of predictive genetic test results being used in insurance premiums. In Canada, there is currently no legislation in place specifically prohibiting genetic discrimination.

Genetics Education

As highlighted throughout this article, there is increasing emphasis on using genetic/genomic information to inform preventive medicine and health promotion on all levels of patient care. Nurses in all areas of clinical practice will play a considerable role in providing the counseling, information, support, and follow-up for individuals identified as being at a higher risk of disease based on their genetic status. Consequently it has been recognized that genetics education is an important requirement for all health professionals, and guidelines for education and competencies have been developed.[64,65] In addition, dedicated genetics education organizations for health professionals have been established in The United States, Europe, and the United Kingdom, offering useful online teaching modules.[65–68] It has been recognized by the UK Department of Health that all nurses must be competent in delivering genomic health care, and that professional leaders should be prioritizing the incorporation of genomics into education and practice.[69] Despite these efforts, genetic/genomic education is still lacking within nursing curricula internationally. Improving genetics education for nurses and all health professionals is vital to full integration of genetic/genomic advances into everyday care and the benefit of patients. However, this is a substantial challenge that should not be underestimated, and will require a significant amount of funding and resources.[9,66,70]

SUMMARY

This article provides an overview of how the understanding and application of genetic/genomic information is changing health care practice, and is becoming an integral part of routine health assessment as well as a standard component of a multidisciplinary approach to the diagnosis and treatment of disease. This integration has implications for health care professionals involved in all aspects of patient care. Primary care practitioners and nurses, in particular, will be at the forefront of using and interpreting genetic test results for the prevention and treatment of common chronic diseases, with only the more complicated cases referred to a genetics specialist. Examples are provided for how both germline and somatic mutations are having an impact on the drugs prescribed to manage diseases. Keeping knowledge current in this rapidly advancing field is a challenge for all health professionals.

The key message for nurses is that they are in a unique position to assist with the integration of genetics into everyday practice. Nurses are ideally placed to help with the interpretation of genetic information and to educate and counsel patients, making information accessible. The fact that nurses have close relationships with both patients and their families offers the opportunity to identify when a disease may have a genetic component. The major challenge for professional leaders is in ensuring that nurses are satisfied they have adequate training and support in learning about genetics, which historically has been poorly covered in the nursing curricula. This shortcoming has been identified as a problem internationally, and it is anticipated that there will be a shift in education over the coming years to accommodate this rapidly evolving change in practice.

ACKNOWLEDGMENTS

The author thanks Theresa Wiseman, Audrey Ardern-Jones, and Ros Eeles for their comments on this article.

REFERENCES

1. Lango H, Weedon MN. What will whole genome searches for susceptibility genes for common complex disease offer to clinical practice? J Intern Med 2008;263(1):16–27.
2. Pearson H. Genetic testing for everyone. Nature 2008;453(7195):570–1.
3. Javitt GH, Hudson K. The right prescription for personalized genetic medicine. Personalized Medicine 2007;4(2):115–8.
4. Zheng SL, Sun J, Wiklund F, et al. Cumulative association of five genetic variants with prostate cancer. N Engl J Med 2007;358:910–9.
5. Human Genomics Strategy Group. Building on our inheritance: genomic technology in healthcare. The Department of Health; 2012. Available at: https://www.gov.uk/government/uploads/system/uploads/attachment_data/file/213705/dh_132382.pdf. Accessed March 1, 2013.
6. Collins F, McKusick V. Implications of the Human Genome Project for medical science. JAMA 2001;285:540–4.
7. Burke W. Genetic testing in primary care. Annu Rev Genomics Hum Genet 2004; 5:1–14.
8. Samani NJ, Tomaszewski M, Schunkert H. The personal genome—the future of personalised medicine? Lancet 2010;375(9725):1497–8.
9. Calzone KA, Cashion A, Feetham S, et al. Nurses transforming health care using genetics and genomics. Nurs Outlook 2010;58(1):26–35.
10. World Health Organisation. 2013. Available at: www.who.int. Accessed March 1, 2013.
11. Hall WD, Mathews R, Morley KI. Being more realistic about the public health impact of genomic medicine. PLoS Med 2010;12(7):10.
12. Van Rijn MJ, van Duijn CM, Slooter AJ. Impact of genetic testing on complex diseases. Eur J Epidemiol 2005;20(5):383–8.
13. Witte JS. Personalized prostate cancer screening: improving PSA tests with genomic information. Sci Transl Med 2010;2(62):55.
14. Mihaescu R, Meigs J, Sijbrands E, et al. Genetic risk profiling for prediction of type 2 diabetes. PLoS Curr 2011;11:3.
15. Cancer Research UK. 2013. Available at: www.cancerresearchuk.org/. Accessed March 1, 2013.
16. Thompson D, Easton DF. Cancer incidence in BRCA1 mutation carriers. J Natl Cancer Inst 2002;94(18):1358–65.
17. Breast Cancer Linkage Consortium. Cancer risks in BRCA2 mutation carriers. J Natl Cancer Inst 1999;91(15):1310–6.
18. Aarnio M, Mecklin JP, Aaltonen LA, et al. Life-time risk of different cancers in hereditary non-polyposis colorectal cancer (HNPCC) syndrome. Int J Cancer 1995;64:430–3.
19. Pharoah PD, Antoniou AC, Easton DF, et al. Polygenes, risk prediction, and targeted prevention of breast cancer. N Engl J Med 2008;358(26):2796–803.
20. Antoniou AC, Easton DF. Models of genetic susceptibility to breast cancer. Oncogene 2006;25(43):5898–905.
21. Feero WG, Guttmacher AE, Collins FS. The genome gets personal—almost. J Am Med Assoc 2008;299:1351–2.

22. Khoury MJ, Gwinn M, Yoon PW. The continuum of translation research in genomic medicine: how can we accelerate the appropriate integration of human genome discoveries into health care and disease prevention? Genet Med 2007; 9:665–74.
23. Offit K. Genomic profiles for disease risk: predictive or premature? J Am Med Assoc 2008;299:1353–5.
24. Pashayan N, Pharoah P. Translating genomics into improved population screening: hype or hope? Hum Genet 2011;130(1):19–21.
25. Pashayan N, Duffy SW, Chowdhury S, et al. Polygenic susceptibility to prostate and breast cancer: implications for personalised screening. Br J Cancer 2011; 104(10):1656–63.
26. Stewart A, Brice P, Burton H, et al. Genetics, health care and public policy. Cambridge (United Kingdom): Cambridge University Press; 2007.
27. Lerman C, Shields AE. Genetic testing for cancer susceptibility: the promise and the pitfalls. Nat Rev Cancer 2004;4(3):235–41.
28. Speicher MR, Geigl JB, Tomlinson IP. Effect of genome-wide association studies, direct-to-consumer genetic testing, and high-speed sequencing technologies on predictive genetic counselling for cancer risk. Lancet Oncol 2010; 11(9):890–8.
29. Pomerantz MM, Freedman ML. Genetics of prostate cancer risk. Mt Sinai J Med 2010;77(6):643–54.
30. Ransohoff DF, Khoury MJ. Personal genomics: information can be harmful. Eur J Clin Invest 2010;40(1):64–8.
31. Bangma CH, Roemeling S, Schröder FH. Overdiagnosis and overtreatment of early detected prostate cancer. World J Urol 2007;25(1):3–9.
32. Independent UK Panel on Breast Cancer Screening. The benefits and harms of breast cancer screening: an independent review. Lancet 2012;380:1778–86.
33. Haga SB, Khoury MJ, Burke W. Genomic profiling to promote a healthy lifestyle: not ready for prime time. Nat Genet 2003;34:347–50.
34. Hunter DJ, Khoury MJ, Drazen JM. Letting the genome out of the bottle—will we get our wish? N Engl J Med 2008;358(2):105–7.
35. Khoury MJ. Genetics and genomics in practice: the continuum from genetic disease to genetic information in health and disease. Genet Med 2003;5: 261–8.
36. Domchek SM, Friebel TM, Singer CF, et al. Association of risk-reducing surgery in BRCA1 or BRCA2 mutation carriers with cancer risk and mortality. JAMA 2010;304(9):967–75.
37. Pruthi S, Gostout BS, Lindor NM. Identification and management of women with BRCA mutations or hereditary predisposition for breast and ovarian cancer. Mayo Clin Proc 2010;85:1111–20.
38. Vogel VG, Costantino JP, Wickerham DL, et al. Update of the National Surgical Adjuvant Breast and Bowel Project Study of Tamoxifen and Raloxifene (STAR) P-2 Trial: preventing breast cancer. Cancer Prev Res (Phila) 2010;3:696–706.
39. National Human Genome Research Institute. Personalized medicine: how the human genome era will usher in a health care revolution. 2005. Available at: http://www.genome.gov/13514107. Accessed March 1, 2013.
40. Kamali F, Wynne H. Pharmacogenetics of warfarin. Annu Rev Med 2010;61: 63–75.
41. Sanderson S, Emery J, Higgins J. CYP2C9 gene variants, drug dose, and bleeding risk in warfarin-treated patients: a HuGEnet systematic review and meta-analysis. Genet Med 2005;7:97–104.

42. McClain MR, Palomaki GE, Piper M, et al. A rapid-ACCE review of CYP2C9 and VKORC1 alleles testing to inform warfarin dosing in adults at elevated risk for thrombotic events to avoid serious bleeding. Genet Med 2008;10(2):89–98.

43. Abdel-Razeq H, Marei L. Current neoadjuvant treatment options for HER2-positive breast cancer. Biologics 2011;5:87–94.

44. Piccart-Gebhart MJ. Adjuvant trastuzumab therapy for HER2-overexpressing breast cancer: what we know and what we still need to learn. Eur J Cancer 2006;42:1715–9.

45. Valachis A, Mauri D, Polyzos NP, et al. Trastuzumab combined to neoadjuvant chemotherapy in patients with HER2-positive breast cancer: a systematic review and meta-analysis. Breast 2011;20(6):485–90.

46. Green MJ, Botkin JR. Genetic exceptionalism in medicine: clarifying the differences between genetic and non-genetic disease. Ann Intern Med 2003;138:571–5.

47. Clark A, Ticehurst F. Living with the genome: ethical and social aspects of human genetics. Basingstoke (United Kingdom): Palgrave Macmillan; 1996.

48. Smerecnik CM, Mesters I, de Vries N, et al. Educating the general public about multifactorial genetic disease: applying a theory-based framework to understand current public knowledge. Genet Med 2008;10(4):251–8.

49. Mesters I, Ausems A, De Vries H. General public's knowledge, interest and information needs related to genetic cancer: an exploratory study. Eur J Cancer Prev 2005;14(1):69–75.

50. Davison C, Macintyre S, Smith GD. The potential social impact of predictive genetic testing for susceptibility to common chronic diseases: a review and proposed research agenda. Sociol Health Illn 1994;16(3):340–71.

51. Calzone KA. Genetic predisposition testing: clinical implications for oncology nurses. Oncol Nurs Forum 1997;24:712–8.

52. Graves KD, Peshkin BN, Luta G, et al. Interest in genetic testing for modest changes in breast cancer risk: implications for SNP testing. Public Health Genomics 2011;14(3):178–89.

53. 23andMe. 2013. Available at: https://www.23andme.com/. Accessed March 15, 2013.

54. DeCODE. 2013. Available at: www.decodeme.com/. Accessed March 15, 2013.

55. Genetic Health. 2013. Available at: www.genetic-health.co.uk/. Accessed March 15, 2013.

56. Prainsack B, Reardon J, Hindmarsh R, et al. Personal genomes: misdirected precaution. Nature 2008;456(7218):34–5.

57. Calzone K, Bowles-Biesecker B. Genetic testing for cancer predisposition. Cancer Nurs 2002;25(1):15–25.

58. O'Daniel J, Haga SB. Public perspectives on returning genetics and genomics research results. Public Health Genomics 2011;14(6):346–55.

59. Koehly LM, Peters JA, Kenen R, et al. Characteristics of health information gatherers, disseminators, and blockers within families at risk of hereditary cancer: implications for family health education interventions. Am J Public Health 2009;99(12):2203–9.

60. Koehly LM, Peters JA, Kuhn N, et al. Sisters in hereditary breast and ovarian cancer families: communal coping, social integration, and psychological well-being. Psychooncology 2008;17(8):812–21.

61. Finlay E, Stopfer JE, Burlingame E. Factors determining dissemination of results and uptake of genetic testing in families with known BRCA1/2 mutations. Genet Test 2008;12(1):81–91.

62. Lerman C, Marshall J, Audrain J, et al. Genetic testing for colon cancer susceptibility: anticipated reactions of patients and challenges to providers. Int J Cancer 1996;69(1):58–61.
63. Billings P, Beckwith J. Genetic testing in the workplace: a view from the USA. Trends Genet 1992;8(6):198–202.
64. American Association of Colleges of Nursing. The essentials of baccalaureate education for professional nursing practice. 2008. Available at: http://www. genome.gov/Pages/Careers/HealthProfessionalEducation/geneticscompetency. pdf. Accessed March 15, 2013.
65. National Coalition for Health Professional Education in Genetics. Core competencies in genetics essential for all health-care professionals. 2007. Available at: http://www.nchpeg.org/. Accessed March 15, 2013.
66. Bancroft EK. Genetic testing for cancer predisposition and implications for nursing practice: narrative review. J Adv Nurs 2010;66(4):710–37.
67. EuroGentest. Harmonising genetic testing across Europe. 2009. Available at: http://www.eurogentest.org/. Accessed March 1, 2013.
68. The National Genetics Education and Development Centre. 2009. Available at: http://www.geneticseducation.nhs.uk. Accessed March 1, 2013.
69. Genetics in Nursing & Midwifery Task and Finish Group. Genetics/genomics in nursing and midwifery: Task and Finish Group report to the Nursing and Midwifery Professional Advisory Board. The Department of Health; 2011. Available at: https://www.gov.uk/government/uploads/system/uploads/attachment_ data/file/215250/dh_131947.pdf. Accessed March 1, 2013.
70. Burke S, Kirk M. Genetics education in the nursing profession: literature review. J Adv Nurs 2006;54(2):228–37.

Hypertrophic Cardiomyopathy

Kim Subasic, BSN, MS, PhD

KEYWORDS

- Hypertrophic cardiomyopathy • Autosomal dominant • Sudden cardiac death

KEY POINTS

- Hypertrophic cardiomyopathy (HCM) is a genetic, cardiovascular disorder associated with mutations in the protein of the cardiac sarcomere.
- HCM has marked genetic and phenotypic heterogeneity and incomplete penetrance and is the most common genetic cardiovascular disorder, with a prevalence of 1:500 persons.
- The silent presentation of HCM masks the unexpected possibility for sudden cardiac death (SCD).
- Genetic testing provides the opportunity for early identification of HCM, prompt treatment, and awareness for people who are genotype positive yet phenotype negative.
- In addition, for those who are found not to have HCM, genetic testing is cost effective when compared with unnecessary life-long monitoring and evaluation.

INTRODUCTION

HCM is a genetic, cardiovascular disorder associated with mutations in the protein of the cardiac sarcomere. This illness has marked genetic and phenotypic heterogeneity and incomplete penetrance. An asymmetric thickness of the left ventricle without association to other cardiac or systemic disorders differentiates HCM from other cardiac illnesses. The hypertrophy occurs most often in the left ventricle but can extend to the septum or apex or may be concentric. HCM is the most common genetic, cardiovascular disorder, with a prevalence of 1:500 persons, and is the most common cause of unexplained SCD, accounting for 36% of all unexplained SCD in high school and college athletes.[1–6] In the general population, the annual risk of SCD due to HCM is approximately 1%.[7,8] For people with HCM, the phenotypic presentation varies, ranging from asymptomatic to symptoms associated with heart failure. The autosomal dominant pattern of inheritance and absence of specific symptoms underscores the need for all first-degree relatives to be evaluated for HCM on confirmation of the illness in another family member.

Funding Sources: None.
Conflict of Interest: None.
Department of Nursing, University of Scranton, Linden Street, Scranton, PA 18510, USA
E-mail address: kimberly.subasic@scranton.edu

Nurs Clin N Am 48 (2013) 571–584
http://dx.doi.org/10.1016/j.cnur.2013.09.001   nursing.theclinics.com

GENETIC ASSOCIATION

HCM was first identified in 1957[9] and a genetic association with HCM found in the 1980s.[10] HCM is inherited from an autosomal dominant gene, which carries the probability of being passed on to 50% of an individual's offspring. Although genetic testing can identify familial HCM in approximately 60% of the probands,[11] obtaining conclusive tests results are associated with more than 1400 mutations on 11 different genes of the cardiac sarcomere.[12] The 4 most common mutations occur on the cardiac β–myosin heavy chain, cardiac troponin T, α-tropomyosin, and the myosin-binding protein C.[1,13]

The cardiac β–heavy chain and myosin-binding protein C mutations account for approximately 80% of HCM mutations, followed by the troponin T and troponin 1.[1,14] Mutations of the cardiac β–myosin heavy chain have been linked with early-onset, extensive hypertrophy and the high risk of sudden death.[1,15] The cardiac troponin T gene has a slower onset, presenting with mild to modest cardiac hypertrophy at approximately 30 years of age. Mutations of the α-tropomyosin and the myosin-binding protein C are slower to manifest, with delayed presentation until middle age or later.[13]

Box 1 depicts clinical research findings associated with common HCM mutations. A specific mutation cannot predict the prognosis of a person with HCM and a need exists for more research before a specific phenotype can be attributed to a specific genotype.[12,16] In addition, Ho[14] recognizes the limited clinical yield and clinical impact with regard to penetrance and predictability.

PATHOPHYSIOLOGY

The distinguishing feature of familial HCM is myocardial fibrosis, an excessive asymmetric hypertrophy of the ventricular septum without association to any other illness or cardiac disease.[14,17] The hypertrophy creates a thickening of the left ventricle but may include the septum or apex or be concentric. The normal width of the left ventricle wall is 10 mm or 12 mm. Hypertrophy of the left ventricular wall greater than or equal to 15 mm is indicative of HCM and left ventricular hypertrophy of 13 mm to 14 mm is consider borderline.[18,19] Left ventricular hypertrophy greater than or equal to 30 mm is considered at risk for SCD.[20] In teenagers and young adults, close examination is needed to rule out that an enlarged heart is a result of HCM versus an enlarged heart that is often present in athletes.[21] The presence of left ventricular hypertrophy to confirm a clinical diagnosis of HCM is difficult prior to adolescence.[14] The diagnosis of HCM in children is determined based on hypertrophy that is "greater than or equal of 2 standard deviation above the mean for age, sex, or body size"[18] (p. 2774).

HCM can be present with or without obstruction. In the obstructive form, two murmurs may be auscultated, the first murmur due to the left ventricular outflow gradient and the second murmur due to mitral valve insufficiency.[15] Hypertrophy along the upper region of the ventricular septum can impair blood flow through the aortic valve, resulting in a decreased cardiac output. An outflow obstruction can also occur due to hypertrophy that interferes with the mitral valve, creating systolic anterior motion resulting in mitral regurgitation.[17]

SYMPTOMS

Varied penetrance and phenotypic presentation make prompt identification and treatment of HCM challenging. There are no unique symptoms solely associated with HCM and, because many of these symptoms are associated with other forms of cardiac

Box 1
Clinical findings associated with the 8 most common HCM gene mutations

- Myosin-binding protein C (MYBPC3)
  - Slow to manifest
  - Presents in middle age or later
- β–Myosin heavy chain (MYH7)
  - Associated with early-onset, extensive hypertrophy
  - Left ventricular hypertrophy noted by second decade of life
  - ↑ Risk sudden death
  - Greater risk for heart failure
- Cardiac troponin T (TNNT2)
  - Penetrance is low in children
  - Mild hypertrophy
  - Abnormal ECG
  - Low risk for SCD
- Cardiac troponin I (TNNT3)
  - Extreme heterogeneity
- α-Tropomyosin (TPM1)
  - Variable prognosis
  - Risk for SCD
- Actin (ACTC1)
  - Apical hypertrophy
- Regulatory myosin light chain (MYL2)
  - Skeletal myopathy
- Essential myosin light chain (MYL3)
  - Skeletal myopathy

Data from Refs.[1,11,19,22–24,30–32]

disease, physicians may easily overlook HCM. Some people with HCM are asymptomatic, as in athletes who die of SCD yet seem physically healthy and in the prime of life. The presentation of HCM varies—some with HCM have no symptoms whereas others have myriad symptoms that correspond to a compromised heart (**Box 2**). Common symptoms include chest pain, shortness of breath, syncope, dizziness, and palpitations.[22] A systolic heart murmur may be heard or can be provoked by having the individual perform the Valsalva maneuver, change positions, or hold his or her breath.[21] The presentation of symptoms often corresponds with the severity of left ventricular hypertrophy and whether or not outflow obstruction exists.[18,25] Symptoms can be triggered or exacerbated by emotional stress, physical exertion, or lying flat after eating meals.[26] Complications associated with HCM are listed in **Box 3**.

Women present with symptoms more frequently than men, although symptom onset occurs at a later age for women.[27–29] Men have the highest frequency of symptom presentation between the ages of 15 and 29, whereas women tend to have a

---

Box 2
Symptoms associated with HCM

Shortness of breath with exertion

Orthopnea

Easily fatigued

Exertional chest pain

Palpitations

Syncope

Arrythmmias

Unexplained heart murmur

---

delayed onset of symptoms until 40 to 50 years of age.[29] SCD occurrs more often in African American men than white men.[30] Men have higher rates of SCD than women; however, girls and women have a higher mortality rate near 10 to 11 years of age and boys and men tend to have a higher incidence of SCD at 15 to 16 years of age.[31,32]

DIAGNOSIS

A thorough screening consisting of a detailed family medical history and physical examination is crucial for early detection of HCM. It is important to screen individuals for a positive family history of premature death or SCD and to take note of unexplained shortness of breath and syncope or dizziness with physical activity. Physical assessment findings may reveal a heart murmur. Differential diagnosis may include hypertensive heart disease or an athlete's heart.

It is possible that early diagnostic tests show no evidence of HCM, but the illness may appear later in life, particularly during puberty or after the age of 50.[1,11,17–19,23,24] Due to the high risk of SCD occurring in children with HCM, it is necessary that regular

---

Box 3
Complications associated with HCM

- Congestive heart failure
- Atrial fibrillation
- Ventricular tachyarrhythmia
- Alterations to the mitral valve
- Myocardial ischemia
- Mitral regurgitation
- Endocarditis
- Heart failure
- Sudden or premature death

Adapted from Gersh BJ, Maron BJ, Bonow RO, et al. 2011 ACCF/AHA guideline for the diagnosis and treatment of hypertrophic cardiomyopathy. A report of the American College of Cardiology Foundation/American Heart Association Task Force on Practice Guidelines. Circulation 2011;124:e783–e831; with permission.

---

screenings, proper diagnosis, early monitoring, individualized treatment, and family education begin as soon as possible. On detection of HCM, patients should be referred to an HCM specialist rather than a cardiologist, who may not be familiar with this disease and the variety of expression that it carries. Due to the inherited nature of HCM, a cardiac evaluation should be performed on first-degree relatives of the identified patient. It is recommended that individuals meet with a genetics counselor to discuss the potential impact of HCM for the family. Suspicion of HCM requires confirmation of the illness through diagnostic testing. Commonly used diagnostic tests include an echocardiogram, ECG, and cardiac MRI.

An abnormal ECG is produced in 75% to 95% of people with HCM.[18] This noninvasive test is useful when HCM is under suspicion or as a screening device but cannot rule out the presence of HCM. Abnormal ECG findings may include a widened QRS complex or alterations in the ST and T wave.[33]

A 2-D Doppler echocardiogram can confirm the presence of HCM and is considered the gold standard in the diagnosis of HCM.[18] This noninvasive test provides color-coded images of the blood flow through the heart and provides for visualization of the heart wall and areas of obstruction or regurgitation.

Cardiac MRI provides high-quality images of the heart and is useful when echocardiogram results are inconclusive. Cardiac MRI allows for better visualization of the apex of the heart and the anterolateral wall. Results from this test can clarify diagnosis based on cardiac morphology.[17]

A Holter monitor is a small portable ECG that a patient wears for 24 to 48 hours. This device records every heartbeat and continuous heart rhythm during a programmed time frame. It is especially helpful to track irregular arrhythmias that a patient may not physically recognize. Arrhythmias common to HCM include atrial fibrillation and ventricular tachycardia.

An exercise stress test is conducted after the diagnosis of HCM to examine the stability of the heart during activity. During the test, heart rate and blood pressure are closely monitored. A decrease in blood pressure or failure of the blood pressure to increase with activity represents instability of the heart. An exercise stress test can be combined with a Doppler echocardiogram to provide views of the blood flow throughout the heart during the exercise stress test.

A transesophageal echocardiogram (TEE) is useful in determining hypertrophy in posterior areas of the heart that are not easily detected with a standard echocardiogram. The TEE can also be useful in detecting obstruction, mitral regurgitation, left ventricular outflow gradient, and myocardial function.[17] Practice guidelines recommend that a TEE be performed prior to a myectomy or alcohol septal ablation.[18]

Coronary arteriography is an invasive procedure used to measure pressure within the heart chambers and to assess cardiac output, outflow obstruction, and function of heart valves. Angiography and tomographic imaging offer an understanding of the hemodynamic status and must be performed prior to an alcohol septal ablation.[18]

A genetic test offers the most definitive diagnosis of this illness; unfortunately, the accuracy of genetic testing is limited to common mutations of HCM and is challenged due to varying genetic mutations.[11,12,34,35] Gersh and colleagues[18] report, however, that, "Experienced clinical laboratories identify the pathogenic HCM mutation in approximately 60%–70% of patients with a positive family history and approximately 10%–50% of patients without a family history"[18] (p. 2776). Genetic testing can identify the presence of genetic strains of HCM that may not have a phenotypic presentation until mid- to- late adulthood. Benefits of genetic testing include early identification and prompt treatment of people who are genotype positive yet phenotype negative, thereby decreasing the possibility of complications associated with the illness or from SCD.[19]

Despite the availability of genetic testing since 2003, recent studies have shown that fewer than 50% of people with HCM undergo genetic testing.[14,36–39] Genetic testing carries a multitude of personal, emotional, behavioral, ethical, and legal implications. Impediments to genetic testing include uncertainty regarding diagnosis and prognosis and the emotional stress of knowing that the mutation has transferred to children.[40] Parents' younger age, higher education level, and knowledge of genetic testing for HCM were associated with a better likelihood of genetic testing for their children.[37,38] Prior to genetic testing, genetic counseling should be encouraged and individuals should review life and disability insurance. Despite protection from the Genetic Information Nondiscrimination Act (GINA), some people with HCM experience legal difficulty regarding insurance coverage.[36] In addition, a decision as to whether or not genetic testing is covered by an insurance plan should be determined prior to genetic testing. The cost of genetic testing for HCM is between $3000 and $5500 for the first person in the family to be tested and $100 and $900 for subsequent family members.[41,42] Despite the high cost or the possibility of inconclusive results, genetic testing is cost effective in the management of HCM because should certain family members test negative for the gene mutation there is no need to evaluate or screen their descendants.[43] In addition to being cost effective, individuals with a family history of HCM can be tested at younger age, thereby guiding effective treatment that decreases the risk for SCD.

TREATMENT

There are no specific treatments for HCM. Rather, treatment is individualized base on symptoms, whether or not obstruction is present, family history, and risk for SCD. Left ventricular outflow obstruction is considered severe when the outflow pressure gradient is greater than or equal to 50 mm Hg at rest.[14] Treatment modalities consist of pharmacologic, surgery, or a combination of both. In severe cases of HCM, a heart transplant may be warranted.

PHARMACOLOGIC STRATEGIES

Pharmacologic therapy is geared toward improving symptoms. Typically, medications are prescribed to help decrease the workload of the heart, to decrease symptoms associated with ineffective pumping of the heart, to improve ventricular filling, or to control arrhythmias. A diuretic may also be ordered. People with HCM should take antibiotics prior to undergoing any dental work or invasive procedure, including tattoos or body piercing, to decrease the risk of endocarditis. **Table 1** depicts various pharmacologic therapies that may be used alone or in combination for the treatment of symptoms associated with HCM and medications that should be avoided.

SURGICAL TREATMENT

Limited surgical options or procedures exist for the treatment of HCM. Treatment decisions are based on the presence of symptoms and whether or not outflow obstruction exists as well as the ability of a person to tolerate the procedure. In the event that surgical options are ineffective, the person with HCM may require a cardiac transplant. The success rate of cardiac transplants for HCM is reported as comparable to transplantation for other cardiac illnesses.[44]

An implantable cardioverter defibrillator (ICD) is recommended for individuals at risk for SCD. An ICD is a small device surgically implanted just below the clavicle and

Table 1 Medications and HCM	
Commonly Prescribed	**Medications to Avoid**
β-Blockers	Vasodilators
• Atenolol	Dihydropyridine calcium channel blockers
• Propranolol	Digitalis
• Metoprolol	Dopamine
Calcium channel blockers	Dobutamine
• Verapmil	Norephrine
• Diltiazem	Angiotensin receptor blockers
Intravenous phenylephrine	Phosphodieterase-5 inhibitors
Antiarrhythmics	Nitrates or β-adrenergic agonists
• Amiodarone	
• Disopyramide	
Low-dose diuretics	
Anticoagulant	
Diltiazem	

Adapted from Gersh BJ, Maron BJ, Bonow RO, et al. 2011 ACCF/AHA guideline for the diagnosis and treatment of hypertrophic cardiomyopathy. A report of the American College of Cardiology Foundation/American Heart Association Task Force on Practice Guidelines. Circulation 2011;124:e783–e831; with permission.

recommended when arrhythmias cannot be controlled by medications or when a person is identified as high risk for SCD. Although this treatment method is effective in preventing SCD in individuals who are high risk for SCD, it is essential that consideration be given to the age of the person receiving the ICD as well as the benefits and risks associated with ICDs. Prior to the insertion of an ICD in a young person, careful consideration must be given to the age, years of anticipated body growth, and significance of associated risk factors for SCD prior to the insertion of an ICD. Consideration must to given to the need for the insertion of new leads as the person grows, complications associated with inappropriate firing of the device or fractures in the leads of the device based on body growth, manufacturer's recall of a device, physical limitations, and the psychosocial impact that may arise as a result of having an ICD.[18] Although this device can be life saving, inappropriate electrical shocks are not uncommon.[45] Therefore, cardiac rehabilitation or counseling should be offered to ease the psychosocial concerns affiliated with an ICD. The primary benefit of an ICD is the prevention or abortion of a life-threatening arrhythmia. Risks and complications associated with an ICD include infection, hematoma, inappropriate firing of the device, pericardial effusion, pneumothorax, arrhythmias, and dislodgement of the leads.[18]

An alcohol septal ablation is a nonsurgical procedure, first used in 1995, that involves injecting a small amount of absolute alcohol into a small branch of the coronary artery that supplies blood to the upper portion of the left ventricular septum.[46] This procedure is best suited for people who experience outflow obstruction, are poor surgical candidates, or are older in age. The injection of a small amount of alcohol creates a localized myocardial infarction that destroys cellular components of the ventricular wall, creating a thinned wall, which decreases the systolic anterior motion of the mitral valve systolic, and improving blood flow through the heart.[18] After an alcohol septal ablation, patients must remain in the hospital for a few days to be closely monitored due to the risk for sustained ventricular arrhythmias and heart block.[18] This procedure is controversial among HCM specialists due to the long-term effects associated with adding injury to an already compromised heart. Although this may be an efficacious procedure for people with obstructive HCM that does not respond to pharmacologic treatment, alcohol ablation carries risks of postoperative complications, including sustained ventricular arrhythmias, cardiac tamponade, the need for a pacemaker, and death.[47] There is a high likelihood that a pacemaker is necessary after an alcohol septal ablation due to the risk the procedure carries for complete heart block. Alcohol septal ablation is not recommended for children because this treatment method involves permanent, intended injury to the heart wall. The benefits of alcohol septal ablation include no surgical incision or need for general anesthesia, shorter recovery time, improved functional capacity, improved quality of life, and decreased presence of angina.[18] Three months after an alcohol septal ablation, improved quality of life and emotional well-being were noted.[48]

A ventricular septal myotomy-myectomy is a surgical procedure in which a small portion of the thickened ventricular septum is removed, yielding improved blood flow through the heart. A myectomy has proved an effective approach for any age group and noted to improve quality of life as well as to offer long-term survival rates and presents with few postoperative complications.[18,49] This surgical procedure was first used in the 1960s and is now considered the preferred treatment due to high success rates, minimal complications, and low mortality.[14,18]

A dual-chamber pacemaker is reserved for individuals who have severe symptoms related to obstructive HCM and is not recommended for people with HCM that is non-obstructive.[18] This is best suited for individuals over age 65 and may be considered necessary after an alcohol septal ablation.

MANAGEMENT OF HCM

The management of HCM focuses on maintaining quality of life and decreasing the presence of symptoms and risk for SCD. Improved screening, treatment options, and management of HCM have led to positive outcomes, as evidenced by a decreased mortality of less than 3%.[7] As a result of effective lifestyle changes, pharmacologic treatment, and surgical options, many people with HCM have normal life expectancies. Screening for HCM should start during childhood for families who have a history of HCM. A detailed family history and a thorough physical assessment are the most-effective screening tools for detecting HCM.[21] A detailed family history identifies whether or not a positive family history of premature death, cardiac arrest, or cardiac disease exists. A physical examination requires a focused assessment on heart sounds. If a murmur is detected or elicited during a physical examination, further cardiac evaluation is recommended.

Those at risk for HCM require monitoring through adulthood due to the silent presentation of the illness. Because HCM carries the possibility of spontaneous or accelerated hypertrophy during adolescence, it is recommended that adolescents be screened annually through early adulthood and then every 5 years due to the risk of a delayed HCM phenotype.[10,14] A physical examination, ECG, and echocardiogram or cardiac MRI are suggested for screening individuals who are genotype positive and phenotype negative.[18] **Box 4** illustrates items considered as part of risk stratification for the prevention of SCD. The number of risk factors is not indicative of a greater risk for SCD but should be taken into consideration in the individualization of treatment for people with HCM.

RISK TO ATHLETES

The United States Sudden Death in Young Athletes Registry has identified that an incident of SCD occurs once every 3 days in the United States during organized youth

---

Box 4
Risk stratification in the prevention of sudden cardiac death

- Personal history of cardiac abnormalities
- Family history of SCD or ventricular arrhythmias
- Unexplained syncope
- 3 or More beats of nonsustained supraventricular tachycardia
- Left ventricular wall thickness greater than or equal to 30 mm
- Abnormal blood pressure response during exercise
- Left ventricular outflow obstruction
- Late gadolinium enhancement on cardiac MRI
- Left ventricular apical aneurysm
- Specific genetic mutation associated with SCD

Adapted from Gersh BJ, Maron BJ, Bonow RO, et al. 2011 ACCF/AHA guideline for the diagnosis and treatment of hypertrophic cardiomyopathy. A report of the American College of Cardiology Foundation/American Heart Association Task Force on Practice Guidelines. Circulation 2011;124:e783–e831; with permission.

---

sporting events.[4] A study by Eckart and colleagues[50] revealed that 13% of SCDs in military recruits ages 18 to 35 years of age are associated with HCM. SCD occurs more frequently in men.[4,30] The incidence of SCD in athletes is 0.61/100,000 persons; however, this may be higher due to the absence of a mandated reporting system.[4,21] In a study of athletes who died of SCD precipitated by exercise, 63% of the deaths occurred between 3 PM and 9 PM, which corresponds with a frequent time period for athletic competition.[51] Preparticipation athletic screenings, however, fail to identify athletes with HCM, confirming that HCM may exist without symptoms.[21,30,51,52] In contrast, Corrado and colleagues[53] found that preparticipation screening programs were effective in identifying athletes at risk for SCD. Individuals thought to have HCM should avoid physical activity that requires sprinting, is excessive in duration, requires high levels of conditioning, or occurs in extreme weather conditions.[54]

PREGNANCY

Women with HCM who are pregnant are considered high risk due to both increased fluid volume within the body and physical strain on their already compromised hearts. Although there is a low mortality rate for women with HCM during pregnancy, complications associated with HCM should be closely monitored. If symptoms of heart failure, sustained arrhythmias, or left ventricular outflow obstruction occur, a cardiologist specialized in HCM should be included as a member of the medical team.[18] There is a 50% likelihood that HCM will be passed onto the offspring. Advances in genetic research may change future-related aspects of living with HCM, however, by offering people with this illness the potential to give birth without transferring the genetic abnormality to offspring. Preimplantation genetic diagnosis (PGD) is a clinical procedure that offers a means of reproduction for those with a genetic illness to have children without transferring the illness to the child.[54] This procedure is a combination of in vitro fertilization and the genetic screening of embryos for the presence of a specific illness prior to the implantation of embryos in the woman. For some, PGD may be perceived as an option to eradicate the illness for future generations.

LIFESTYLE CHANGES

Lifestyle changes may be necessary depending on the severity of hypertrophy, outflow obstruction, or presentation of symptoms for people living with HCM. These changes may include withdrawal from competitive sports and avoidance of intense physical activity. People with HCM need to engage in physical activity that is moderate enough to allow for conversation during the activity.[14] Health recommendations for people with HCM are similar to those associated with other forms of cardiac disease. These include refraining from smoking, monitoring cholesterol, avoiding hot tubs and saunas, maintaining a healthy weight, abstaining from a sedentary lifestyle, and avoiding dehydration or overexhaustion. People with HCM are not able to engage in occupations that involve the use of commercial motor vehicles or in aviation.[55] Lastly, those with HCM should avoid extreme weather conditions and refrain from high altitudes.

PSYCHOSOCIAL CONCERNS

Uncertainty of being at risk for SCD places limitations on daily life and generates an emotional or psychological burden on people living with HCM.[40] The quality of life and psychological well-being are negatively altered in people who have HCM.[26,56] Similarly, quality of life within the domains of general health and sleep quality were found lower for persons with HCM compared with individuals with other inherited cardiac arrhythmias.[57,58] Additional concerns of living with this illness are associated with the financial impact of needing specialized medical care and future-related concerns of "Will I be able to…"[38] The physical, emotional, and financial challenges for persons with HCM can be overwhelming. The psychosocial impact can be decreased when individuals with HCM engage in a support group.[38,43] A national support group, the Hypertrophic Cardiomyopathy Association, a nonprofit organization, serves as resource and advocacy group for individuals who have HCM, their family members, and their health care providers.

Physical restrictions limit the potential for people with HCM to maintain social engagements. The pychosocial aspects of having HCM are not limited to persons with HCM but include other family members. Spouses learn about and experience HCM alongside the person with HCM, including shared concern about children having HCM. Bratt and colleagues[59] noted that parents who have a child with HCM experience lifestyle changes that affect the family.

LEGAL CONSIDERATIONS

The GINA, a federal law enacted in 2008, protects individuals from genetic discrimination and misuse of genetic information as it relates to employment and health insurance.[60] The protection of genetic information expands up to and includes fourth-degree relatives as well as a fetus or embryo. It is now illegal for health insurers or employers to require or request an individual to have genetic testing. This law does not provide protection of genetic information associated with life insurance, disability insurance, or long-term health care insurance. An employer with fewer than 15 employees is exempt from the legal mandates that fall under GINA. In addition, GINA is not applicable to active-duty military personnel. Genetic information cannot be used to underwrite health insurance policies. Survivors of genetic illness (for example, genetic breast and ovarian cancer) and persons who have physical symptoms related to a genetic illness do not qualify for legal protection offered through GINA; however, the Health Insurance Portability and Accountability Act and the Americans with Disabilities Act can provide some legal protection.

SUMMARY/DISCUSSION

In summary, HCM is an autosomal dominant, genetic, cardiovascular disorder associated with mutations on the proteins of the cardiac sarcomere. The prevalence of HCM is 1:500 and commonly linked with SCD of athletes. A distinguishing feature of HCM is myocardial fibrosis or an excessive asymmetric thickening of the left ventricle, septum, or apex; or it may be concentric. This hypertrophy can create an outflow obstruction in the heart and impair function of the heart valves. There are no specific symptoms directly related to HCM, thereby posing challenges for prompt identification and treatment. Genetic testing offers the most definitive diagnosis but is challenged due to numerous mutations on multiple genes of the cardiac sarcomere. HCM has marked genetic and phenotypic heterogeneity and incomplete penetrance. As a result, treatment is individualized based on the presence of symptoms or risk for SCD.

HCM resources
  Hypertrophic Cardiomyopathy Association http://www4hcma.org
  Parent Heart Watch http://www.parentheartwatch.org
  The Cardiomyopathy Association http://www.cardiomyopathy.org

Genetic testing
  http://www.ncbi.nlm.nih.gov/sites/GeneTests/?db=GeneTests

GINA of 2008
  http://www.genome.gov/10002328

REFERENCES

1. Barsheshet A, Brenyo A, Moss AJ, et al. Genetics of sudden cardiac death. Curr Cardiol Rep 2011;13:364–76.
2. Maron BJ. Medical progress: sudden death in young athletes. N Engl J Med 2003;349:1064–75.
3. Maron BJ, Doerer JJ, Haas TS, et al. Profile and frequency of sudden death in 1463 young competitive athletes: from a 25 year U.S. national registry: 1980–2005. Circulation 2006;114:830–8.
4. Maron BJ, Doerer JJ, Haas TS, et al. Sudden deaths in young competitive athletes: analysis of 1866 deaths in the United States, 1980–2006. Circulation 2009; 118:1085–92.
5. Morita H, Larson MG, Barr SC, et al. Single-gene mutations and increased left ventricular wall thickness in the community: the framingham heart study. Circulation 2006;113:2697–705.
6. Van Camp SP, Bloor CM, Mueller FO, et al. Nontraumatic sports death in high school and college athletes. Med Sci Sports Exerc 1995;27:641–7.
7. Elliot PM, Gimeno JR, Thamna R, et al. Historical trends in reported survival rates in patients with hypertrophic cardiomyopathy. Heart 2006;92:785–91.
8. Meyer L, Stubbs B, Fahrenbruch C, et al. Incidence, causes, and survival trends from cardiovascular-related sudden cardiac arrest in children and young adults 0–35 years of age: a 30 year review. Circulation 2012;126:1363–72.
9. Teare D. Asymmetrical hypertrophy of the heart in young adults. Br Heart J 1958;20:1–8.
10. Elliot P, McKenna J. Hypertrophic cardiomyopathy. Lancet 2004;2004(363): 1881–91.

11. Ho CY. Genetics and clinical destiny: improving care in hypertrophic cardiomy-opathy. Circulation 2010;122:2430–40.
12. Maron MS. A Paradigm shift in our understanding of the development of the hy-pertrophic cardiomyopathy phenotype? Not so fast! Circulation 2013;127:10–2.
13. Seidman C. Hypertrophic cardiomyopathy: from man to mouse. J Clin Invest 2000;106:9–13.
14. Ho CY. Hypertrophic cardiomyopathy in 2012. Circulation 2012;125:1432–8.
15. Roberts R, Sigwart U. New concepts in hypertrophic cardiomyopathies, part 1. Circulation 2001;104:2113–6.
16. Jensen MK, Havndrup O, Christiansen M, et al. Penetrance of hypertrophic car-diomyopathy in children and adolescents: a 12 year follow-up study of clinical screening and predictive genetic testing. Circulation 2013;127:48–54.
17. Desai MY, Ommen SR, McKenna WJ, et al. Imaging phenotype versus genotype in hypertrophic cardiomyopathy. Circ Cardiovasc Imaging 2011;4:156–8.
18. Gersh BJ, Maron BJ, Bonow RO, et al. 2011 ACCF/AHA guideline for the diag-nosis and treatment of hypertrophic cardiomyopathy. A report of the American College of Cardiology Foundation/American Heart Association Task Force on Practice Guidelines. Circulation 2011;124:2761–96.
19. Maron BJ, Niimura H, Casey SA, et al. Development of left ventricular hypertro-phy in adults with hypertrophic cardiomyopathy caused by cardiac myosin-binding protein C gene mutations. J Am Coll Cardiol 2001;38:315–21.
20. Spirito P, Bellone P, Harris K, et al. Magnitude of left ventricular hypertrophy and risk of sudden death in hypertrophic cardiomyopathy. N Engl J Med 2000;342:1778–85.
21. Maron BJ, Thompson PD, Ackerman MJ, et al. Recommendations and consid-erations related to preparticipation screening for cardiovascular abnormalities in competitive athletes: 2007 update: a Scientific Statement from the American Heart Association council on ntrition, physical activity, and metabolism: endorsed by the American College of Cardiology Foundation. Circulation 2007;115:1643–55.
22. Bashyam MD, Savithri GR, Kumar MS, et al. Molecular genetics of familial hyper-trophic cardiomyopathy. J Hum Genet 2003;48:55–64.
23. Pasquale F, Syrris P, Kaski JP, et al. Long-term outcomes in hypertrophic cardio-myopathy caused by mutations in the cardiac troponin T gene. Circ Cardiovasc Genet 2012;5:10–7.
24. Wang L, Seidman JG, Seidman C. Narrative review: harnessing molecular ge-netics for the diagnosis and management of hypertrophic cardiomyopathy. Ann Intern Med 2010;152:513–20.
25. Ho CY, Lopez B, Coelho-Filho O, et al. Myocardial fibrosis as an early manifes-tation of hypertrophic cardiomyopathy. N Engl J Med 2010;363:552–63.
26. Lampert R, Salberg L, Burg M. Emotional stress triggers symptoms in hypertro-phic cardiomyopathy: a survey of the Hypertrophic Cardiomyopathy Associa-tion. Pacing Clin Electrophysiol 2010;33:1047–53.
27. Adabag AS, Kuskowski MA, Maron BJ. Determinants for clinical diagnosis of hy-pertrophic cardiomyopathy. Am J Cardiol 2006;98:1507–11.
28. Brimacombe M, Walter D, Salberg L. Gender disparity in a large nonreferral-based cohort of hypertrophic cardiomyopathy patients. J Womens Health (Larchmt) 2008;17:1629–34.
29. Dimitrow PP, Czarnecka D, Jaszcz KK, et al. Sex differences in age at onset of symptoms in patients with hypertrophic cardiomyopathy. J Cardiovasc Risk 1997;4:33–5.

30. Maron BJ, Carney KP, Lever HM, et al. Relationship of race to sudden cardiac death in competitive athletes with hypertrophic cardiomyopathy. J Am Coll Cardiol 2003;41:974–80.
31. Drezner JA, Chun J, Harmon KG, et al. Survival trends in the United States following exercise-related sudden cardiac arrest in high school and college athletic programs: 2000–2006. Heart Rhythm 2008;5:794–9.
32. Ostman-Smith O, Wettrell G, Keeton B, et al. Age and geneder specific mortality rates in childhood hypertrophic cardiomyopathy. Eur Heart J 2008;29:1160–7.
33. Popjes ED, St John Sutton M. Hypertrophic cardiomyopathy; pathophysiology, diagnosis, and treatment. Geriatrics 2003;58:41–6.
34. Bos JM, Ommen SR, Ackermann MJ. Genetics of hypertrophic cardiomyopathy: one, two or more diseases? Curr Opin Cardiol 2007;22:193–9.
35. Ghosh N, Haddad H. Recent progress in the genetics of cardiomyopathy and its role in the clinical evaluation of patients with cardiomyopathy. Curr Opin Cardiol 2011;26:155–64.
36. Christiaans I, Kok TM, van Langen IM, et al. Obtaining insurance after DNA diagnostics: a survey among hypertrophic cardiomyopathy mutation carriers. Eur J Hum Genet 2010;18:251–3.
37. Fitzgerald- Butt SM, Byrne L, Gerhardt CA, et al. Parental knowledge and attitudes toward hypertrophic cardiomyopathy genetic testing. Pediatr Cardiol 2010;31:195–202.
38. Subasic K. Living with hypertrophic cardiomyopathy. J Nurs Scholarsh 2013. [Epub ahead of print].
39. Van Driest SL, Ommen SR, Jamil Tajik A, et al. Yield of genetic testing in hypertrophic cardiomyopathy. Mayo Clin Proc 2005;80:739–44.
40. Smart A. Impediments to DNA testing and cascade screening for hypertrophic cardiomyopathy and long QT syndrome: a qualitative study of patient experiences. J Genet Couns 2010;19:630–9.
41. Deo RC, MacRae CA. Clinical screening and genetic testing. Heart Fail Clin 2010;6:231–8.
42. Tester DJ, Ackerman MJ. Genetic testing for potentially lethal, highly treatable inherited cardiomyopathies/channelopathies in clinical practice. Circulation 2011;123:1021–37.
43. Ingles J, McGaughran J, Scuffman PA, et al. A cost-effective model of genetic testing for the evaluation of families with hypertrophic cardiomyopathy. Heart 2012;98:625–30.
44. Maron MS, Kaismith BM, Udelson JE, et al. Survival after cardiac transplantation in patients with hypertrophic cardiomyopathy. Circ Heart Fail 2010;3:574–9.
45. Schinkel AF, Vriesendorp PA, Sijbrands EJ, et al. Outcome and complications after implantable cardioverter defibrillator therapy in hypertrophic cardiomyopathy. Circ Heart Fail 2012;5:552–9.
46. Sigwart U. Non-surgical myocardial reduction for hypertrophic obstructive cardiomyopathy. Lancet 1995;346:211–4.
47. Sorajja P, Valeti U, Nishimura RA, et al. Outcome of alcohol septal ablation for obstructive hypertrophic cardiomyopathy. Circulation 2008;118:131–9.
48. Serber ER, Sears SF, Nielsen CD, et al. Depression, anxiety, and quality of life in patients with obstructive hypertrophic cardiomyopathy three months after alcohol spetal ablation. Am J Cardiol 2007;100:1592–7.
49. Ommen SR, Maron BJ, Olivotto I, et al. Long-term effects of surgical septal myectomy on survival in patients with obstructive hypertrophic cardiomyopathy. J Am Coll Cardiol 2005;46:470–6.

50. Eckart RE, Scoville SL, Campbell CL, et al. Sudden death in young adults: a 25 year review of autopsies in military recruits. Ann Intern Med 2004;141: 829–34.
51. Maron BJ, Shirani J, Poliac L, et al. Sudden death in young competitive athletes: clinical, demographic, and pathological profiles. JAMA 1996;276:199–204.
52. Pfister GC, Puffer JC, Maron BJ. Preparticipation cardiovascular screening for US collegiate student-athletes. JAMA 2000;283:1597–9.
53. Corrado D, Basso C, Pavei A, et al. Trends in sudden cardiovascular death in young competitive after implementation of a preparticipation screening program. JAMA 2006;296:1593–601.
54. Kuliev A, Pomerantseva E, Polling D, et al. PGD for inherited cardiac diseases. Reprod Biomed Online 2012;24:443–53.
55. Maron BJ, Chaitman BR, Ackerman MJ, et al. AHA scientific statement: recommendations for physical activity and recreational sports participation for young patients with genetic cardiovascular diseases. Circulation 2004;109:2807–16.
56. Cox S, O'Donoghue AC, McKenna WJ, et al. Health related quality of life and psychological wellbeing in patients with hypertrophic cardiomyopathy. Heart 1997;78:182–7.
57. Hamang A, Eide GE, Nordin K, et al. Health status in patients at risk of inherited arrhythmias and sudden expected death compared to the general population. BMC Med Genet 2010;11:27. Available at: http://www.biomedcentral.com/1471-2350/11/27. Accessed January 5, 2013.
58. Pedrosa RP, Lima SG, Drager LF, et al. Sleep quality and quality of life in patients with hypertrophic cardiomyopathy. Cardiology 2010;117:200–6.
59. Bratt E, Ostman-Smith I, Sparud-Lundin C, et al. Parents' experiences of having an asymptomatic child diagnosed with hypertrophic cardiomyopathy through family screening. Cardiol Young 2011;21:8–14.
60. Lieb JR, Hoodfar E, Haidle JL, et al. Washington update: the new genetic privacy law. Community Oncol 2008;5:351–4.

The Impact of Genomics on Oncology Nursing

Laura Curr Beamer, DNP, AOCNP, APNG[a,b],
Lauri Linder, PhD, APRN, CPON[b,c], Bohua Wu, MD[d],
Julia Eggert, PhD, GNP-BC, AOCN®[d,e,*]

KEYWORDS

- Cancer genetics • Genomics • Oncology nursing
- Genetic Information Nondiscrimination Act (GINA) • Epigenetics

KEY POINTS

- Nurses and patients younger than age 66 years of age have received little formalized education in genetics and genomics.
- Completion of the human genome in 2003 has led to personalized medicine for oncology patients for the continuum of care in prevention, diagnosis, prognosis, and treatment of cancer.
- Collection of a detailed and accurate family history enables the nurse to generate a helpful cancer risk assessment.
- Application of ethics and policy to families with a genetic mutation has implications for storage of the family history in the electronic medical record.
- Oncology nurses require a knowledge base of genetics and genomics to anticipate the physical and education needs of the patient and their family.

INTRODUCTION: NATURE OF THE PROBLEM

The completion of the human DNA sequence by the Human Genome Project (HGP) in 2003 has proved to be a foundation for research in cancer.[1] Also viewed as the

Funding Sources: None (L. Linder, J. Eggert); American Cancer Society, Doctoral Cancer Nursing Scholarship, 121293-DSCN-11-197-01-SCN (L.C. Beamer).
Conflict of Interest: None (L.C. Beamer, L. Linder, J. Eggert).
[a] School of Nursing & Health Studies, College of Health & Human Sciences, Northern Illinois University, 1240 Normal Road, DeKalb, IL 60115, USA; [b] College of Nursing, University of Utah, 10 South 2000 East, Salt Lake City, UT 84112, USA; [c] Cancer Transplant Service Line, Primary Children's Medical Center, 100 North Mario Capecchi Drive, Salt Lake City, UT 84113, USA; [d] Healthcare Genetics Doctoral Program, School of Nursing, Health, College of Education and Human Development, Clemson University, St Francis Boulevard, Clemson, SC 29634, USA; [e] Cancer Risk, Screening Program, Bon Secours St. Francis Hospital, Greenville, SC 29601, USA
* Corresponding author. School of Nursing, College of Health, Education and Human Development, Clemson University, Clemson, SC 29634.
E-mail address: jaegger@clemson.edu

groundwork for technology development, the HGP used gel electrophoresis, gas chromatography-mass spectrometry, and radiation-hybrid mapping to map the human genome enabling more sensitive technology to be built for laboratory use, leading to greater understanding of normal molecular signaling and how it is altered not only in cancer but also specific types of these malignancies.[2] Growing awareness and understanding at the gene and molecular signaling levels has affected the prevention, early detection, diagnosis, and treatment of cancers.[2] New genomic knowledge across the oncology care continuum has required specialized nurses in these settings to increase their knowledge of genetics and genomics and how to apply this knowledge to achieve the goals of better patient outcomes. The Oncology Nursing Society (ONS) position statement on "application of cancer genetics and genomics through the oncology care continuum" and the American Nurses Association (ANA), 2009, *Essentials of Genetic and Genomic Nursing: Competencies, Curricula Guidelines, and Outcome Indicators* provide guidance to oncology nurses on key genetic and genomic competencies related to their practice.[3–5]

A typical patient who has cancer has almost no genetic and genomic knowledge. Their oncology nurse providers most likely have a similar genetic inform and genomication deficit. The average age for a person with a cancer diagnosis is 66 years, so in 2013, people diagnosed with cancer were born in 1946.[6] **Table 1** compares the progressive years and steps of some genetic discoveries considering the average age of patients and nurses today (personal conversation with Robert Lightfoot, MS High School biology instructor 1968–2009, Peace Lutheran High School, Aurora, CO).[3–16]

In 2007, when these Baby Boomers reached 60 years of age, they had received little formalized genetic education; most of their knowledge was obtained through the news, magazines, or the Internet. Therefore, most have limited genetic knowledge on which to build an understanding about potentially life-threatening disease caused by genetic damage, diagnosed by technology that reveals mutated genes, and treated with therapies, many personalized, that can target altered molecular pathways directed by damaged genes.[15]

Oncology nurses are the frontline caregivers of persons diagnosed with a malignancy and they must be prepared for the impact of genomics on the diagnosis, detection, and treatment of cancer. Today, the nursing workforce is aging; the average nurse is approaching 50 years of age and approximately one-third of this group are more than 50 years of age.[16] Of the 33,323 active members of the ONS who indicated an age range on their membership application, 15,735 (47%) self-identified as aged 50 years or older.[17] Much like that of patients with cancer, the early and professional education of oncology nurses did not include much detail about genetics beyond Mendel's laws of inheritance.[18] Most applications of genetics to oncology patient care and other specialties has occurred since 2003. Even with the focus on and intensification of genetic and genomic education by nurse leaders in genetics, there is still much content to be learned and applied when taking care of a patient with a cancer diagnosis, and their family.

Review of Normal Genetics and Cancer Genetics

The central dogma of molecular biology, with DNA replicated to DNA, DNA transcribed to RNA, and RNA translated to protein is well known to nurses, however the DNA packaging, epigenetics, molecular signaling, and targeting inherent in oncology today is a new frontier to many in this specialty.[19] **Fig. 1** depicts the chromosome structure and packaging of the DNA.[20]

As the double strand of DNA is tightly wound around multiple histones (group of proteins used to coil DNA like a thread on a spool) to form a chromosome, histone tails

Table 1
Projected lifetime level of genetic knowledge for average age of oncology nurse and an individual diagnosed with cancer born in 1946

Born in 1946	Patient Age (y), Education Level (BS)	Average Age of Oncology Nurse, Education Level (BSN)	Genetic Discovery
1946	Born	—	—
1953	7	—	Chemical structure of DNA
1957	11	—	Central dogma of molecular biology hypothesized
1960	14, high school sophomore	—	Discovery of mRNA
1961	15, high school	—	Genetic code cracked Theory of gene activation and suppression developed
1967	21	—	Role of reverse transcriptase in RNA to DNA Genetic engineering discipline implemented
1969	22, graduated college or early career	Born	Mendel
1977	31	8, 4th grade	Gilbert and Sanger devise techniques for DNA sequencing
1979	33	10, elementary school	Little genetic information in high school or college textbooks
1986	40	17, high school	Sequencing of the human genome was initiated
1990	44, career development	22, graduated from college	—
2003	57	40	Completion of the human genome sequencing announced
2006	60	43	Little formalized genetic education available or obtained
2008–2010	—	47	American Association of Critical Care Nursing Essentials published requiring genetics education in Baccalaureate nursing curricula and graduate nursing education Oncology Nursing Society position statement on "application of cancer genetics and genomics through the oncology care continuum" American Nurses Association, *Essentials of Genetic and Genomic Nursing: Competencies, Curricula Guidelines, and Outcome Indicators* AACN undergraduate and AACN graduate
2012	66	49	Average age of cancer diagnosis and average age of nursing workforce Genetics used in diagnosis, and treatment of cancer with much personalization based on tumor profiling
2013	—	50, average age of oncology nurse	—

Data from Refs.[3–16]

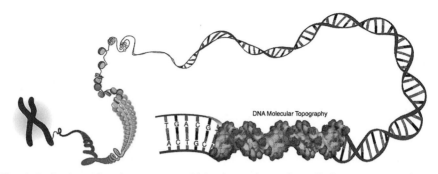

DNA Molecular Topography

Fig. 1. Packaging of a chromosome within the nucleus of a cell. (*Courtesy:* Darryl Leja, National Human Genome Research Institute. Available at: http://www.genome.gov/dmd/img.cfm?node=Photos/Graphics&id=85341. Accessed November 01, 2013.)

and DNA methylation are identified. When a gene is transcribed the DNA thread around the histone loosens, the DNA sequence opens up allowing the nucleotide sequence to be read by RNA, ultimately producing a normal protein. On completion of the protein building, the reverse sequence occurs. The structures associated with epigenetics are depicted in **Fig. 2**.[21]

Each individual has 23 pairs of chromosomes, 22 pairs of autosomes (non–sex chromosomes) and 1 pair of sex chromosomes. After replication, each identical half of the chromosome is identified as a chromatid.[22] The parts of a chromosome are depicted in **Fig. 1**, with the addition of telomeres at each end of the chromatid. Telomeres normally stabilize the chromosome with shortening as the individual ages. The process of carcinogenesis is known to prevent the telomeres from shortening, thereby facilitating the immortalization of the cancer cell.

Each chromatid comprising the chromosome is composed of duplicate genes, some with multiple alleles (alternative form of a gene). A common alleleic example is the ABO blood group, with 3 alleles. A normal chromosome expresses only 2 (phenotype) at a time such as AB, OO, or AO. In cancer, 1 allele may be normal (wild type) and the other allele may be a mutation.[23]

The chromosomes consist of 2 tightly coiled strands of DNA, composed of multiple nucleotides. Each nucleotide includes a nitrogenous base along with a sugar and a phosphate group. The 2 DNA strands form a double helix, held together with hydrogen bonds. There are 2 types of nitrogenous bases, purines and pyrimidines. The purines are double-ringed and include adenine (A) and guanine (G.) The pyrimidines are single-ringed and include thymine (T) and cytosine (C). Ribonucleic acid (RNA) differs from DNA in that it is a single-stranded nucleotide chain. Within the RNA molecule, thymine (T) is replaced by uracil (U). The RNA molecule has been intensively studied and is becoming a research target for the diagnosis and treatment of disease. **Table 2** presents the multiple types of RNA involved in the regulation of gene products (proteins).[24–27]

Tumor Genetics

Changes in the DNA or RNA can result in polymorphisms (common changes in DNA) and/or mutations (disease-causing changes in DNA). The most common gene (allele) type is termed the wild type.[28] Mutations can occur in protooncogenes (*ras*, *v-src*), allowing them to be activated into oncogenes with continued cell proliferation. Mutations also can occur in tumor suppressor genes (*Rb*, *p53*, *WT1*, *BRCA1*, *BRCA2*, *VHL*,

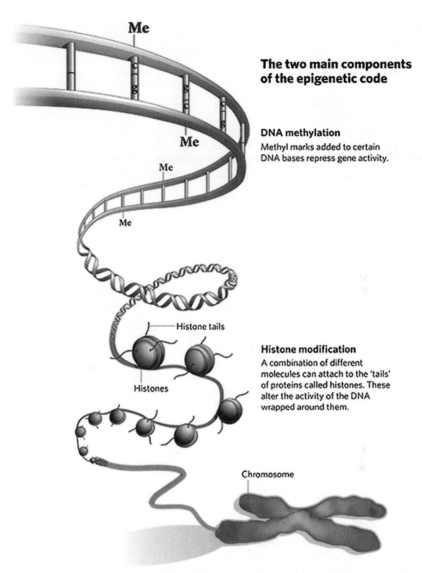

The two main components of the epigenetic code

DNA methylation
Methyl marks added to certain DNA bases repress gene activity.

Histone modification
A combination of different molecules can attach to the 'tails' of proteins called histones. These alter the activity of the DNA wrapped around them.

Fig. 2. Mechanisms of epigenetics. (*From* Qiu J. Unfinished symphony. Nature 2006;441(11):144–5; Reprinted by permission from Macmillan Publishers Ltd.)

APC, *NF-1*, *NF-2*, and *MTS-1*), preventing the occurrence of normal cell processes such as promoting programmed cell death (apoptosis).[29] With mutations in these 2 regulatory gene types there is continued proliferation and immortalization of the cells and the ultimate development into malignancy (**Table 3**).[30–38]

Mutations are caused by a variety of dramatic and less dramatic changes to the DNA. These can include translocations, such as Philadelphia chronic myelocytic leukemia (CML) and the 9:22 exchange, 2-hit mutations as seen with the *BRCA* genes and breast cancer or, mismatch repair changes found with colon cancer. Once a malignancy is diagnosed, the mutation(s), which provided a growth or survival advantage to the cancer cells or are necessary to maintain their malignant status (driver

Table 2 Types of RNA	
RNA	Function
Transfer RNA (tRNA)	Brings amino acids to site of protein synthesis
Messenger RNA (mRNA)	Orders nucleotides into amino acids for protein expression
Ribosomal RNA (rRNA)	Structural support for the protein
MicroRNA (miRNA)	Short noncoding RNA that inhibits mRNA so there is decreased gene expression
Piwi-interacting RNA (piRNA)	Epigenetic and posttranscriptional gene silencing in germline cells, especially spermatogenesis
Small interfering RNA (siRNA)	Gene silencing

Data from Refs.[24–27]

mutations), are present in all the cancer cells.[38] **Table 4** includes some types of mutations and other chromosomal changes.[39–42]

Although the human genome strives to be mostly static, the epigenome is easily altered by environmental influences such as ultraviolet light. As seen in **Fig. 2**, in the typical genome there are many areas of normal hypermethylation that are found to be hypomethylated in the cancer genome. In areas of the normal genome containing regulatory regions of gene clusters of CpG islands, there are groups of paired cytosines (C) and guanines (G) present. During a disease process such as cancer, this region can become hypermethylated causing transcriptional silencing of genes, especially tumor suppressor genes. Note the methylated C and G nucleotides, identified in **Fig. 2**.

The tails that protrude from the small histone proteins, seen in **Fig. 2**, assist to tightly package the DNA and prevent transcription. These tails can be changed by small chemical groups such as acetyl, methyl, and phosphoryl, or peptides such as ubiquitin. One such molecule, small ubiquitin-like modifier, can open or elongate the strands between histones, allowing transcription. These mechanisms of epigenetics are now being targeted for cancer therapies.[43–46]

Signaling pathways are also being targeted for personalized treatments of cancers. A variety of genes and their products (proteins) are affected as the molecular level signaling pathways are turned off and on. Apoptosis is 1 of the most important normal mechanisms that is altered with malignant transformation. Three primary biochemical changes affect the process of programmed cell death. These include (1) activation of a group of specialized proteins (caspases) with the ability to cut proteins at specific sites to promote cell death, (2) DNA and protein breakdown, and (3) recognition by phagocytic cells for engulfment and destruction.[47,48] These biochemical changes lead to an organized destruction of the cell components and membrane leading to programmed cell death. Normally, these processes eliminate cancer cells but, with the evolution of cancer, there is a disrupted balance of proapoptotic and antiapoptotic proteins (Bcl-2 family), causing an evasion of apoptosis allowing immortalization of the cell (**Fig. 3**).[49]

Other signaling pathways initiated by genes also affect or support malignant transformation. These include (1) the p13Ka pathway believed to be specific to the epidermal growth factor receptor (EGFR)/epidermal receptor family of receptors (ERBB), which includes Her2/neu; (2) the mTOR (mechanistic target of rapamycin) pathway, which can be activated by oncogenes to allow cancer cell growth, survival, and proliferation of cancers; or (3) the PARP (poly[ADP] ribose polymerase) pathway, which stimulates changes in gene expression, amounts of available RNA and protein, and the site and activity of proteins that mediate signaling responses.[50–52] Each of

Table 3
Examples of oncogenes and tumor suppressor genes with some associated cancers

Regulatory Gene Types	Normal Function	Cancer Type(s)
Oncogenes		
BRAF	Produces protein for RAS/MAPK pathway to regulate proliferation of cells, differentiation, migration, and apoptosis	Somatic mutations causing melanoma, colon, rectum, ovary and thyroid cancer
Ras family (*H-Ras*, *N-Ras* and *K-Ras*)	Actin cytoskeletal integrity, cell proliferation, differentiation and apoptosis	Pancreatic cancer
HER2/*neu*	Epidermal growth factor	Breast cancer
MMR genes (*MLH1*, *MSH2*, *MSH6*, *PMS2*)	Maintain fidelity of DNA during replication	—
Myc	Regulator gene that codes for a transcription factor and regulates global chromatic structure by regulating histone acetylation	Burkitt lymphoma
hTERT	Maintains telomere ends so associated with immortalization of cells	Not specific
Src	Participates in engagement of various members of tyrosine kinase families. Part of immune response signaling pathways	Colon cancer, breast cancer, prostate cancer, metastasis
BCL-2	Helps regulate apoptosis (antiapoptosis)	Chronic lymphocytic leukemia B-cell, non-Hodgkin lymphoma, breast cancer, follicular lymphoma, B-cell lymphoma
Tumor Suppressor Genes		
APC	Acts as a tumor suppressor. Helps control cell division, attachment to other cells in tissue, and if a cells moves within or away from a tissue	Colon, intestinal, familial adenomatous polyposis (FAP) syndrome
BRCA	DNA repair, transcription and ubiquitination	Breast, ovarian, prostate, melanomas, and pancreatic cancers
MEN1	Role in repression of telomerase expression. Chromatin regulation	Multiple endocrine neoplasia type 1 parathyroid cancer, carcinoid tumors, pancreatic cancer, or endocrine tumors such as a pituitary tumor
TP53	Conserves stability of the genome, apoptosis and inhibits, angiogenesis, activates DNA repair proteins	Colon, breast, and lung cancer, leukemias, lymphomas and sarcomas. Li-Fraumeni syndrome
PTEN	Promotes apoptosis, negatively regulates the AKT/PKB signaling pathway	Cowden syndrome, breast cancer, thyroid cancer, head and neck cancer, glioma type 2, prostate cancer, and endometrial cancer

Data from Refs.[30–38]

Table 4
Some examples of mutations and other chromosome abnormalities found with cancer

Type of DNA Change	Description	Example of Cancer Type
Polymorphisms	Changes in the DNA sequence of a gene that are not disease related, occur at variable frequency, and are associated with individualization in the general population. A single nucleotide polymorphism (SNP, pronounced as snip) is a DNA change in 1 nucleotide	Not disease related
Mutations		
Frameshift	One or more bases added or deleted from the normal DNA sequence causing altered form of expected protein	Colorectal cancer
Missense	Single base pair change results in substitution of 1 amino acid for another in the protein being built. Some of the substitutions could cause a malfunctioning or no appropriate protein	Seen in somatic mutations *BRAF V600 E* (non-Hodgkin lymphoma, colorectal cancer, papillary thyroid cancer, non–small cell lung cancer, and adenocarcinoma of the lung), KRAS G12D (colorectal cancer and pancreatic cancer, and EGFR L858 R lung cancer)
Nonsense	Change an "amino acid adding signal" to "stop adding amino acids" for a growing protein. Causes a truncated, presumably nonfunctional protein	—
RNA negative	Result in absence of RNA transcribed from a gene copy	Human papilloma virus–associated cancers
Splicing	Occurs when DNA that should be removed from the coding sequence is retained, or DNA that should not be added is spliced in, resulting in frameshift mutations	—
Chromosomal Alterations		
Translocation	Segments of 1 chromosome that break off and attach themselves to other chromosomes resulting in altered protein production	Chronic myelocytic leukemia (Philadelphia chromosome)
Aneuploidy	Abnormal number of chromosomes	Leukemia, multiple myeloma
Loss of heterozygosity	Loss of a segment of both copies of a chromosome	—
Microsatellite instability	Repetitive pieces of DNA scattered throughout the genome in noncoding regions (introns). Marker of germline abnormality in MMR genes or hypermethylation in sporadic cases	Lynch syndrome

Data from Refs.[39–42]

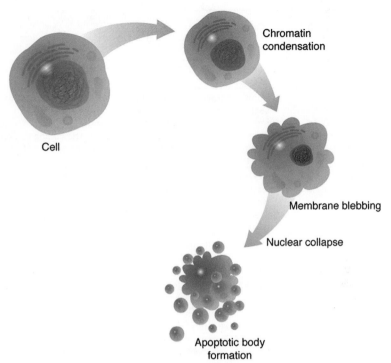

Chromatin condensation

Cell

Membrane blebbing

Nuclear collapse

Apoptotic body formation

Fig. 3. Apoptosis. (*Courtesy:* National Human Genome Research Institute. Available at: http://www.genome.gov/Glossary/index.cfm?p=viewimage&id=10. Accessed September 10, 2013.)

these (as well as other signaling pathways) is associated with different cancers including *MET* amplifications with lung cancer, advanced renal cell carcinoma, or ovarian and breast cancer, respectively. Inhibition of these and other signaling pathways are being targeted to impede the survival of profiled tumors.[50–52]

METHODS OF GENETIC ANALYSIS AND GENE DISCOVERY

Many times patients ask what is happening to their blood or malignant tumor when there is testing for predisposition or profiling for diagnosis, treatment guidance, or prognosis. **Table 5** includes some of the genetic testing technologies and a description of what can be identified through these mechanisms.[53–56] Nurses can help allay anxiety of patients with a brief and simple explanation.

CANCER SYNDROMES

Knowledge of genetic mutations that cause hereditary cancer syndromes influence plans to prevent or treat cancer. It is imperative that oncology nurses have at least a basic understanding of hereditary cancer syndromes. Information about common hereditary cancer syndromes is provided in **Table 6**.[57–83]

GENETIC HISTORY
Children and Adolescents

The health history for children and adolescents should include the prenatal and neonatal history as well as the child's subsequent growth and development. For

Table 5
Examples of methods of genetic analysis and gene discovery

Method	Analysis
Allele specific oligonucleotide	Detects 1 single specific mutation that involves a short sequence of DNA
Direct sequencing	Determines the sequence of the gene being tested and detects sequence changes in the regions being analyzed Direct sequencing detects sequence changes in the regions being analyzed but can miss mutations outside the coding region or mutations that are large genomic rearrangements or large deletions
Genome-wide association studies	Surveys the entire genome for small nucleotide alterations Detects SNPs or small mutations to determine association with disease Reviews for changes with specific disease (cancer type) vs genomes of persons without the disease
High-throughput genome sequencing	Techniques designed to offer faster and cheaper ways to obtain genetic data with potential impact on personalized profiling for diagnosis, pharmacogenomics, and disease monitoring
Large genomic rearrangements	Detects large rearrangements, deletions, and duplications (like pages or paragraphs missing or rearranged in a mystery novel) Used to identify *BRCA1* family mutations
Microarray	Technique attaches large numbers (hundreds to thousands) of DNA, RNA, protein, or tissue segments to slides in a specific location, followed by application of a fluorescent label. The biosample is processed so that the genetic material of the sample binds to the genetic material on the slide. The slide is scanned to measure the brightness of each fluorescent dot. The brighter the dot, the greater the fluorescent activity Microarray is used for mutation detection and gene expression
Sequential analysis of gene expression	Provides a picture of the mRNA population in a cancer sample
Single strand confirmation polymorphism analysis (SSCP)	A sequence change of DNA alters the size and/or shape of a DNA fragment, detected by SSCP on a gel. An altered gene produces a gel band different from normal gene SSCP easily detects insertions or deletions of 4 or more bases of DNA; however, mutations exchanging 1 base for another without altering the length of the DNA fragment are difficult to detect. In this technique, gel electrophoresis separates different conformations of the strands before sequencing
Next generation DNA sequencing (second-generation sequencing)	New lower cost and higher efficiency techniques to target the whole genome, whole exome, and whole transcriptome. Detects somatic cancer genome alterations of the nucleotide (substitutions, small insertions, deletions, variations in copy number)
Protein truncation assay	Analysis of coding DNA, directly translated in the laboratory into protein Shortened proteins detected on a gel, based on mobility differences between larger and smaller proteins Sensitive for detection of mutations in which the sequence change results in a shortened form of the protein Does not detect other types of mutations

(continued on next page)

Table 5 *(continued)*	
Method	**Analysis**
Techniques to identify chemical modification or packaging of DNA	Reviews methylation across the entire genome (methylome) Identifies the addition of methyl groups to GC -rich region of DNA Hypomethylation with removal of methyl groups causing inactivation of a gene Methylation pattern of genes by tissue type
Transcriptome sequencing	Analyzes coding RNA molecules and noncoding RNA sequences in 1 or specific population of cells[55]
Whole exome sequencing or targeted exome capture	Low-cost alternative technique to sequence exon (gene to protein coding regions) pieces of the genome Identifies area of protein function change in Mendelian and common diseases

Data from Refs.[53–56]

example, children with Beckwith-Wiedemann syndrome, which is associated with growth asymmetry resulting from abnormalities on the short arm (p) of chromosome 11 (11p), have an increased risk of Wilms tumor and hepatoblastoma.[84] Review of the developmental history may also provide information relating to delays in achievement of developmental milestones or loss of developmental milestones that may provide clues to the development of cancer.[85]

The provider should identify and document the presence of any constitutional chromosomal abnormalities, that is, those chromosomal abnormalities present in every cell of the body. The presence of these abnormalities increases the child's risk of developing a malignancy. These abnormalities include abnormalities in number, such as trisomy 21, or structure, such as the presence of a ring chromosome. As an example, children with trisomy 21 have a 20-fold increased risk of developing acute lymphoblastic leukemia and require more intense therapy to treat their disease compared with otherwise previously healthy children.[86] Approximately 3% to 10% of neonates with trisomy 21 are at increased risk of developing transient myeloproliferative disorder, which may resolve spontaneously without antineoplastic therapy. Of these children, around 15% to 20% of cases result in early death and another 13% to 33% progress to acute megakaryoblastic leukemia, a subtype of acute myeloid leukemia.[86]

The health history also should identify and document the presence of congenital and acquired immunodeficiency states, autoimmune disorders, and neurofibromatosis. Immunodeficiency states may be associated with genomic instability, which can increase the risk of cancer development.[87,88] Chronic immunosuppressive therapy is associated with an increased risk of lymphoproliferative conditions.[89] Autoimmune and chronic inflammatory conditions may result in the generation of free radicals that can increase the risk of carcinogenesis.[90] Neurofibromatosis is associated with an increased risk of sarcomas, brain tumors, optic gliomas, and leukemia.[91]

The family history for children and adolescents also should address the presence of cancer in other family members, including other childhood cancers. Although only 5% to 10% of childhood cancers can be attributed to a familial cancer syndrome, this aspect of the health history should not be overlooked.[92]

Adults

Similar to children and adolescents, a family history of cancer is an important consideration in determining the presence of a hereditary or familial cancer syndrome in an

Table 6
Common hereditary cancer syndromes

Genetic Syndrome (Common Acronym)	Gene(s)	Typical Age at Onset	Most Common Cancers/Cancer Sites in Syndrome	Additional Findings
Ataxia telangiectasia	ATM	1–4 y	Leukemia, lymphoma	Oculomotor apraxia, choreoathetosis, telangiectasias of the conjunctivae, immunodeficiency, frequent infections
Beckwith-Wiedemann syndrome	IC1, IC2, CDKN1C, may have 2 copies of a section of father's chromosome 11p15.5	Signs may be present during pregnancy; cancer onset 2–5 y	Wilms tumor (kidney), hepatoblastoma, neuroblastoma, rhabdomyosarcoma	Macrosomia, macroglossia, visceromegaly, omphalocele, neonatal hypoglycemia, ear creases/pits, adrenocortical cytomegaly, renal medullary dysplasia, nephrocalcinosis, medullary sponge kidney, nephromegaly
Birt-Hogg-Dubé syndrome	FLCN	Skin lesions occur in the 30s to 40s; renal cancer typically by age 48 y	Oncocytoma hybrid, chromophobe and clear cell renal carcinoma	Fibrofolliculomas, trichodiscomas/angiofibromas, perifollicular fibromas, and acrochordons (skin tags); bilateral and multifocal pulmonary cysts, pneumothoraces
Bloom syndrome	BLM	Benign findings start in utero. Age of typical cancer onset depends on type, but ranges between 1 and 34 y	Lymphoma, lower gastrointestinal tract, skin, acute myelogenous leukemia, upper gastrointestinal and respiratory tracts, urogenital, liver, breast, acute lymphoblastic leukemia, lower respiratory, sarcoma, germ cell, brain, retinoblastoma	Severe intrauterine and postnatal growth restriction, sparse subcutaneous tissue, short stature, sun-sensitive facial lesions, gastroesophageal reflux, upper and lower respiratory tract infections, premature menopause, male infertility, chronic obstructive pulmonary disease, diabetes mellitus

Syndrome	Gene	Clinical onset	Associated cancers	Other findings
Cowden (PTEN hamartoma tumor) syndrome	PTEN	Benign findings typically appear by the 20s; cancer onset in the 30s to 40s	Breast, endometrial, papillary thyroid; less often colon and renal cell carcinoma	Major: multiple gastrointestinal hamartomatas or ganglioneuromas, macrocephaly, macular pigmentation of the glans penis, trichilemmonas, acral and palmar keratoses, papillomatous and mucosal lesions. Minor: autism spectrum disorder; esophageal glycogenic acanthosis; lipomas, intellectual disability (IQ$\leq$75), thyroid nodules, adenoma, or goiter; vascular anomalies
Familial adenomatous polyposis (FAP)	APC	Polyps may appear by 7 y, colon cancer typically occurs by 39 y	Colon, hepatoblastoma	100s to 1000s of colon polyps, gastric fundus polyps, duodenal polyps, osteomas, dental anomalies, congenital hypertrophy of the retinal pigment epithelium (CHRPE), soft tissue tumors, desmoid tumors. Attenuated FAP shows 10–99 polyps or $\geq$100 polyps with onset at 35 y or later
Gardner syndrome	—	—	Colon	Colon polyps plus osteomas, epidermoid cysts, fibromas, desmoid tumors
Turcot syndrome in FAP	—	—	Colon, medulloblastoma	Colon polyps plus tumors of the central nervous system
Familial atypical multiple mole melanoma (FAMMM)	CDKN2A	Average age of onset of melanoma is 42 y	Melanoma, pancreatic	Typically >50 melanocytic nevi

(continued on next page)

Table 6
(continued)

Genetic Syndrome (Common Acronym)	Gene(s)	Typical Age at Onset	Most Common Cancers/Cancer Sites in Syndrome	Additional Findings
Hereditary breast cancer syndromes	BRCA1	Typically before 50 y, especially before 45 y	Breast (female or male), ovary (especially serous epithelial), primary peritoneal, pancreatic	—
	BRCA2	—	Breast (female or male), ovary (especially serous epithelial), primary peritoneal, pancreatic, prostate, melanoma, fallopian tube, gallbladder and bile duct	Fanconi anemia
	CHEK2	—	Breast (female or male), potentially: thyroid, prostate, colon, kidney	—
	PALB2	—	Breast, pancreas, esophagus, stomach	Fanconi anemia
Hereditary leiomyomatosis and renal cell cancer (HLRCC)	FH	Skin findings typically appear by age 25 y, uterine fibroids by age 30 y, renal cancer by age 44 y	Renal cell carcinoma	Cutaneous leiomyomata, uterine leiomyomata
Hereditary diffuse gastric cancer (HDGC)	CDH1	Typically before 40 y, possibly by 14 y	Diffuse gastric, lobular breast	—
Hereditary neuroblastoma (NBL)	ALK, PHOX2B	Infancy to 3 y	Malignant neuroblastoma, ganglioneuroblastoma, ganglioneuroma	Benign neuroblastoma, ganglioneuroblastoma, ganglioneuroma
Hereditary paraganglioma-pheochromocytoma syndrome (HPP/HPC)	SDHA, SDHB, SDHC, SDHD, SDHAF2, MAX	Before 45 y	Malignant paragangliomas and pheochromocytomas	Benign paragangliomas and pheochromocytomas
Hereditary retinoblastoma	RB1	Before 5 y	Bilateral (more likely) and unilateral (less likely) retinoblastomas, pinealomas, osteosarcomas, soft tissue sarcomas, melanomas	Absent red reflex (leukoria), glaucoma, orbital cellulitis, uveitis, hyphema, or vitreous hemorrhage

Syndrome	Gene(s)	Age/polyp notes	Associated cancers	Additional features
Juvenile polyposis syndrome (JPS)	BMPR1A, SMAD4	Can occur in infancy; polyps typically occur by age 20 y, juvenile refers to polyp type, not age of onset	Most common: colon Less common: stomach, esophagus, pancreas	Benign hamartomatous polyps in the stomach, small intestine, colon, and rectum. May occur concurrently with hereditary hemorrhagic telangiectasia when SMAD4 mutation present
Li-Fraumeni syndrome (LFS)	p53	Dependent on cancer type; see cancers in syndrome for typical age of onset	Core cancers: soft tissue sarcoma (average age of onset age 14 y), osteosarcoma (not Ewing sarcoma; average age of onset age 15 y), brain (astrocytomas, glioblastomas, medulloblastomas, choroid plexus; average age of onset age 16 y), breast (average age of onset age 33 y), adrenocortical (typically by age 3 y); Less common: acute leukemia lymphoma; colorectal endometrial, esophageal, germ cell, bronchoalveolar lung cancer, ovarian, pancreatic, prostate, stomach, thyroid, kidney, and skin cancers (including melanoma); and neuroblastoma	—
Lynch syndrome (LS)	MLH1, MLH3, MSH2, MSH6, PMS1, PMS2, EPCAM, MYH	—	Colon, uterus (endometrial), renal collecting system, biliary collecting system, ovary, breast, gastric (not diffuse), small bowel, pancreatic	—
Turcot in Lynch syndrome	—	—	Lynch syndrome cancers plus glioblastoma multiforme	—
Muir-Torre syndrome	—	—	Lynch syndrome cancers plus sebaceous carcinoma	Sebaceous adenomas, sebaceous epitheliomas, keratoacanthomas

(continued on next page)

Table 6
(continued)

Genetic Syndrome (Common Acronym)	Gene(s)	Typical Age at Onset	Most Common Cancers/Cancer Sites in Syndrome	Additional Findings
Multiple endocrine neoplasia type 1 (MEN-1)	MEN1	—	Pituitary macroadenomas (rare), gastrinoma (usually malignant), bronchial and thymic carcinoid tumors, adrenalcortical tumor may be malignant if >1 cm	Benign parathyroid tumors causing hypercalcemia, prolactinoma, gastrinoma (rarely benign), insulinoma, glucagonoma, vasoactive intestinal peptide-secreting tumor, adrenocortical tumor (usually benign), facial angiofibromas, collagenomas, lipomas, meningiomas, ependymomas, leiomyomas
Multiple endocrine neoplasia type 2	—	Medullary thyroid cancer onset	—	—
MEN 2A	RET	Early adulthood	Medullary thyroid, pheochromocytoma	Parathyroid adenoma or hyperplasia
Familial medullary thyroid carcinoma (FMTC)	RET	Middle adulthood	Medullary thyroid, pheochromocytoma (less common)	—
MEN 2B	RET	Early childhood	Medullary thyroid, pheochromocytoma	Mucosal neuromas of the lips and tongue, enlarged lips, gastrointestinal ganglioneuromatosis, asthenic marfanoid body habitus
Neurofibromatosis type 1 (NF-1)	NF1	Benign findings may be present at birth and progress over the lifespan	Malignant peripheral nerve sheath tumors, optic nerve gliomas, astrocytoma, breast	Multiple café-au-lait spots, axillary and inguinal freckling, multiple cutaneous neurofibromas, iris Lisch nodules, learning disabilities, plexiform neurofibromas, optic nerve, gliomas, scoliosis, tibial dysplasia, and vasculopathy (renal, brain, aorta, heart), unidentified bright objects on brain magnetic resonance imaging

Syndrome	Gene	Onset	Associated cancers	Features
Nevoid basal cell carcinoma (Gorlin) syndrome	PTCH	Benign findings in the 20s; skin cancer in the 30s, medulloblastoma by age 2 y	Skin (basal cell before age 30 y or >5 in a lifetime), medulloblastoma	Multiple jaw keratocysts, plantar and palmar pits, macrocephaly, bossing of the forehead, coarse facial features, facial milia, bifid ribs, wedge-shaped vertebrae, premature calcification of the falx cerebri (<20 y), ovarian fibromas, cardiac fibromas (rare)
Peutz-Jeghers syndrome (PJS)	STK11 (LKB1)	Gastrointestinal symptoms typically begin by age 10 y	Colorectal, gastric, pancreatic, breast, ovarian, adenoma malignum of the cervix (rare)	Hamartomatous polyps in the jejunum, ileum, duodenum, stomach, large bowel, and nasal passages; anemia, bowel obstruction, and intussusception; dark blue to dark brown macules around the mouth, eyes, and nostrils, in the perianal area, and on the buccal mucosa; hyperpigmented macules on the fingers; sex cord tumors with annular tubules (women); Sertoli cell testicular tumors causing gynecomastia
Rhabdoid tumor predisposition syndrome (RTPS)	SMARCB1	Before age 2 y	Renal or extrarenal rhabdoid tumors; choroid plexus carcinoma, medulloblastoma, central primitive neuroectodermal tumors	—
von Hippel-Lindau (VHL)	VHL	Retinal changes may occur by age 1 y	Clear cell renal carcinoma	Hemangioblastomas of the cerebellum, spinal cord, and retina; renal cysts; pheochromocytoma, pancreatic cysts, and neuroendocrine tumors; endolymphatic sac tumors; epididymal and broad ligament cysts
X-linked lymphoproliferative (Duncan) syndrome (XLP)	SH2D1A, XIAP (BIRC4)	Infancy to 45 y	Lymphoma (especially high-grade B-cell lymphoma of the intestine)	Male gender because X-linked, hemophagocytic lymphohistiocytosis, dysgammaglobulinemia, hepatitis, hepatic necrosis, profound bone marrow failure

Data from Refs.[57-83]

adult. Approximately 5% to 10% of cancers are hereditary, 75% to 80% of cancers are sporadic leaving approximately 10% of cancers to be familial.[93,94] Family members with cancer at a typical age of onset, such as breast cancer at age 80 y, are likely to have a sporadic cancer, whereas cancer onset in a young adult is a red flag for a cancer syndrome.[94,95] A history of cancer during childhood or adolescence may increase the risk of developing cancer during adulthood. For example, the treatment of Hodgkin lymphoma with mantle radiation may lead to breast cancer onset as soon as 5 years later.[95,96]

In addition to possessing a genome, every individual has an epigenome. Chemical compounds in the epigenome regulate gene activation and inactivation, but are not part of the DNA.[96,97] The epigenome can be passed on during cell division and between generations.[96,97] Family members often share a common environment, similar values, and accepted lifestyle behaviors that lead to favorable or unfavorable epigenetic changes in addition to inherited genes.[97]

Lifestyle behaviors such as diet low in fruits and vegetables[98] or high in processed meats[99] or well done red meat,[99,100] level of physical activity,[99,101] percent of body fat,[99,102] tobacco use,[103] and alcohol intake[99,104] may lead to epigenetic changes that increase or decrease the risk of developing some types of cancer.

It is crucial to confirm the diagnosis of unknown or uncertain cancers whenever possible to help with understanding the health history. For example, abdominal cancer could represent gastric, uterine, ovarian, colon, pancreatic cancer, or uterine fibroids. Pathology reports or death certificates can help clarify uncertain cancer diagnoses. When these scientific documents are unavailable, family-reported treatment of cancer, such as chemotherapy or radiotherapy, suggests the illness was cancer. Accurate historical knowledge of familial cancer incidence helps care providers discern the risk for a genetic syndrome.

Geriatric

Although genetic syndromes can also occur in the geriatric population, most malignancies in elders are sporadic cancers caused by DNA damage acquired over a life time. These cancers are caused by somatic mutations, found only in a few cells within the body. In contrast, germline mutations are present at conception and located in every cell in the body.

With normal aging, much like genetic changes associated with carcinogenesis, there is also diminished DNA repair and defects in tumor suppressor genes in conjunction with life-long exposure to environmental carcinogens.[105] An enzyme, telomerase, is known to replace the short pieces of DNA at the end of chromosomes (telomeres) and prevent aging. Without telomerase, the telomeres lose nucleotides with each replication, becoming shortened and contributing to chromosomal instability of somatic cells. With cancer, telomerase activity is increased and sustained; thus associated with longevity of life of cancer cells.[106] During the anaphase of mitosis, the fused chromosomes are randomly torn apart causing mutations and other abnormalities of chromosomes leading to the development of genetic diseases including cancer.[107] These acquired genetic changes lead to more sporadic cancers than inherited via germline mutations and cause the development of more malignancies in the elderly.

Epigenetic changes also induce sporadic cancers. The CpG islands (discussed earlier) are located close to promoter genes along the DNA strand. In normal cells, these regions are typically unmethylated allowing gene transcription. In many tumors, the CpG islands are methylated, preventing gene transcription, often of important tumor suppressor genes like p53. Histone modifications are also common.[108]

These epigenetic modifications are believed to precede cancer-associated mutations in the noted tumor suppressors, protooncogenes, and other areas of genomic instability.[109,110]

Genetic alterations associated with cancer in the elderly can lead to a variety of phenotypic traits that can be similar to normal changes of aging. Oncology nurses need to be aware of these changes and help their patients know when to see their oncologist. These signs and symptoms are compared in **Table 7**.

PEDIGREE

A family pedigree is an excellent graphic tool to help the oncology nurse determine whether the client and family require a referral for genetic care. Standard guidelines for creating a pedigree were created by members of the National Society of Genetic Counselors (NSGC) and were adopted by NSGC and the American College of Medical Genetics.[111] The nurse should construct a family pedigree with at least 3 generations using the standardized symbols, lines, and a legend. A list of key elements to include in a pedigree are provided in **Box 1**. Confirmation of the diagnosis of unknown or uncertain cancers helps to discern the risk for a genetic syndrome. For example, abdominal cancer could represent gastric, uterine, ovarian, colon, pancreatic cancer, or uterine fibroids. Pathology reports or death certificates can be helpful in clarifying uncertain cancer diagnoses. Accurate knowledge helps discern the risk for a genetic syndrome.

The family history may not reveal cancer in other members. This happens for a variety of reasons. A new mutation may have occurred. Mutation carriers may not have cancer when penetrance is not complete. Penetrance refers to the percentage of individuals who carry a mutation that develops the related disease. Also, the family structure may be limited.[112] Within the context of *BRCA* mutations, Weitzel and colleagues[113] defined limited family structure as "fewer than 2 first- or second-degree female relatives surviving past age 45 years in either lineage" (p. 2588). When a *BRCA* mutation occurs in the paternal lineage and at-risk women are absent or died at an early age, the pattern of inheritance may not be readily seen in the pedigree. The paternal lineage seen in the pedigree in **Fig. 4** illustrates this concept.

REVIEW OF SYSTEMS

The review of systems evaluates the past and present health status of the individual by body system.[114] This review should include a thorough discussion of all body systems not just those associated with the presenting symptoms. This aspect of the patient

Table 7 Ambiguous phenotypes with cancer versus aging	
Cancer	**Aging**
Increased skin pigment	Age spots
Rectal bleeding	Hemorrhoids
Constipation	Old age
Dyspnea	Getting old, out of shape
Decrease in urinary stream	Dribbling, benign prostatic hyperplasia
Fatigue	Normal atrophy, fibrosis
Breast changes	Loss of energy due to aging
Bone pain	Arthritis

Box 1
Constructing a pedigree

Include at least 3 generations including the patient's first-degree, second-degree, and third-degree relatives including the maternal and paternal lineage

Identify the patient

Use the standard symbols and relationship lines recommended by the American College of Medical Geneticists and National Society of Genetic Counselors to distinguish affected and unaffected individuals

Include the ethnic background for each grandparent

Ethnicity may relate to an increased or decreased risk for a given cancer syndrome

List the current age, age at diagnosis (if applicable), cause of and age at death (if applicable) for each individual in the pedigree

Provide relevant health information for each individual (such as history of colonoscopy and colon polyps in a family with colon cancer)

Include a legend of all symbols used in the pedigree

Adapted from Bennett RL, French KS, Resta RG, et al. Standardized human pedigree nomenclature: update and assessment of the recommendations of the National Society of Genetic Counselors. J Genet Couns 2008;17:424–33. http://dx.doi.org/10.1007/s10897-008-9169-9; with permission.

---

history allows the provider to ask questions about other symptoms that the patient (or parents) may not have recognized or deemed important. The provider should pay special attention to phenotypic traits that indicate the potential presence of a genetic disorder, for example, cancer occurring in paired organs such as breasts, kidneys, or eyes. The provider should also determine whether the cancers occurred simultaneously (ie, synchronous tumors) or at different times (ie, metachronous tumors).[115,116] Responses provided during the review can further guide the physical examination and provide clues regarding the possibility of a familial cancer syndrome.

PHYSICAL ASSESSMENT

The client of any age is examined for the clinical signs of the suspected syndrome as described previously (see **Table 5**).

For the common hereditary cancer syndromes, the physical assessment for children and adolescents should focus on the suspected diagnosis; however, attention to aspects of normal growth and development should not be overlooked. Accurate height and weight measurements should be plotted on the appropriate growth chart. Body mass index should be calculated and plotted for all children beginning at 24 months of age. Occipital frontal circumference (OFC) measurements should be obtained for all children 24 months of age and younger and plotted on the appropriate growth curve.[117] The OFC measurement should also be obtained on any child with questionable head size. Similarly, the OFC is measured on adults suspected of having Cowden (PTEN hamartoma tumor) syndrome and plotted on the graph created by Bushby in 1992.[118] An individual with an OFC more than the 98th percentile for the appropriate gender has macrocephaly, a potential sign of Cowden syndrome.[119,120] Whenever possible, growth measurements should be compared with previous measurements to identify growth failure or abnormalities that may be associated with the cancer development and/or an underlying genetic condition.

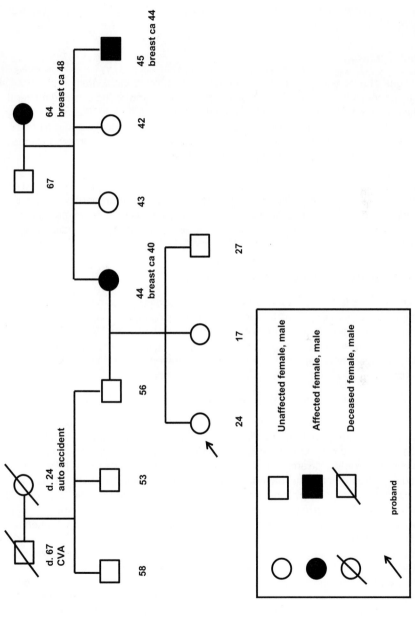

Fig. 4. Paternal lineage pedigree.

The initial impression should attend to the child's general appearance and the extent to which the child behaves in an age-appropriate manner. The provider should conduct a developmental assessment, with attention to age-related milestones. During the conduct of the head-to-toe physical assessment, the provider should attend to the presence of major and minor malformations that may indicate the presence of an underlying genetic condition associated with a given cancer syndrome (**Fig. 5**).

MEDICAL IMAGING

The signs of a hereditary cancer syndrome may be found incidentally during routine health screenings or diagnostic examinations. Case examples include finding keratocystic odontogenic tumors on routine dental panorex radiographs (**Fig. 6**), keratocystic odontogenic tumor and bifid ribs or vertebrae on chest radiographs, all findings seen in Cowden syndrome. Conversely, medical imaging can be ordered to specifically look for signs of a hereditary cancer syndrome.

Certain genetic mutations, such as *TP53*, which causes Li-Fraumeni syndrome and *ATM*, which causes ataxia telangiectasia, cause abnormal sensitivity to ionizing radiation.[57,74] Diagnostic imaging with ionizing radiation or therapeutic radiotherapy should be avoided when reasonably possible in individuals with these mutations.[57,74] A mastectomy is the preferred treatment over segmentectomy plus radiotherapy for breast cancer in an individual with a TP53 or ATM mutation.

ADDITIONAL USES OF GENETIC TESTING

Genetic testing is now used to determine predisposition for an inherited cancer, the genetic profile of a specific tumor for diagnosis, staging and prognosis, or pharmacogenomic management for personalization of the treatment. **Table 8** shows the germline cancers with their designated genetic mutations that can be identified through predisposition testing, if there is chemoprevention, or if surveillance is available for a person who has never had a diagnosis of cancer.[121–125]

Diagnosis, Personalized Treatment, and Prognosis

Several multigene panels offer genetic testing results to providers to more specifically personalize treatment of patients diagnosed with early-stage breast or colon cancer. These are used to predict recurrence risk and assist in treatment decisions for adjuvant chemotherapy. Current clinical trials incorporate these tests to assist in assigning patients to treatment arms based on tumor markers. Hundreds of breast cancer tumors have undergone genome sequencing to compare the somatic DNA changes in the tumor with the normal DNA present in the patients' cells. Some of these changes have led to discoveries that tumors with increased numbers of point mutations and chromosomal translocations occur more commonly in aromatase inhibitor-resistant estrogen receptor positive (ER+) cancers and the HER2 negative and positive breast cancer subtypes. The effect of neoadjuvant aromatase inhibitors in patients with certain somatic mutations is also an outcome of research focused on multigene tests on breast cancer tumors. The ultimate goal is that this type of genome sequencing will someday be able to identify molecular changes that can be used as targets for new therapies in multiple types of cancers.[126] Understanding both the meaning of the tests at the molecular level and how the results can affect the patients' treatment and side effects enables the oncology nurse to inform the patient/family about anticipatory needs and use for focused assessments.

Patient ID sticker   Date _____

Concerns *Intrusive Thoughts?* No Yes _____

Right Breast | **Left Breast**

Right = WNL   **Left** = WNL
Nipple w/out   **Nipple** w/out
dimpling, discharge,   dimpling, discharge,
retraction   retraction
Breast: **Breast:**
mild   mild
moderate   moderate
dense   dense
glandular   glandular
fibrocystic   fibrocystic
fibroglandular   fibroglandular
post-radiation   post-radiation
changes   changes
healing biopsy   healing biopsy
lumpectomy   lumpectomy
mastectomy   mastectomy

BSE Instruction Yes No

Working Diagnosis _____

Recommendations
Surveillance: Mammogram yearly now ☐ or at age: _____
supplement w/ U/S MRI CBE q 6 months BSE monthly
Surgery: Completion mastectomy RRM bil RRM RRSO
Prevention:
Tamoxifen Raloxifene Grapeseed Other _____

Notes from F/U appt _____

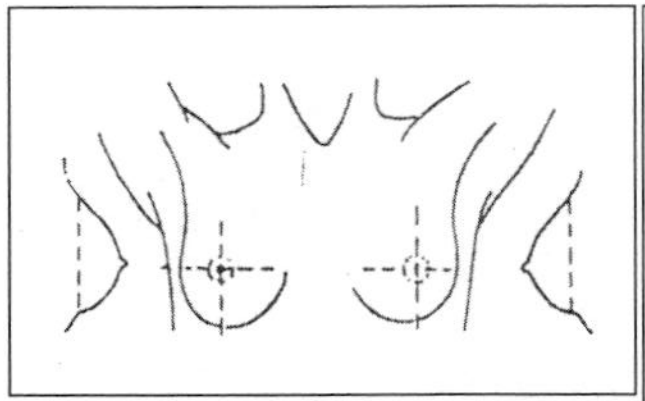

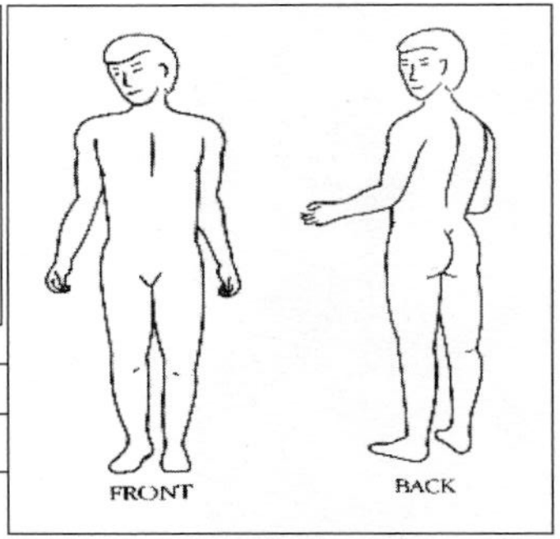

Physical Examination By Whom: _____
General: well- developed, no acute distress other: _____
Weight: _____ Height: _____
VS: B/P _____ Pulse _____ Resp. _____ Temp. _____
Skin: no suspicious lesions freckles tan moles other: _____
HEENT: HC _____ cm. Alopecia Oropharynx clear Tongue smooth
Neck: supple thyromegaly nodularity other: _____
Chest: CTA percussion wheezes crackles bilateral other: _____
CV: RRR w/out murmur, rub, or gallop other: _____
Breasts: no areas of concern/no dominant masses
ABD: Soft non-tender Normal BS other: _____
Lymph: No adenopathy: axillary cervical supraclavicular inguinal
Extremities: W/out edema other: _____
Neuro: grossly intact other: _____
Additional comments: _____

FRONT   BACK

Fig. 5. Physical assessment form. (*Courtesy of Department of Clinical Cancer Genetics, City of Hope National Medical Center, Duarte, CA; with permission.*)

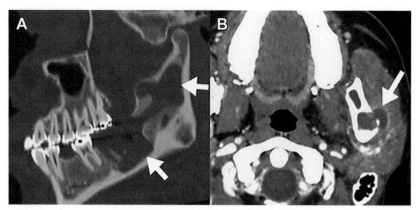

Fig. 6. Keratocystic odontogenic tumors of the mandible (*arrows*). (*From* Devenney-Cakir B, Subramaniam RM, Reddy SM, et al. Cystic and cystic-appearing lesions of the mandible: review. AJR Am J Roentgenol 2011;196:WS66–77. http://dx.doi.org/10.2214/AJR.09.7216. Available at: http://www.ajronline.org/doi/full/10.2214/AJR.09.7216. Accessed September 9, 2013; with permission.)

PHARMACOGENOMICS

Pharmacogenomics refers to the variations within an entire genome that result in variability in drug response, including how drugs are absorbed, metabolized, distributed, and excreted.[127] This term is in contrast to pharmacogenetics, which refers to genetic influences on therapeutic responses.[128] **Table 9** presents a list of medications commonly used in oncology care along with the associated pharmacogenomic implication(s), and related nursing considerations.[129–136]

Pharmacokinetics

Pharmacokinetics refers to how a given drug is absorbed, metabolized, distributed, and excreted. Metabolism is an enzyme-mediated process that occurs in 2 phases. During phase 1 metabolism, which occurs primarily through oxidation, the given drug is inactivated, or, in the case of a prodrug, converted to its active form. During phase 2, the metabolites formed in phase 1 are conjugated with other endogenous chemicals through processes including glucuronidation, sulfation, and acetylation, which allows them to be more readily excreted.[137]

Phase 1 metabolism is largely regulated via cytochrome P450 (CYP450) enzymes, a group of more than 40 enzyme families. These enzymes account for approximately 75% of drug metabolism with the CYP1, CYP2, and CYP3 families playing key roles in the process.[138] Each of these families includes multiple genes, which in turn have multiple alleles that influence individual variations in drug metabolism. A table identifying medications with pharmacokinetics influenced by CYP genes is accessible online through the Indiana University Division of Clinical Pharmacology at: http://medicine.iupui.edu/clinpharm/ddis/table.aspx.[139]

Polymorphisms and Drug Metabolism

Consequences of polymorphisms in genes coding for enzymes affecting drug metabolism are varied and may necessitate changes in drug dosing to avoid toxicity or even lack of a desired therapeutic effect. Polymorphisms in individual alleles may result in the capacity for normal metabolism, loss of function, or increased metabolic activity.

Table 8
Predisposition testing for inherited cancers: gene, prevention, and surveillance

Inherited Cancer Predisposition	Gene Mutation	Prevention	Surveillance
Breast	BRCA1/2	Tamoxifen Bilateral total mastectomy Bilateral salpingooophorectomy	Clinical breast examination every 6 mo with annual mammography and magnetic resonance imaging
Cervical	Human papilloma virus (HPV) 16/18 genotypes	HPV vaccination for girls aged 11–12 y and 13–18 y to catch up missed vaccine or complete the vaccination series	Cytology testing every 3–5 y depending on age of client HPV contesting every 5 y for women aged 30–65 y
Central nervous system	Lynch syndrome (LS) MLH1 and MSH2 carriers	No data to support	Annual physical examination starting at 25–30 y
Colon	LS, MLH1 and MSH2 carriers Attenuated FAP, APC	No data to support	Colonoscopy at age 20–25 y or 2–5 y before the earliest colon cancer before age 25 y and repeat every 1–2 y Colonoscopy every 1–2 y
Endometrial	LS, extracolonic MLH1 and MSH2 carriers	Prophylactic hysterectomy and bilateral salpingooophorectomy after childbearing is completed (National Comprehensive Cancer Network, LS-2)	Annual endometrial sampling is an option, but no clear evidence for endometrial screening with LS
Ovarian	BRCA1/2 LS, MLH1 and MSH2 carriers	Prophylactic bilateral salpingooophorectomy for carriers of BRCA1/2, MLH1, or MSH2 after completing childbearing	BRCA1/2: consider transvaginal ultrasonography and CA-125 every 6 mo starting at age 30 or 5–10 y before the earliest case in family, if prophylactic bilateral salpingooophorectomy was not done (National Comprehensive Cancer Network, HBOC-A, p 1) LS: no evidence to support surveillance
Pancreatic	LS; MLH1 and MSH2 carriers	No data to support	No data to support routine surveillance
Prostate	BRCA	—	No data to support routine surveillance
Stomach (gastric) and small bowel	LS; extracolonic MLH1 and MSH2 carriers	No data to support	No evidence for routine surveillance except Asian descent may consider esophagogastroduodenoscopy with extended duodenoscopy to distal duodenum or into the jejunum every 3–5 y beginning at age 30–35 y
Urolitheal	LS: extracolonic MLH1 and MSH2 carriers	No data to support	LS: consider annual urinalysis commencing at age 25–30 y

Data from Refs.[123–127]

Table 9
Selected medications used in cancer care, associated pharmacogenomic implication(s), and nursing considerations

Medication	Associated Pharmacogenomic Implication(s)	Nursing Considerations
5-Fluorouracil (5-FU)	Dihydropyimidine dehydrogenase (DPD) enzyme is responsible for catalyzing rate-limiting step of 5-FU breakdown Point mutation occurring in DPYD*2A allele leads to inability to deactivate 5-FU leading to increased toxicity	No genotyping currently available Monitor patients for signs of toxicity Oral uracil breath test capable of distinguishing between individuals with normal DPD activity and those with DPD deficiency
6-Mercaptopurine	SNP in drug-metabolizing enzyme, thiopurine methyltransferase (TPMT) resulting in enzyme deficiency	Individuals homozygous for 2 nonfunctional alleles at very high risk for severe hematologic toxicity TMPT genotyping with dosing guidelines based on genotype available Monitor complete blood count values closely
Codeine	Polymorphisms in CYP2D6 enzyme can: Prevent conversion of the prodrug to the active drug, resulting in lack of pain relief Result in ultrametabolism, increasing the risk of overdose	Monitor pain response carefully in individuals receiving codeine CYP2D6 genotyping available; avoid prescribing codeine to known poor or ultrarapid metabolizers
Irinotecan	UGT1A1*28 allele with 7 TATA repeats (wild type allele contains 6 repeats) in the promoter region associated with increased irinotecan toxicity in homozygotes and heterozygotes	UGT1A1 genotyping available and recommended on package insert for irinotecan Monitor absolute neutrophil count and bilirubin levels on individuals receiving irinotecan Individuals homozygous for the UGT1A1*28 allele may require decreased dosing
Methotrexate	Methylenetetrahydrofolate reductase enzyme involved in folate metabolism, DNA repair, and protein synthesis Individuals with 677T polymorphism are at increased risk for hyperhomocysteinuria which increases the risk for blood clots and stroke	Monitor patients for development of blood clots Educate patients regarding signs and symptoms of blood clots and stroke 677T polymorphism occurs more frequently among whites
Tamoxifen	Active metabolite is produced by CYP2D6 enzyme Medications that block the activity of CYP2D6 may reduce the effectiveness of tamoxifen	Review drug history for medications that inhibit CYP2D6 For patients receiving selective serotonin reuptake inhibitors that are strong CYP2D6 inhibitors, such as fluoxetine or paroxetine, change to a medication that is not a CYP2D6 inhibitor

Data from Refs.[131–138]

Individuals identified as homozygous for wild type alleles with normal metabolic activity are designated as extensive or effective metabolizers. An individual who is heterozygous, possessing at least 1 wild type allele, is regarded as an intermediate metabolizer. Individuals homozygous for nonfunctional alleles are designated as poor metabolizers and are at increased risk for toxicity for drugs administered in their active form. If the drug is a prodrug, however, poor metabolizers experience no response. Individuals who are designated as ultrametabolizers have increased enzyme activity. These individuals experience decreased drug activity from medications administered in their active form yet are at increased risk of toxicity from prodrugs.[140]

Pharmacodynamics

Pharmacodynamics may be regarded as what the drug does to the body. In addition to the physiologic and biochemical effects on the body, pharmacodynamics encompasses the relationship between drug concentration and drug effect. As with pharmacokinetics, genetic variation can influence pharmacodynamics.[140] Pharmacodynamics is largely influenced by cell surface and nuclear receptors. Polymorphisms in these receptors may alter the uptake of a given medication and prevent the drug from having an effect. As an example, polymorphisms in topoisomerase 1 (TOP1), which is the target of irinotecan, as well as other downstream effectors, tyrosyl DNA phosphodiesterase (TDP1), and X-ray crosscomplementation factor (XRCC1), have been related to grade 3 and 4 neutropenia associated with irinotecan as well as response to this medication.[141]

TREATMENT

Cancer treatment is also experiencing a paradigm shift created by genetic testing of an individual's (germline) buccal cells or blood, and/or the tumor tissue (somatic).[142] Over the past 2 decades, tamoxifen use has moved from treatment of breast cancer to prevention of breast cancer for women with a previous diagnosis of breast cancer and those never diagnosed. Traditionally, tamoxifen treatment was based on cancer staging; however, tumor hormone status is more commonly used as the standard. The National Cancer Coalition Network guidelines now indicate that women who have tested positive for a BRCA1/2 mutation can be treated with tamoxifen as chemoprevention. A substudy of women participating in the National Surgical Adjuvant Breast Project P-1 with the BRCA2 mutation and receiving tamoxifen had a 62% decrease risk of breast cancer compared with those women who took the placebo. Because the study had a small number of participants, the results were not generalizable.[143] Consideration of tumor markers for determining breast cancer treatment has continued to be included using the second-generation estrogen antagonists and aromatase inhibitors. Treatment of other solid tumors, such as advanced non–small cell lung cancer (NSCLC), also uses biomarker status to determine if targeted therapy (geftinib) holds promise for individualized treatment of EGFR-positive NSCLC. Other markers include KIT (CD117)-positive malignant gastrointestinal tumors (GIST), or bcr-abl–positive CML.[144]

Biomarkers also aid in the determination of use for the next generation of hormone-directed therapies against breast cancer. In ER+ breast cancer, such therapies include second-generation estrogen antagonists such as fulvestrant and third generation aromatase inhibitors such as anastrozole, letrozole, and exemestane. Approved recently for advanced NSCLC, tumor profiling is used to guide therapy and its use in earlier disease. Tumor profiling with gene panels (Mammaprint, OncotypeDX) is currently used to determine the need for chemotherapy in ER+ breast cancers.

Presence of the *BRCA2* mutation in ovarian cancer has been correlated with a better outcome than tumors with a wild type *BRCA* gene. These results suggest better survival, improved chemotherapy response but a mutator phenotype with more mutations than the *BRCA* wild type. For women with high-grade serious ovarian cancer, these results can offer hope for better outcomes even though the effect of more mutations is difficult to explain.[145]

As these new models of profiling and treatment determination become main stream, even more robust strategies are required to evaluate target status in clinical studies to facilitate the evaluation and positioning of novel targeted therapies. The success of the current genetic profiling tests has led to a call for the development of more personalized tests. Although some are currently available, most are still in the research phase and are using experimental processes. Since 2008, 3 commercial companies have introduced tests that provide genomic profiles of a tumor with treatment suggestions. Because these tests on tumor tissues are performed in Clinical Laboratory Improvement Amendments (CLIA) certified laboratories, the tests do not require US Food and Drug Administration approval when they are sold. The results are provided directly to the physicians but there is limited range of use by the oncologists. The tests have limited evidence-based results and none from randomized clinical trials. Until such clinical testing occurs, there are questions regarding their usefulness and if they lead to better outcomes. Advertised on the Internet, many patients can access the content and ask questions that may be difficult for oncology nurses and providers to answer. Some questions could include the cost of the testing ($3400–35,000), number of genes examined (~100 to whole genome or whole exome), validation (limited, with 2 of 3 only a pilot feasibility study and no scholarly sharing of information, to only an abstract or 1 article published) and turnaround time (<10 business days to >3 weeks based on what molecular sequence is being examined). For oncology professionals with limited genetic education and research knowledge, the result is that these questions will remain unanswered or poorly explained to patients, offering limited understanding of the process and/or patient outcomes associated with this commercial testing. Although any testing might be better than no testing, science directs that use of these tests to personalize treatment should optimally be done with a randomized clinical trial so that all variables are controlled and the patient's safety is held to the highest standard.[146]

The use of radiation for both early detection and treatment of cancer damages DNA and places the individual at a higher risk for developing a cancer. This is especially true for young women with developing breasts who receive mantle radiation therapy for Hodgkin lymphoma. Guidelines for the follow-up management of these young women, including the optimal time for initiation of screening, are included in **Table 10**.[147,148]

The *ATM* gene, ataxia telangiectasia mutated, regulates cellular responses to DNA damage induced by ionizing radiation. Specifically, the gene helps to control the rate of cellular growth and proliferation and division. In addition, the protein it produces assists in recognition of damaged or broken strands and coordination of DNA repair to maintain genomic stability. A small percentage of the US population (1%) carries a mutated copy of the *ATM* gene, making them at higher risk for developing breast cancer.[149] If women who carry this deleterious *ATM* variant receive radiation therapy as part of their treatment of a breast cancer diagnosis, they have an increased risk for a contralateral breast cancer.[150]

Patients with Li-Fraumeni syndrome have germline *p53* mutations and are at higher risk for developing several types of cancer at earlier ages during childhood or as young adults. Clinical observations revealed that persons with known *p53* mutations were at higher risk of secondary malignancies if treated with radiation for a first primary

Table 10	
National Comprehensive Cancer Network guidelines for women at high risk of breast cancer because of previous thoracic irradiation	
Age	**Screening Follow-up[a]**
Initiate 8–10 y after therapy, or age 40 y, whichever comes first, if chest or axillary radiation	Annual breast screening
	Breast magnetic resonance imaging in addition to mammography for women who received irradiation to the chest between ages 10 and 30 y
	Monthly self-breast examination
	Annual breast examination by a health care professional

[a] Women should be familiar with their breasts and promptly report changes to their health care provider. Periodic, consistent breast self-examination may facilitate breast self-awareness. Premenopausal women may find breast self-examination most informative when performed at the end of menses.

Adapted from Alm El-Din MA, El-Badawy SA, Taghian AG. Breast cancer after treatment of Hodgkin's lymphoma: general review. Int J Radiat Oncol Biol Phys 2008;72(5):1291–7; with permission.

cancer. One study identified that in 8 patients treated for breast cancer, 6 were treated with postoperative radiation. For these 6 individuals, there were 3 ipsilateral breast recurrences, 3 contralateral breast cancers, 2 radiation-induced cancers, and 3 new primaries. The investigators suggest that these significant observations support the need for bilateral mastectomy as the initial treatment and the avoidance of radiotherapy.[151]

The use of screening radiation at an early age is a growing concern for young women who are at a high risk of breast cancer as a result of identification as a *BRCA* mutation carrier or who have a lifetime risk of more than 20% defined by models that use family history. Current national guidelines indicate that women who are *BRCA* mutation carriers begin mammographic and magnetic resonance imaging (MRI) surveillance at the age of 25 years, or the age of 30 years if there is a lifetime risk of greater than 20% defined by models using family history.[152] Of interest, 1 study reported in 2012 identified that alternating diagnostic mammography (DM)/MRI every 6 months starting at age 25 years provided the highest life expectancy (*BRCA1*, 72.52 years, *BRCA2*, 77.63 years). With the inclusion of radiation risk, a small proportion of new breast cancers were attributed to radiation exposure (*BRCA1*, <2%; *BRCA2*, <4%). When radiation risk was considered, alternating the DM/MRI at age 25 years or only an annual MRI at age 25 years then delayed alternating with DM at age 30 years was the most effective treatment. The highest number of false-positive screens per woman (*BRCA1*, 4.5 *BRCA2*, 8.1) was associated with the alternating DM/MRI starting at age 25 years. Because these results are in conflict with the current National Comprehensive Cancer Network screening guidelines for high-risk women, once again the importance that health care providers be knowledgeable in genetics and possess an ability to properly discuss with the women what is best for their personal plan of surveillance, needs to be emphasized (**Table 11**).[151,153]

ETHICAL ASPECTS OF GENETIC TESTING

Because the results of genetic testing for hereditary cancers have consequences for the entire family, ownership of these test results is a matter of debate. The principle of respect for autonomy refers to self-governance.[154] Applied to cancer genetics, the recipient of a genetic test is the owner of the results. Some medical ethicists and

Table 11
NCCN guidelines for women at risk of breast cancer with >20% lifetime risk defined by models based on family history

Age	Screening Follow-up[a]
Begin at age 30 y	Annual mammogram breast screening plus clinical breast examination every 6–12 mo
	Consider annual breast magnetic resonance imaging, or individualized based on earliest age of onset in family
	Monthly self-breast examination
	Annual breast examination by a health care professional

[a] Women should be familiar with their breasts and promptly report changes to their health care provider. Periodic, consistent breast self-examination may facilitate breast self-awareness. Premenopausal women may find breast self-examination most informative when performed at the end of menses.

Adapted from Heymann S, Delaloge S, Rahal A, et al. Radio-induced malignancies after breast cancer postoperative radiotherapy in patients with Li-Fraumeni syndrome. Radiat Oncol 2010;5:104; with permission.

health care providers believe autonomy is the most important ethical principle; but others disagree.[155]

The ideal of first do no harm is attributed to the Hippocratic Oath and is highly valued throughout health care.[156] This ideal relates to the ethical principle of nonmaleficence, which holds that, "one ought not to inflict evil or harm."[154]

The principle of beneficence focuses on doing good, preventing harm, and removing harm.[154] The primary purpose of doing a genetic test is to do good, such as provide an explanation for illness in an individual or family and to prevent or reduce harm by facilitating disease prevention among unaffected individuals.

Cancer genetics health care providers frequently encounter ethical dilemmas. For example, some individuals wish to decline sharing genetic test results with potentially at-risk relatives. This problem might be mitigated by discussing disclosure of results before genetic testing. An anonymous letter can be written stating that a relative tested positive for a given mutation and encouraging the recipient to pursue genetic counseling and care. This process may infringe on the recipient of the letter's right to decline learning about risk for genetic disease. Occasionally, the individual receiving testing may change his or her mind about learning the test results. This is problematic when the result is a deleterious mutation.

Another issue occurs when some members of a family wish to have genetic testing but others do not wish to learn their mutation status. An obligate carrier is an untested individual who directly exists between 2 first-degree relatives who have a mutation for a disease transmitted through autosomal dominant inheritance (**Fig. 7**). Obligate carrier pedigree depicts a young woman who inherited the same mutation in *BRCA1* as her maternal grandmother. The untested and unaffected mother is the first-degree relative connecting the young women to her grandmother. Therefore, the mother must also have the known mutation in *BRAC1*. She is an obligate carrier of the known mutation. An ethical dilemma may result if the mother does not wish to know her *BRCA1* mutation status. Conversely, the client may not wish to share results with at-risk family members. In both of these scenarios, the health care provider is confronted with competing duties to respect the autonomy of the client or relative and to warn or rescue at-risk individuals.

Testing minor children for genetic disorders should be based on the best interest of the child. This means that genetic test results are clinically actionable and will help

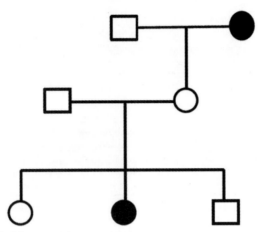

Fig. 7. Pedigree of obligate carrier.

guide the health care of the child.[157] Diagnostic testing for a child who currently exhibits symptoms of a genetic disease is supported by the American Academy of Pediatrics and American College of Medical Genetics.[158] Both organizations agree that presymptomatic testing should not be performed to determine carrier status for disorders that do not occur in childhood.[158] Presymptomatic testing is permissible when the disorder manifests symptoms in childhood. For example, children with a mutation in *APC* require enhanced screening including α-fetoprotein tumor marker screening and liver ultrasonography from birth to 5 years old to monitor for hepatoblastoma, followed by colonoscopy starting between age 8 and 10 years of age for known carriers of a mutation.[63] Unaffected children can be spared these measures. Conducting tissue typing on a child to assess compatibility to serve as a stem cell donor for a sibling is permissible after assessing the physical, emotional, and psychosocial implications on the donor child.[158] A dispassionate advocate should be assigned to ensure the donor child is not being coerced to donate stem cells.[158]

DNA banking is available for individuals with a poor prognosis based on their diagnostic work-up. The purpose of DNA banking is to save a specimen until an appropriate genetic test that does not currently exist becomes available.[159] The results of the test may be vital to the progeny of the dying patient. Although health care insurance does not typically cover DNA banking, the cost is often a few hundred dollars or less and may provide valuable information at some time in the future. Participation in a hereditary cancer genetic research registry is another option to help family members and other individuals.

HEALTH POLICY AND GENETICS

Three laws afford protection against genetic discrimination in the United States. First, the Americans with Disabilities Act of 1990 (ADA) provides protection against discrimination among individuals with a symptomatic genetic disorder, but not for those with presymptomatic genetic disorders.[160] Second, the Health Insurance Portability & Accountability Act of 1996 (HIPAA) applies only to insurance that is employer based and group health insurance that is commercially issued.[160] HIPAA prohibits group health plans from using genetic information to deny coverage or charge a higher premium and the use of presymptomatic genetic test results as a preexisting condition.[160] The third law is the Genetic Information Nondiscrimination Act of 2008 (GINA). This law

Table 12	
Protection under the Genetic Information Nondiscrimination Act (GINA)	
Protected	**Not Protected**
Medical history of families	Symptomatic genetic illness
Genetic testing for carrier status	Access to life, disability, and long-term disability insurance
Prenatal genetic testing	Members of the military
Presymptomatic (susceptibility) testing	Veterans who receive care via the Veterans Administration
Tissue and tumor testing	Individuals who receive care via the Indian Health Service Federal employees who receive care via the Federal Employees Health Benefits program

Adapted from Genetic Alliance, Johns Hopkins University, and National Coalition for Health Professional Education in Genetics. A discussion guide for clinicians, 2010. Available at: www.nchpeg.org/documents/GINA_discussion-guide-2june10.pdf. Accessed April 5, 2013; with permission.

was created to remove barriers of access to genetic care by providing protection against misuse of an individual's genetic information.[161] A comparison of what is and is not covered by GINA is provided in **Table 12**. Members of the military, clients of the Veterans Administration system, and federal employees are protected by other policies or rules.[161]

CONFIDENTIALITY AND THE GENETIC HEALTH RECORD

The confidentiality of genetic information is protected by the HIPAA.[162] One special concern regarding genetic information including pedigrees in the common health record is that pedigrees contain information on family members who have not given consent to the health care provider or institution to access their information. Some institutions restrict access to genetic information in electronic health records, others maintain a separate hard copy of the genetic health record, and others are confident about the protection of genetic information provided by the HIPAA.

SUMMARY

Since 2003, genetics and genomics information has led to exciting new diagnostics, prognostics, and treatment options in oncology practice to offer novel personalized care to patients diagnosed with cancer. Cancer care is evolving to a highly specific targeted approach that effects the molecular biology of a malignancy. Profiling of cancers offers providers insight into treatment and prognostic factors to share with the patient and their families. Germ line testing provides an individual with information for surveillance or therapy that may help prevent cancer in their lifetime and options for family members as yet untouched by malignancy. This testing also can alert parents to begin colonoscopies for surveillance of their young children if the child carries an *APC* mutation. Understanding genetics and the implications of a mutation can offer hope to a patient and family dealing with a new cancer diagnosis. There is a need for oncology nurses and other oncology health care providers to become comfortable with incorporating education about genetics/genomics into their clinical practice and patient education. Although genetics/genomics information was not included in the formal education of patients and their nurses or other health care providers, it is becoming an everyday component of cancer care. Whether the genetic cause of cancer is germline or sporadic, it still has a devastating effect that the oncology nurse needs to address to help the family cope. The focus is not only on the diagnosis; it is part of early detection, prevention, diagnosis, treatment, and survivorship emphasizing the ONS position statement on "application of cancer genetics and genomics through the oncology care continuum."[3]

REFERENCES

1. National Human Genome Research Institute. The Human Genome Project completion: frequently asked questions. 2010. In: National Human Genome Research Institute. Available at: http://www.genome.gov/11006943. Accessed January 11, 2013.
2. Palmer A. The foundation for cancer research – the human genome project. Academic Excellence Showcase, 2013; Paper 5. Available at: http://digitalcommons.wou.edu/aes_event/2013/chem/5. Accessed September 28, 2013.
3. Oncology Nursing Society. Oncology nursing: the application of cancer genetics and genomics throughout the oncology care continuum. Oncol Nurs Forum 2013;40(1):10–1.
4. American Nurses Association. Essentials of genetic and genomic nursing: competencies, curricula guidelines, and outcome indicators. 2nd edition. Silver Spring (MD): American Nurses Association; 2009.
5. American Association of Colleges of Nursing. The essentials of Master's education. In: American Association of Colleges of Nursing. 2011. Available at: http://www.aacn.nche.edu/education-resources/MastersEssentials11.pdf. Accessed September 28, 2013.
6. Schiller JS, Lucas JW, Peregoy JA. Summary health statistics for U.S. adults: National Health Interview Survey. National Center for Health Statistics. Vital Health Stat 10 2012;252:1–207. Available at: http://seer.cancer.gov/csr/1975_2003/results_single/sect_01_table.11_2pgs.pdf. Accessed January 11, 2013.
7. Watson JD, Crick FH. Molecular structure of nucleic acids: a structure for deoxyribose nucleic acid. Nature 1953;171:737–8.
8. 1957 Francis H. C. Crick (1916-2004) sets out the agenda of molecular biology. In: Genetics and genomics timeline. Available at: http://www.genomenewsnetwork.org/resources/timeline/1957_Crick.php. Accessed September 28, 2013.
9. 1960 The discovery of messenger RNA (mRNA) by Sydney Brenner (1927-), Francis Crick (1916-), Francois Jacob (1920-) and Jacques Monod (1910-1976). In: Genetics and genomics timeline. Available at: http://www.genomenewsnetwork.org/resources/timeline/1960_mRNA.php. Accessed September 28, 2013.
10. 1961 Marshall Nirenberg (1927-) cracks the genetic code. In: Genetics and genomics timeline. Available at: http://www.genomenewsnetwork.org/resources/timeline/1961_Nirenberg.php. Accessed September 28, 2013.
11. 1967 Mary Weiss and Howard Green. Available at: http://www.genomenewsnetwork.org/resources/timeline/1967_Weiss_Green.php. Accessed September 28, 2013.
12. 1977 Walter Gilbert (1932-) and Frederick Sanger (1918-) devise techniques for sequencing DNA. In: Genetics and genomics timeline. Available at: http://www.genomenewsnetwork.org/resources/timeline/1977_Gilbert.php. Accessed September 28, 2013.
13. 1986-1990 Launching the effort to sequence the human genome. In: Genetics and genomics timeline. Available at: http://www.genomenewsnetwork.org/resources/timeline/1986_Hood.php. Accessed September 28, 2013.

14. The essentials of Baccalaureate education for professional nursing practice. In: American Association of Colleges of Nursing. 2008. Available at: http://www. aacn.nche.edu/education-resources/baccessentials08.pdf.   Accessed September 28, 2013.
15. American Recovery & Reinvestment Act at NCI. Personalized cancer care/drug development platform. Available at: http://www.cancer.gov/aboutnci/recovery/ recoveryfunding/personalized. Accessed September 28, 2013.
16. US Department of Health and Human Services. HRSA (released April 2013) The US nursing workforce: trends in supply and education. 2010. Available at: http:// bhpr.hrsa.gov/healthworkforce/reports/nursingworkforce/index.html. Accessed September 28, 2013.
17. Rishel C. Succession planning in oncology nursing: a professional must-have. Oncol Nurs Forum 2013;40(2):114–5.
18. Mendel G. 1866. Versuche über Plflanzenhybriden. Verhandlungen des naturfor-schenden Vereines in Brünn, Bd. IV für das Jahr 1865, Abhandlungen, 3–47. Available at: http://www.ub.uni-frankfurt.de/. Accessed September 28, 2013.
19. Crick FH. Nucleic acids. Sci Am 1957;197:188–200.
20. Medical physiology/cellular physiology/DNA and reproduction. In: Wikibooks. 2013. Available at: http://en.wikibooks.org/wiki/Medical_Physiology/Cellular_ Physiology/DNA_and_Reproduction. Accessed June 16, 2013.
21. Qiu J. Unfinished symphony. Nature 2006;441(11):144–5.
22. Chromatid. In: Genetics home reference: your guide to understanding genetic conditions. 2013. Available at: http://ghr.nlm.nih.gov/glossary=chromatid. Ac-cessed September 28, 2013.
23. Allele. In: National Cancer Institute dictionary of genetic terms. Available at: http:// www.cancer.gov/geneticsdictionary?cdrid=339337. Accessed September 28, 2013.
24. Ghildiyal M, Zamore P. Small silencing RNAs: an expanding universe. Nat Rev Genet 2009;10(2):94–108.
25. Ritchier W, Gao D, Rasko JE. Defining and providing robust controls for micro-RNA. Bioinformatics 2012;28(8):1058–61.
26. Siomi MC, Sato K, Pezic D, et al. PIWI-interacting small RNAs: the vanguard of genome defense. Nat Rev Mol Cell Biol 2011;12(4):246–58.
27. Whitehead KA, Dahlman JE, Langer RS, et al. Silencing or stimulation? SiRNA delivery and the immune system. Annu Rev Chem Biomol Eng 2011;2: 77–96.
28. Wild-type. In: NCI dictionary of genetics terms. Available at: http://www.cancer. gov/geneticsdictionary?cdrid=44805. Accessed September 28, 2013.
29. Lodish H, Berk A, Zipursky SL, et al. Proto-oncogenes and tumor-suppressor genes. In: Molecular cell biology. 4th edition. New York: WH Freeman; 2000. Section 24.2. Available at: http://www.ncbi.nlm.nih.gov/books/NBK21662/. Ac-cessed September 28, 2013.
30. Malumbres M, Barbacid M. RAS oncogenes; the first 30 years. Nat Rev Cancer 2003;3(6):459–65.
31. Cotterman R, Jin VX, Krig SR, et al. N-Myc regulates a widespread euchromatic program in the human genome partially independent of its role as a classical transcription factor. Cancer Res 2008;68(23):9654–62.
32. Friedenson B. The BRCA1/2 pathway prevents hematologic cancers in addition to breast and ovarian cancers. BMC Cancer 2007;7:152.
33. MEN1. In: GeneCards. 2013. Available at: http://www.genecards.org/cgibin/ carddisp.pl?gene=MEN1&search=men+1. Accessed September 28, 2013.

34. Thakker RV. Multiple endocrine neoplasia type 1 (MEN1). Best Pract Res Clin Endocrinol Metab 2010;24(3):355–70.
35. Glukhov AI, Svinareva LV, Severin SE, et al. Telomerase inhibitors as novel antitumour drugs. Appl Biochem Microbiol 2011;47(7):655–60.
36. BCL2. In: GeneCards. 2013. Available at: http://www.genecards.org/cgi-bin/carddisp.pl?gene=BCL2. Accessed September 28, 2013.
37. PTEN. In: GeneCards. 2013. Available at: http://www.genecards.org/cgi-bin/carddisp.pl?gene=PTEN&search=pten. Accessed September 28, 2013.
38. Turner NC, Reis-Filho JS. Genetic heterogeneity and cancer drug resistance. Lancet Oncol 2012;13(4):e178–85.
39. Watanabe Y, Castoro RJ, Kim HS, et al. Frequent alteration of MLL3 frameshift mutations in microsatellite deficient colorectal cancer. PLoS One 2011;6(8): e23320.
40. Hon LS, Kaminker JS, Xhang Z. Computational approaches for predicting causal missense mutations in cancer genome projects. Curr Bioinform 2008;3:46–55.
41. Jung AC, Briolat J, Millon R, et al. Biological and clinical relevance of transcriptionally active human papillomavirus (HPV) infection in oropharynx squamous cell carcinoma. Int J Cancer 2009;126(8):1882–94.
42. Rajagopalan H, Lengauer C. Aneuploidy and cancer. Nature 2004;432:338–41.
43. Feramisco JD, Casey RL, Tsao H. Recent updates on genetics: teaching old dogmas new tricks. Pediatr Dermatol 2008;25(1):99–108.
44. Bernstein BE, Meissner A, Lander ES. The mammalian epigenome. Cell 2007; 128(4):669–81.
45. Wossidlo M, Nakamura T, Lepikhov K, et al. 5-Hydroxymethylcytosine in the mammalian zygote is linked with epigenetic reprogramming. Nat Commun 2011;2:241.
46. Milosavljevic A. Emerging patterns of epigenomic variation. Trends Genet 2011; 27(6):242–50.
47. Lefers M. Caspase. In: Department of Molecular Biosciences, Northwestern University. 2004. Available at: http://groups.molbiosci.northwestern.edu/holmgren/Glossary/Definitions/Def-C/caspase.html. Accessed September 28, 2013.
48. Wong R. Apoptosis in cancer: from pathogenesis to treatment. J Exp Clin Cancer Res 2011;30:87.
49. Apoptosis. In: National Human Genome: talking glossary of genetic terms/apoptosis. Available at: http://www.genome.gov/Glossary/index.cfm?p=viewimage&id=10. Accessed September 28, 2013.
50. Engelman JA, Zejnullahu K, Mitsudomi T, et al. MET amplification leads to gefitinib resistance in lung cancer by activating ERBB3 signaling. Science 2007; 316(5827):1039–43.
51. Laplante M, Sabatini DM. mTOR signaling in growth control and disease. Cell 2012;149(2):274–93.
52. Gibson BA, Kraus WL. New insights into the molecular and cellular functions of poly(ADP-ribose) and PARPs. Nat Rev Mol Cell Biol 2012;13(7):411–24.
53. Engert S, Wappenschmidt B, Betz B, et al. MLPA screening in the BRCA1 gene from 1,506 German hereditary breast cancer cases: novel deletions, frequent involvement of exon 17, and occurrence in single early-onset cases. Hum Mutat 2008;29(7):948–58.
54. Meyerson M, Gabriel S, Getz G. Advances in understanding cancer genomes through second-generation sequencing. Nat Rev Genet 2010;11:685–96.
55. Soon WW, Hariharan M, Snyder MP. High-throughput sequencing for biology and medicine. Mol Syst Biol 2013;9:640.

56. Tuna M, Amos CI. Genomic sequencing in cancer. Cancer Lett 2012. http://dx.doi.org/10.1016/j.canlet.2012.11.004. Accessed September 28, 2013.

57. Gatti R, Ataxia-Telangiectasia. In: Pagon RA, Bird TD, Dolan CR, et al, editors. GeneReviews. Seattle (WA): University of Washington; 2010. Available at: http://www.ncbi.nlm.nih.gov/books/NBK26468/. Accessed March 17, 2013.

58. Shuman C, Beckwith JB, Smith AC, et al. Beckwith-Wiedemann syndrome. In: Pagon RA, Bird TD, Dolan CR, et al, editors. GeneReviews. Seattle (WA): University of Washington; 2010. Available at: http://www.ncbi.nlm.nih.gov/books/NBK1394/. Accessed March 17, 2013.

59. Toro JR. Birt-Hogg-Dubé syndrome. In: Pagon RA, Bird TD, Dolan CR, et al, editors. GeneReviews. Seattle (WA): University of Washington; 2008. 2010. Available at: http://www.ncbi.nlm.nih.gov/books/NBK1522/. Accessed March 17, 2013.

60. Sanz MM, German J. Bloom's syndrome. In: Pagon RA, Bird TD, Dolan CR, et al, editors. GeneReviews. Seattle (WA): University of Washington; 2010. Available at: http://www.ncbi.nlm.nih.gov/books/NBK1398/. Accessed March 17, 2013.

61. Eng C. PTEN hamartoma tumor syndrome (PHTS). In: Pagon RA, Bird TD, Dolan CR, et al, editors. GeneReviews. Seattle (WA): University of Washington; 2010. Available at. http://www.ncbi.nlm.nih.gov/books/NBK1488/. Accessed March 17, 2013.

62. Pilarski R, Stephens JA, Noss R, et al. Predicting PTEN mutations: an evaluation of Cowden syndrome and Bannayan–Riley–Ruvalcaba syndrome clinical features. J Med Genet 2011;48:505–12. http://dx.doi.org/10.1136/jmg.2011.088807.

63. Jasperson KW, Burt RW. APC-associated polyposis conditions. In: Pagon RA, Bird TD, Dolan CR, et al, editors. GeneReviews. Seattle (WA): University of Washington; 2011. Available at: http://www.ncbi.nlm.nih.gov/books/NBK1345/. Accessed March 17, 2013.

64. Hamilton SR, Liu B, Parsons RE, et al. The molecular basis of Turcot's syndrome. N Engl J Med 1995;332:839–47. http://dx.doi.org/10.1056/NEJM199503303321302.

65. Mize DE, Bishop M, Resse E, et al. Familial atypical multiple mole melanoma syndrome. In: Riegert-Johnson DL, Boardman LA, Hefferon T, et al, editors. Cancer syndromes. Bethesda (MD): National Center for Biotechnology Information; 2009. Available at: http://www.ncbi.nlm.nih.gov/books/NBK7030/. Accessed March 17, 2013.

66. Petrucelli N, Daly MB, Feldman GL. BRCA1 and BRCA2 hereditary breast and ovarian cancer. In: Pagon RA, Bird TD, Dolan CR, et al, editors. GeneReviews. Seattle (WA): University of Washington; 2010. Available at: http://www.ncbi.nlm.nih.gov/books/NBK1247/. Accessed March 17, 2013.

67. Inheritance in Man, OMIM®. Partner and localizer of BRCA2; PALB2. Baltimore (MD): Johns Hopkins University; 2012. MIM number: 6 610355. Available at: http://www.omim.org/entry/610355. Accessed March 17, 2013.

68. Pithukpakorn M, Toro JR. Hereditary leiomyomatosis and renal cell cancer. In: Pagon RA, Bird TD, Dolan CR, et al, editors. GeneReviews. Seattle (WA): University of Washington; 2010. Available at: http://www.ncbi.nlm.nih.gov/books/NBK1252/. Accessed March 17, 2013.

69. Kaurah P, Huntsman DG. Hereditary diffuse gastric cancer. In: Pagon RA, Bird TD, Dolan CR, et al, editors. GeneReviews. Seattle (WA): University of Washington; 2011. Available at: http://www.ncbi.nlm.nih.gov/books/NBK1139/. Accessed March 17, 2013.

70. Johnson RH, Park JR. ALK-related neuroblastoma susceptibility. In: Pagon RA, Bird TD, Dolan CR, et al, editors. GeneReviews. Seattle (WA): University of

Washington; 2012. Available at: http://www.ncbi.nlm.nih.gov/books/NBK24599/. Accessed March 17, 2013.

71. Kirmani S, Young WF. Hereditary paraganglioma-pheochromocytoma syndromes. In: Pagon RA, Bird TD, Dolan CR, et al, editors. GeneReviews. Seattle (WA): University of Washington; 2012. Available at: http://www.ncbi.nlm.nih.gov/books/NBK1548/. Accessed March 17, 2013.

72. Lohmann DR, Gallie BL. Retinoblastoma. In: Pagon RA, Bird TD, Dolan CR, et al, editors. GeneReviews. Seattle (WA): University of Washington; 2010. Available at: http://www.ncbi.nlm.nih.gov/books/NBK1452/. Accessed March 17, 2013.

73. Haidle JL, Howe JR. Juvenile polyposis syndrome. In: Pagon RA, Bird TD, Dolan CR, et al, editors. GeneReviews. Seattle (WA): University of Washington; 2011. Available at: http://www.ncbi.nlm.nih.gov/books/NBK1469/. Accessed March 17, 2013.

74. Schneider K, Zelley K, Nichols KE, et al. Li-Fraumeni syndrome. In: Pagon RA, Bird TD, Dolan CR, et al, editors. GeneReviews. Seattle (WA): University of Washington; 2013. Available at: http://www.ncbi.nlm.nih.gov/books/NBK1311/. Accessed July 9, 2013.

75. Kohlmann W, Gruber SB. Lynch syndrome. In: Pagon RA, Bird TD, Dolan CR, et al, editors. GeneReviews. Seattle (WA): University of Washington; 2012. Available at: http://www.ncbi.nlm.nih.gov/books/NBK1211/. Accessed March 17, 2013.

76. Giusti F, Marini F, Brandi ML. Multiple endocrine neoplasia type 1. In: Pagon RA, Bird TD, Dolan CR, et al, editors. GeneReviews. Seattle (WA): University of Washington; 2012. Available at: http://www.ncbi.nlm.nih.gov/books/NBK1538/. Accessed March 17, 2013.

77. Moline J, Eng C. Multiple endocrine neoplasia type 2. In: Pagon RA, Bird TD, Dolan CR, et al, editors. GeneReviews. Seattle (WA): University of Washington; 2013. Available at: http://www.ncbi.nlm.nih.gov/books/NBK1257/. Accessed March 17, 2013.

78. Friedman JM. Neurofibromatosis 1. In: Pagon RA, Bird TD, Dolan CR, et al, editors. GeneReviews. Seattle (WA): University of Washington; 2012. Available at: http://www.ncbi.nlm.nih.gov/books/NBK1109/. Accessed March 17, 2013.

79. Evans DG, Farndon PA. Nevoid basal cell carcinoma syndrome. In: Pagon RA, Bird TD, Dolan CR, et al, editors. GeneReviews. Seattle (WA): University of Washington; 2013. Available at: http://www.ncbi.nlm.nih.gov/books/NBK1151/. Accessed March 17, 2013.

80. Amos CI, Frazier ML, Wei C, et al. Peutz-Jeghers syndrome. In: Pagon RA, Bird TD, Dolan CR, et al, editors. GeneReviews. Seattle (WA): University of Washington; 2011. Available at: http://www.ncbi.nlm.nih.gov/books/NBK1266/. Accessed March 17, 2013.

81. Inheritance in Man, OMIM. Rhabdoid tumor predisposition syndrome 1. Baltimore (MD): Johns Hopkins University; 2010. MIM number: 609322. Available at: http://www.omim.org/entry/609322?search=number%3A%28601607%20OR%20609322. Accessed March 17, 2013.

82. Frantzen C, Links TP, Giles RH. Von Hippel-Lindau disease. In: Pagon RA, Bird TD, Dolan CR, et al, editors. GeneReviews. Seattle (WA): University of Washington; 2012. Available at: http://www.ncbi.nlm.nih.gov/books/NBK1463/. Accessed March 17, 2013.

83. Filipovich A, Johnson J, Zhang K, et al. Lymphoproliferative disease, X-Linked. In: Pagon RA, Bird TD, Dolan CR, et al, editors. GeneReviews. Seattle (WA): University of Washington; 2011. Available at: http://www.ncbi.nlm.nih.gov/books/NBK1406/. Accessed March 17, 2013.

84. Slavin TP, Wiesner GL. Developmental defects and childhood cancer. Curr Opin Pediatr 2009;21(6):717–23.

85. Leonard M. Nursing implications of diagnostic and staging procedures. In: Baggott C, Fochtman D, Foley GV, et al, editors. Nursing care of children and adolescents with cancer and blood disorders. 4th edition. Glenview (IL): Association of Pediatric Hematology/Oncology Nurses; 2011. p. 236–67.

86. Seewald L, Taub JW, Maloney KW, et al. Acute leukemias in children with Down syndrome. Mol Genet Metab 2012;107(1–2):25–30.

87. Mueller BU, Pizzo PA. Cancer in children with primary or secondary immunodeficiencies. J Pediatr 1995;126(1):1–10.

88. Salavoura K, Kolialexi A, Tsangaris G, et al. Development of cancer in patients with primary immunodeficiencies. Anticancer Res 2008;28(2B): 1263–9.

89. Tiede C, Maecker-Kolhoff B, Klein C, et al. Risk factors and prognosis in T-cell posttransplantation lymphoproliferative diseases: reevaluation of 163 cases. Transplantation 2013;95(3):479–88.

90. Franks AL, Slansky JE. Multiple associations between a broad spectrum of autoimmune diseases, chronic inflammatory diseases, and cancer. Anticancer Res 2012;32(4):1119–36.

91. Korf BR. Malignancy in neurofibromatosis type 1. Oncologist 2000;5(6):477–85.

92. D'Orazio JA. Inherited cancer syndromes in children and young adults. J Pediatr Hematol Oncol 2010;32(3):195–228.

93. Garber J, Offit K. Hereditary cancer predisposition syndromes. J Clin Oncol 2005;23(2):276–92.

94. National Coalition of Healthcare Provider Education in Genetics. (n.d.). Genetic red flags: quick tips for risk assessment. Available at: http://www.nchpeg.org/index.php?option=com_content&view=article&id=59&Itemid=75. Accessed May 6, 2013.

95. Alm El-Din MA, Hughes KS, Finkelstein DA, et al. Breast cancer after treatment of Hodgkin's lymphoma: risk factors that really matter. Int J Radiat Oncol Biol Phys 2009;73:69–74.

96. National Human Genome Research Institute. Epigenomics, 2012. Available at: http://www.genome.gov/27532724. Accessed March 17, 2013.

97. Genetics home reference: your guide to understanding genetic conditions. Inheriting genetic conditions: inheritance patterns and understanding risk. 2013. Available at: http://ghr.nlm.nih.gov/handbook/inheritance?show=all. Accessed March 17, 2013.

98. Bofetta P, Couto E, Wichmann J, et al. Fruit and vegetable intake and overall cancer risk in the European Prospective Investigation into Cancer and Nutrition (EPIC). J Natl Cancer Inst 2010;102:529–37. http://dx.doi.org/10.1093/jnci/djq072.

99. World Cancer Research Fund/American Institute for Cancer Research. Continuous update project report. Food, nutrition, physical activity, and the prevention of colorectal cancer, 2011. Available at: http://www.dietandcancerreport.org/cancer_resource_center/downloads/cu/Colorectal-Cancer-2011-Report.pdf. Accessed July 9, 2013.

100. Brevik A, Joshi AD, Corral R. Polymorphisms in base excision repair genes as colorectal cancer risk factors and modifiers of the effect of diets high in red meat. Cancer Epidemiol Biomarkers Prev 2010;19:3167–73.

101. Wolin KY, Yan Y, Colditz GA, et al. Physical activity and colon cancer prevention: a meta-analysis. Br J Cancer 2009;100:611–6.

102. World Cancer Research Fund/American Institute for Cancer Research. Continuous update project report. Food, nutrition, physical activity, and the prevention of pancreatic cancer, 2012. Available at: http://www.dietandcancerreport.org/cancer_resource_center/downloads/cu/Pancreatic-Cancer-2012-Report.pdf. Accessed July 9, 2013.

103. Zhao J, Halfyard B, Roebothan B, et al. Tobacco smoking and colorectal cancer: a population-based case-control study in Newfoundland and Labrador. Can J Public Health 2010;101:281–9.

104. World Cancer Research Fund/American Institute for Cancer Research. Continuous update project report. Food, nutrition, physical activity, and the prevention of breast cancer, 2010. Available at: http://www.dietandcancerreport.org/cancer_resource_center/downloads/cu/Breast-Cancer-2010-Report.pdf. Accessed July 9, 2013.

105. Kennedy BJ. Aging and Cancer. In: Balducci L, Lyman GH, Ershler WB, et al, editors. Comprehensive geriatric oncology. Boca Raton (FL): Taylor & Francis; 2004. p. 3–10.

106. Blackburn EH. Structure and function of telomeres. Nature 1991;350(6319): 569–73.

107. Muraki K, Nyhan K, Han L, et al. Mechanisms of telomere loss and their consequences from chromosome instability. Front Oncol 2012;2:135.

108. Rodriguez-Paredes M, Esteller M. Cancer epigenetics reaches mainstream cancer. Nat Med 2011;17(3):330–9.

109. Feinberg AP. Cancer epigenetics is no Mickey Mouse. Cancer Cell 2005;8(4): 267–8.

110. Esteller M. Epigenetics in cancer. N Engl J Med 2008;358(11):1148–59.

111. Bennett RL, French KS, Resta RG, et al. Standardized human pedigree nomenclature: update and assessment of the recommendations of the National Society of Genetic Counselors. J Genet Couns 2008;17:424–33. http://dx.doi.org/10.1007/s10897-008-9169-9.

112. National Cancer Institute. Cancer genetics risk assessment and counseling (PDQ). National Institutes of Health; 2013. Available at: www.cancer.gov/cancertopics/pdq/genetics/risk-assessment-and-counseling/HealthProfessional/page1. Accessed September 28, 2013.

113. Weitzel JN, Lagos VI, Cullinane CA, et al. Limited family structure and BRCA gene mutation status in single cases of breast cancer. JAMA 2007;297(23): 2587–95. http://dx.doi.org/10.1001/jama.297.23.2587.

114. Jarvis C. Physical examination & health assessment. Philadelphia: WB Saunders; 2012.

115. Alkner S, Bendahl P-O, Ferno M, et al. Prediction of outcome after diagnosis of metachronous contralateral breast cancer. BMC Cancer 2011;11:114.

116. Hartman M, Czene K, Reilly M, et al. Incidence and prognosis of synchronous and metachronous bilateral breast cancer. J Clin Oncol 2007;25: 4210–6.

117. American Academy of Pediatrics. Recommendations for preventive pediatric health care. 2008. Available at: http://brightfutures.aap.org/pdfs/AAP%20Bright%20Futures%20Periodicity%20Sched%20101107.pdf. Accessed April 4, 2013.

118. Bushby KMD, Cole T, Matthews JNS, et al. Centiles for adult head circumference. Archives of Disease in Childhood 1992;67:1286–7. Available at. http://adc.bmj.com/content/67/10/1286.full.pdf.

119. Kelly P. Hereditary breast cancer considering Cowden syndrome: a case study. Cancer Nursing 2003;26(5):370–5.

120. Mester JL, Tilot AK, Rybicki LA, et al. Analysis of prevalence and degree of macrocephaly in patients with germline PTEN mutations and of brain weight in PTEN knock-in murine model. Eur J Hum Genet 2011;19:763–8.
121. NCCN guideline. Breast cancer risk reduction version 1.2013. In: National Comprehensive Cancer Network. 2013. Available at: http://www.nccn.org/professionals/physician_gls/pdf/breast_risk.pdf. Accessed September 28, 2013.
122. NCCN guidelines. Cervical cancer screening version 2.2012. In: National Comprehensive Cancer Network. 2013. Available at: http://www.nccn.org/professionals/physician_gls/pdf/cervical_screening.pdf. Accessed September 28, 2013.
123. Saslow D, Solomon D, Lawson HW, et al. American Cancer Society, American Society for Colposcopy and Cervical Pathology, and American Society for Clinical Pathology screening guidelines for the prevention and early detection of cervical cancer. Am J Clin Pathol 2012;137(4):516–42.
124. Saslow D, Castle P, Cox T, et al. American Society guideline for human papillomavirus (HPV) vaccine use to prevent cervical cancer and its precursors. CA Cancer J Clin 2007;57(1):7–28.
125. NCCN guidelines. Lynch syndrome version 2.2013. In: National Comprehensive Cancer Network. 2013. Available at: http://www.nccn.org/professionals/physician_gls/pdf/colorectal_screening.pdf. Accessed September 28, 2013.
126. Goncalves R, Bos R. Using multigene tests to select treatment for early-stage breast cancer. J Natl Compr Canc Netw 2013;11(2):174–82 [quiz: 182]. Available at: http://education.nccn.org/node/11346. Accessed September 28, 2013.
127. Roden DM, Altman RB, Benowitz NL, et al. Pharmacogenomics: challenges and opportunities. Ann Intern Med 2006;145(10):749–57.
128. Roses AD. Pharmacogenomics and the practice of medicine. Nature 2000; 405(6788):857–65.
129. Lee W, Lockhart AC, Kim RB, et al. Cancer pharmacogenomics: powerful tools in cancer chemotherapy and drug development. Oncologist 2005;10(2):104–11.
130. Mattison LK, Fourie J, Hirao Y, et al. The uracil breath test in the assessment of dihydropyrimidine dehydrogenase activity: pharmacokinetic relationship between expired 13CO2 and plasma [2-13C] dihydrouracil. Clin Cancer Res 2006;12(2):549–55.
131. Yates CR, Krynetski EY, Loennechen T, et al. Molecular diagnosis of thiopurine S-methyltransferase deficiency: genetic basis for azathioprine and mercaptopurine intolerance. Ann Intern Med 1997;126(8):608–14.
132. Relling MV, Gardner EE, Sandborn WJ, et al. Clinical Pharmacogenetics Implementation Consortium guidelines for thiopurine methyltransferase genotype and thiopurine dosing. Clin Pharmacol Ther 2011;89(3):387–91.
133. Lanfear DE, McLeod HL. Pharmacogenetics: using DNA to optimize drug therapy. Am Fam Physician 2007;76(8):1179–82.
134. Pangilinan J, Khan G, Zalupski M. Irinotecan pharmacogenetics: an overview for the community oncologist. Commun Oncol 2008;5(2):99–103.
135. Toffoli G, Russo A, Innocenti F, et al. Effect of methylenetetrahydrofolate reductase 677–>T polymorphism on toxicity and homocysteine plasma level after chronic methotrexate treatment of ovarian cancer patients. Int J Cancer 2003; 103(3):294–9.
136. Consortium on Breast Cancer Pharmacogenomics. 2008. Drug interactions with tamoxifen: a guide for breast cancer patients and physicians. 2008. Available at: http://medicine.iupui.edu/clinpharm/COBRA/Tamoxifen%20and%202D6v7.pdf. Accessed April 4, 2013.

137. Shenfield GM. Genetic polymorphisms, drug metabolism, and drug concentrations. Clin Biochem Rev 2004;25(4):203–6.

138. Guengerich FP. Cytochrome P450 and chemical toxicology. Chem Res Toxicol 2007;21(1):70–83.

139. Indiana University, Department of Medicine, Division of Clinical Pharmacology. P450 drug interaction table. 2009. Available at: http://medicine.iupui.edu/clinpharm/ddis/table.aspx. Accessed April 4, 2013.

140. Evans WE, McLeod HL. Pharmacogenomics – Drug disposition, drug targets, and side effects. N Engl J Med 2003;348(6):538–49.

141. Hoskins JM, Marcuello E, Altes A, et al. Irinotecan pharmacodynamics: influence of pharmacodynamic genes. Clin Cancer Res 2008;14(6): 1788–96.

142. Hanke JH, Hughes LR. Targeted therapies for cancer–from tamoxifen to gefitinib ('Iressa'). Drug Discov Today Ther Strat 2004;1(4):411–6.

143. King MC, Wiend S, Hale K, et al. Tamoxifen and breast cancer incidence in women who inherited mutations in BRCA1 and BRCA2. National Surgical Adjuvant Breast and Bowel Project (NSABP P-1) Breast Cancer Prevention Trial. JAMA 2001;286(18):2251–6. Available at: http://www.ncbi.nlm.nih.gov/pubmid/12559863. Accessed March 17, 2013.

144. Mealing S, Barcena L, Hawkins N, et al. The relative efficacy of imatinib, dasatinib and nilotinib for newly diagnosed chronic myeloid leukemia: a systematic review and network. Exp Hematol Oncol 2013;2(1):5.

145. Yang D, Khan S, Sun Y, et al. Association of BRCA1 and BRCA2 mutations with survival, chemotherapy sensitivity, and gene mutator phenotype in patients with ovarian cancer. JAMA 2011;306(14):1557–65.

146. Garber K. Ready or not: personal tumor profiling tests take off. J Natl Cancer Inst 2011;103(2):84–6.

147. Alm El-Din ·MA, El-Badawy SA, Taghian AG. Breast cancer after treatment of Hodgkin's lymphoma: general review. Int J Radiat Oncol Biol Phys 2008;72(5): 1291–7.

148. NCCN guidelines. Hodgkin lymphoma version 2.2013 HODG-15. In: National Comprehensive Cancer Network. 2013. Available at: http://www.nccn.org/professionals/physician_gls/pdf/hodgkins.pdf. Accessed January 2013.

149. ATM. In: Genetics home reference. US National Library of Medicine. 2013. Available at: http://ghr.nlm.nih.gov/gene/ATM. Accessed January 2013.

150. Bernstein JL, Haile RW, Stovall M, et al. Radiation exposure, the ATM gene, and contralateral breast cancer in the Women's Environmental Cancer and Radiation Epidemiology Study. J Natl Cancer Inst 2010;102:475–83.

151. National Comprehensive Cancer Network (NCCN). NCCN Guidelines Version 2.2013. Breast Cancer Screening and Diagnosis 2013;BSCR-2. Available at: http://www.nccn.org/professionals/physician_gls/pdf/breast-screening.pdf. Accessed September 28, 2013.

152. NCCN. Breast cancer screening and diagnosis version 2.2013. In: National Comprehensive Cancer Network. 2013. Available at: http://www.nccn.org/professionals/physician_gls/pdf/breast-screening.pdf. Accessed September 28, 2013.

153. Lowry KP, Lee JM, Kong CY, et al. Annual screening strategies in BRCA1 and BRCA2 gene mutation carriers. A comparative effectiveness analysis. Cancer 2012;118(8):2021–30.

154. Beauchamp TL, Childress JF. Principles of biomedical ethics. New York: Oxford University Press; 2009.

155. Gillon R. Ethics needs principles—four can encompass the rest—and respect for autonomy should be "first among equals". J Med Ethics 2003;29:307–12. Available at: http://jme.bmj.com/content/29/5/307.full. Accessed September 28, 2013.
156. The Hippocratic oath. US National Library of Medicine, 2012. Available at: www.nilm.nih.gov/hmd/greek/greek+oath.html. Accessed March 17, 2013.
157. Caga-anan EC, Smith L, Sharp R, et al. Testing children for adult-onset genetic diseases. Pediatrics 2012;129(1):163–7. http://dx.doi.org/10.1542/peds.2010-3743.
158. Committee on Bioethics, Committee on Genetics, American College of Medical Genetics, et al. Ethical and policy issues in genetic testing and screening of children. Pediatrics 2013;131:620–2.
159. Quillin JM, Bodurtha JN, Siminoff LA, et al. Physician's current practices and opportunities for DNA banking of dying patients with cancer. J Oncol Pract 2011;7:184–7.
160. US Department of Energy Genome Programs. Genetics privacy and legislation. Human Genome Project Information, 2008. Available at: www.ornl.gov/TechResources/Human_Genome/elsi/legistat.html. Accessed February 26, 2013.
161. Genetic Alliance, Johns Hopkins University, National Coalition for Health Professional Education in Genetics. A discussion guide for clinicians, 2010. Available at: www.nchpeg.org/documents/GINA_discussion-guide-2june10.pdf. Accessed April 5, 2013.
162. McGuire AL, Caulfield T, Cho MK. Research ethics and the challenge of whole-genome sequencing. Nat Rev Genet 2008;9:152–6.

Genetics' Influence on Patient Experiences with a Rare Chronic Disorder

A Photovoice Study of Living With Alpha-1 Antitrypsin Deficiency

Pamela Holtzclaw Williams, JD, PhD, RN[a,b,]*, Lucinda Shore, MS[b],
Marvin Sineath[b], Jim Quill[b], Barbara Warner[b], Jamila Keith[b],
Deirdre Walker[b], Sara Wienke, MS, CGC[b], Susan Flavin, MSN, RN[b],
Charlie Strange, MD[b]

KEYWORDS

• Photovoice • Chronic diseases • Genetics

KEY POINTS

- The Medical University of South Carolina Alpha-1 Community Research Partnership succeeded in data collection and analysis because of the mixed methods and use of technology in addressing the needs of this geographically distant rare disease community.
- The process of infusing the study with online technology and communication, including private webinars, secured drop boxes, e-mails, digital cell phone and camera photos, and digital audio narratives that can be sent via online technology kept the study exciting for the participants and allowed remote individuals to feel empowered.
- The authors have been able to demonstrate the feasibility of collecting qualitative research using voices and images of patients, caregivers, and community members living with this genetically inherited chronic condition.
- The partnership was able to develop themes from the narrative and photographic content that help prioritize future community-based participatory research initiatives, which will be used to shape future research and disseminate these conclusions to other populations living with a genetically inherited chronic health condition.

Grant Support: This study was supported by the South Carolina Clinical & Translational Research (SCTR) Institute, with an academic home at the Medical University of South Carolina, NIH/NCATS TL1 TR000061.
[a] College of Nursing, University of Arkansas for Medical Sciences, 4301 West Markham Street, #529, Little Rock, AR 72205-7199, USA; [b] Alpha-1 Community Research Partnership, Medical University of South Carolina, 96 Jonathan Lucas St, MSC 630, Charleston, SC 29425, USA
* Corresponding author.
E-mail address: wilpame@musc.edu

INTRODUCTION

Patients with rare chronic disorders and their caregivers increasingly form communities to support and exchange social experiences. Because up to 10% of the United States population is affected by one of 5000 to 6000 rare disorders, efforts to understand both the individuals and affected communities are important. The current study was conducted using community-based participatory research (CBPR) approaches within a community of patients and caregivers living with alpha-1 antitrypsin deficiency (AATD). This relatively rare inherited condition creates a chronic protein deficiency that predisposes to obstructive lung or liver disease. Patient populations at some risk for lung transplant include individuals who smoked cigarettes and patients who underwent liver transplant in infancy and later adulthood due to accumulation of misfolded alpha-1 antitrypsin (AAT) within hepatocytes. The approaches, methods, and conclusions described here have implications for future research in other rare genetic disease communities that deal with disabling disorders.[1,2]

CBPR partnerships historically emerged to address socially driven health-related needs and policy.[3] The needs are framed by social experiences. For purposes of this article, "social experiences" refer to events not driven by physiologic symptoms. These experiences are influenced by public and social systems, health care infrastructure, and societal norms. Examples of social experiences include those shaped by public resource allocation, health care delivery systems and providers, public awareness and attitudes, and health related policy. Therefore, the social themes in this rare disease community potentially generate universal messages.

The participants in the present study were asked to use their digital cameras and audio recorders to describe the social experiences related to living with ATTD. The aims focused on, but were not limited to, the patients' social experiences related to the genetic component of the disorder. The content of the photographs, narratives, and focus groups reflects themes of burden and resiliency that hold promise to advance knowledge about ATTD and for other rare genetic disorder communities.

METHODS

Community identity framed around a shared genetic risk can generate CBPR approach challenges. The approaches require partnership and community members to share a wide range of perspectives with each other. However, rare disease patients are often geographically dispersed. Some community members protect themselves from identification related to genetic test results because of perceived threats to employment or insurance challenges.[4,5] Therefore, this rare disorder community partnership found it necessary to tailor special strategies to systematically gather community members' input.

The described strategies and methods hold equal interest to the themes that emerged from this CBPR initiative. Few publications describe successful strategies for tailoring collection of community input when there is geographic isolation, disabilities that restrict mobility, or privacy concerns that limit public self-identification. This report describes use and results of mixed methods and technologies to engage community participation. This CBPR partnership, run by and for persons living with AATD and their caregivers, was established with an early goal to prioritize problems to address by research.

Formative Steps of CBPR

Under a memorandum of understanding, 5 patients and community members joined 5 academic clinicians and scientific personnel and became the Medical University of

South Carolina (MUSC) Alpha-1 Community Research Partnership ("the partnership"). The MUSC Clinical and Translational Science Award (CTSA) was leveraged for resources to define research priorities. Community leaders expressed interest in using photovoice methodology found in the literature.[6] Traditional focus groups were added to the design to enhance depth of the inquiry.[7] The MUSC institutional review board (IRB) approved this study to identify and describe the social experiences within the AATD community.

Recruitment

Acting as a community partner, the Alpha-1 Foundation Research Registry is a rare disease registry located at MUSC supported by the nonprofit Alpha-1 Foundation. All recruitment of community member participation in the methods described subsequently was conducted through the e-mail or mailed invitations sent by this registry. This recruitment process assured that the identity of persons living with AATD was protected until he or she made the choice to participate and interface with the partnership's process. Throughout the process, the choice was given to participants whether they wanted to share their identity with other participants, or participate to the extent possible under an anonymous status.

Data Collection

The data was collected during several phases.

Photovoice methods

Twenty-nine enrolled participants attended an online webinar that included a power point presentation and interactive time for questions and discussion. The webinar communicated steps to using cell phone photographic technology, digital cameras, and audio recordings to describe experiences and burdens associated with AATD. Participants could choose to participate in the webinar anonymously. Specific instructions included privacy and confidentiality safeguards for photographic and online communication and content. In addition to contributing photographic images, participants also were instructed to record a digital audio file to further describe the meaning of the photograph's content. The content of the audio files was transcribed for thematic content analysis. The photographs were sorted by theme for dissemination and also imported into NVivo software for content thematic analysis.

The focus group

After all the photographs and audio files were collected, the partners examined the content to select 5 participants for additional communication. Selection was designed to assure diversity of age and geography and included a caregiver. An online focus group was held by anonymous webinar to explore the perceptions invoked by the entire set of photographs and audio files. For example, some participants took turns responding to probes through the webinar microphone, while others used the chat box to type in their responses to probes. The audio portion of the session was transcribed. The transcript and text box narrative were imported into qualitative analysis software for thematic content analysis.

Data Analysis

The coding and analysis of the transcripts and material were imported into NVivo software to support the qualitative analysis. The photos were also imported into NVivo in coordination with the participants' comments about them, to assure the context of the transcribed statements remained intact and paired with the subjects' composed photographs. An inductive approach was applied to assembling a coding framework and coding for conceptual themes.[8] Themes emerged from the iterative steps of coding and text review.[9] The partners met to audit the coding, and an audit trail was maintained in NVivo.

In addition, NVivo supports analysis of word content in a data set by creating a visual graphic referred to as a word cloud. This visual graphic shows key word frequency. Such graphic images add visual support for drawing conclusions and communicating the context of content. **Fig. 1** reflects the word cloud derived by using the transcribed text from the audio files and focus group content.

RESULTS

The enrolled participants (n = 29) represented a wide range of geographic locations, multiple AATD-related genotypes, and ages ranging from early to late adulthood. A diverse community experience was captured by individuals with lung and/or liver symptoms, asymptomatic individuals who were carriers of an abnormal allele with affected young children, individuals who learned of their genetics from affected parents, and individuals disabled at a young age by the condition.

Fifty-five photographs and audio files were submitted. One participant asked permission to write his photo content explanations because of lack of knowledge and access to digital recording hardware. The photographs were taken by a diverse range of cell phone applications and digital cameras. **Table 1** describes the themes that emerged and their meanings and provides exemplar quotes from the qualitative thematic analysis of the content from the audio narratives and focus group discussion.

DISCUSSION OF RESULTING THEMES
Genetic Etiology Influences Family Dynamics

A wide range of images and narrative comments focused on family dynamics affected by the shared genetic risks. Issues around the extent of genetic disclosure to

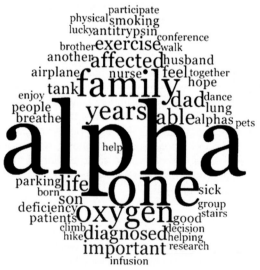

Fig. 1. Word cloud derived by using the transcribed text from the audio files and focus group content.

extended family, family planning for future generations, and numbers of family members currently affected by symptoms and disability were prominent. The study of impact of genetic conditions on relationships, activities, and behaviors within generations of families is in its infancy, with the most study within the inherited cancers.[10,11] The dominance of this theme from most of this study's participants highlights this priority topic for future research.

Genetic Susceptibility to Environmental Exposures

AATD is a disease in which genetic risk is linked to environmental exposures to cause clinical disease. The genetic interaction with environmental exposure risks is best understood in the context of cigarette smoke. However, some data suggest other particulates and fumes may be harmful.[12] Very little study has been done on patients' perceptions and accuracy in understanding inhalant-related health risks associated with any positive genetic test result.[13] Genetic susceptibility to environmental inhalants such as secondhand smoke, pet dander, perfumes, and cleaning products has not been well defined. Therefore, in the absence of data, variability in lifestyles is extreme. Although avoidance of smoking cigarettes is universally advocated, research is needed to clarify which airway irritants cause future lung damage and if these risks are universal in the community.

Genetics Impose Testing Decisions for Immediate, Extended, and Future Family

Families are burdened by the impact of genetics on reproductive decisions, individuals' genetic testing decisions, sibling disclosures and testing decision-making, and parental decisions whether to test children. This decisional burden is common to many genetic disorders, particularly when a genetic test is technologically available to predict future risk of symptoms. Testing decision burden within families with genetic risks and carrier status for inherited chronic conditions has been studied in inherited cardiac conditions,[14] including Fragile X[15] and sickle cell.[16] The emergence of this theme in this population is consistent with those descriptive studies and warrants future research to develop interventions that mitigate the decisional burdens.

Perceiving Judgment by Others

Diseases that cause disability sometimes generate secondary social experiences. Examples of behaviors in response to perceived judgment included choosing to use/not use disability parking, hiding or avoiding medical equipment use to avoid others feeling uncomfortable, and choosing not to disclose prenatal in vitro services for family planning. For lung disease that lacks outward signs of disability, the invisibility can contribute to lack of public support and awareness. This phenomenon is not unique to genetic conditions, as it has been reported by persons living with chronic obstructive pulmonary disease (COPD) unrelated to AATD.[17]

Resilience

Finding the theme of resiliency in the content is consistent with study of other patient communities.[18,19] This community uses physical activity to improve self-efficacy in symptom management and social support through pulmonary rehabilitation, an evidence-based outlet for organized patient mobility that generates quality of life improvement. The community also embraces advocacy and adaptation as personalized health behaviors in response to genetic information.[20]

Table 1
Results of thematic analysis of photovoice data: photographs, audio narratives, and focus groups

Theme and Its Abstracted Meaning	Representative Quotations from Narrative Data	Representative Photograph (www.alphaoneregistry.org)
Genetic Etiology Influences Family Dynamics Learning the chronic condition is based on genetic influences, emotions, and relational dynamics between siblings, parent and child, and spouses/partners; the genetic component can mean that many members of the same family, across generations, are affected at the same time, creating stressful health care costs to family households that affect family budget dynamics	• "I believe my parents felt guilty when we found out that I had alpha (ATTD)." • "The disease has 11 persons affected in my family so far, my sister had double lung transplant." • "My husband and I wonder when we have more children how many of them will have alpha one. It is a definite stressor in family planning." • "The suggestion to my extended family to get tested caused great strife among my family and ended up splitting some of the extended family apart from my immediate family."	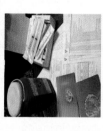
Perceived Genetic Susceptibility to Environmental Exposures in Social Settings Participants understand ATTD as a genetic condition creating susceptibility to risks and triggers from environmental exposures; the heightened awareness modifies their social behavior and raises awareness that past behaviors (eg, smoking) contributed to outcomes	• "I won't go to workout centers just because of the exposure. We bought an exercise bike for home." • "Haven't had to modify too much yet, but in the future I see going to one floor home." • "This (picture of ashtray) represents 2 packs of cigarettes I smoked for over 30 years until I quit."	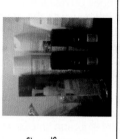
Genetic Inheritance Carries Decision Burden for Immediate, Extended and Future Family The ATTD family history or genetic test result places burdens to decide how and when to disclose to family members, family planning, testing recommendations, and exposure and living environment decisions	• "Decisions to keep your pets are ones alpha patients have to make on their own." • "My 18-month-old daughter is the one with the AATD genotype. My mother smokes and refuses to quit, so I had to make the hard decision to limit my daughter's time with her, and when they see each other it is at places she cannot smoke." • "Some of my family members chose not to get tested (for AATD genes)."	

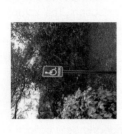

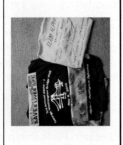

Judged By Others
- Content reflects perceptions of being judged by others, and this influences their social behaviors
- Content reflects apprehension that the invisibility of their disability contributes to lack of public support and awareness

- "I get so embarrassed when I have to use my handicapped parking placard. People look at me like what's the matter with you."
- "I feel like I have to hide the supplies when we have company so nobody feels uncomfortable."
- "After our first son was born we learned we were both carriers of the alpha (AATD) gene. We decided that we did not want to risk having another baby born with the condition. So, we decided to do in vitro fertilization. We usually choose not to discuss our treatment with anyone besides family members, because it can be controversial."

Resilience Strategies Modify Social Impact
Collectively, content indicates actions to reduce psychosocial burden and risk associated with patients' genetic-based condition
- Physical activity with others
- Advocacy with others
- Adaptations to reduce isolation

- "I feel it (gathering with group for physical therapy) is necessary to my physical well-being, and it also stimulates my emotional well-being."
- "Research is so important to alpha-1 (AATD) patients. It is very important to my family and me to participate in fund raisers, research studies and donate to the alpha-1 foundation."
- "Backpack (oxygen tank in backpack picture) makes it easier for dad to maneuver through grocery store."

LIMITATIONS OF STUDY

Although the data were rich in embedded themes, it must be acknowledged that the sample size was small, and there was no randomization in selection. The sample cannot be represented as representative of the entire population of persons with AATD. Ongoing directions of this partnership toward identifying a wider range of the experiences with the AATD community include 2 ongoing studies with significantly larger sample sizes, geographic distribution, and range of social experiences.

SUMMARY

The MUSC Alpha-1 Community Research Partnership succeeded in data collection and analysis because of the mixed methods and use of technology in addressing the needs of this geographically distant rare disease community. The process of infusing the study with online technology and communication, including private webinars, secured drop boxes, e-mails, digital cell phone and camera photos, and digital audio narratives that can be sent via online technology kept the study exciting for the participants and allowed remote individuals to feel empowered. The authors have been able to demonstrate the feasibility of collecting qualitative research using voices and images of patients, caregivers, and community members living with this genetically inherited chronic condition. Importantly, the authors were able to simultaneously address the challenges of geographic distance and privacy in communications between each other.

Additionally, the authors' partnership was able to develop themes from the narrative and photographic content that help prioritize future CBPR initiatives. The CBPR partnership will use these themes to shape future research and disseminate these conclusions to other populations living with a genetically inherited chronic health condition. Finding 5 themes from this relatively small study indicates more research is warranted to advance clinical and public health interventions that mitigate social burden and support resiliency for living with a chronic condition that is genetically inherited and rare.

IMPLICATIONS FOR NURSES, GENETIC COUNSELORS, PROVIDERS, AND CLINICAL SETTINGS

The results and conclusions from this study imply suggestions for improved public health services and clinical delivery of care for persons living with chronic disorders with inherited genetic etiology.

One should recognize the social impact of living with an inherited genetic-based disorder in developing public health services, clinical care, and treatment plans; maintaining a referral resource list to community support options is also important. Additionally, should consider partnering with patient support or research advocacy groups to:

Maintain social engagement and support networks

Contribute to and/or maintain a genetic disorder patient registry that supports communication of research developments and support future recruitment in research participation

Facilitate research to identify and describe[21] patient-centered priorities in advancing intervention development responding to the patient community's psychosocial needs

Promote public awareness and tolerance and educate regarding the need for mobility and social support among patients with chronic illness

One should additionally adapt traditional support group communication, patient education, and research methodology with Web-based technology to overcome geographic distances, privacy concerns, and mobility limitations.

REFERENCES

1. Forman J, Taruscio D, Llera VA, et al. The need for worldwide policy and action plans for rare diseases. Acta Paediatr 2012;101(8):805–7.
2. Haffner ME, Whitley J, Moses M. Two decades of orphan product development. Nat Rev Drug Discov 2002;1(10):821–5.
3. Landy DC, Brinich MA, Colten ME, et al. How disease advocacy organizations participate in clinical research: a survey of genetic organizations. Genet Med 2012;14(2):223–8.
4. Powell A, Chandrasekharan S, Cook-Deegan R. Spinocerebellar ataxia: patient and health professional perspectives on whether and how patents affect access to clinical genetic testing. Genet Med 2010;12(Suppl 4):S83–110.
5. Joly Y, Ngueng Feze I, Simard J. Genetic discrimination and life insurance: a systematic review of the evidence. BMC Med 2013;11:25.
6. Catalani C, Minkler M. Photovoice: a review of the literature in health and public health. Health Educ Behav 2010;37(3):424–51.
7. Cooper CM, Yarbrough SP. Tell me—show me: using combined focus group and photovoice methods to gain understanding of health issues in rural Guatemala. Qual Health Res 2010;20(5):644–53.
8. Elo S, Kyngas H. The qualitative content analysis process. J Adv Nurs 2008; 62(1):107–15.
9. Bradley EH, Curry LA, Devers KJ. Qualitative data analysis for health services research: developing taxonomy, themes, and theory. Health Serv Res 2007; 42(4):1758–72.
10. Hadley DW, Ashida S, Jenkins JF, et al. Generation after generation: exploring the psychological impact of providing genetic services through a cascading approach. Genet Med 2010;12(12):808–15.
11. Morris BA, Hadley DW, Koehly LM. The role of religious and existential well-being in families with lynch syndrome: prevention, family communication, and psychosocial adjustment. J Genet Couns 2013;22(4):482–91.
12. Mayer AS, Stoller JK, Bucher Bartelson B, et al. Occupational exposure risks in individuals with PI*Z alpha(1)-antitrypsin deficiency. Am J Respir Crit Care Med 2000;162(2 Pt 1):553–8.
13. Saukko PM, Ellard S, Richards SH, et al. Patients' understanding of genetic susceptibility testing in mainstream medicine: qualitative study on thrombophilia. BMC Health Serv Res 2007;7:82.
14. Ormondroyd E, Oates S, Parker M, et al. Pre-symptomatic genetic testing for inherited cardiac conditions: a qualitative exploration of psychosocial and ethical implications. Eur J Hum Genet 2013. [Epub ahead of print].
15. Raspberry KA, Skinner D. Negotiating desires and options: how mothers who carry the fragile X gene experience reproductive decisions. Soc Sci Med 2011; 72(6):992–8.
16. Smith M, Aguirre RT. Reproductive attitudes and behaviors in people with sickle cell disease or sickle cell trait: a qualitative interpretive meta-synthesis. Soc Work Health Care 2012;51(9):757–79.
17. McMillan Boyles C, Hill Bailey P, Mossey S. Chronic obstructive pulmonary disease as disability: dilemma stories. Qual Health Res 2011;21(2):187–98.

18. Hall H, Neely-Barnes S, Graff J, et al. Parental stress in families of children with a genetic disorder/disability and the resiliency model of family stress, adjustment, and adaptation. Issues Compr Pediatr Nurs 2012;35(1):24–44.

19. Karlson CW, Leist-Haynes S, Smith M, et al. Examination of risk and resiliency in a pediatric sickle cell disease population using the psychosocial assessment tool 2.0. J Pediatr Psychol 2012;37(9):1031–40.

20. McBride CM, Koehly LM, Sanderson SC, et al. The behavioral response to personalized genetic information: will genetic risk profiles motivate individuals and families to choose more healthful behaviors? Annu Rev Public Health 2010;31(1):89–103.

21. Valenzuela JM, Vaughn LM, Crosby LE, et al. Understanding the experiences of youth living with sickle cell disease: a photovoice pilot. Fam Community Health 2013;36(2):97–108.

Nursing and Genetic Biobanks

Jennifer E. Sanner, PhD, RN[a],*, Erica Yu, PhD, RN, ARNP[b],
Malini Udtha, PhD[c], Pamela Holtzclaw Williams, JD, PhD, RN[d]

KEYWORDS

- Biobanking • Biobanks • Genetics • Research • Nursing

KEY POINTS

- Genetic biobanks are a key resource in studying the genetic components of complex and rare diseases leading to new approaches in genetic research.
- The involvement of nurses in genetic biobanks signifies a need to develop a unique set of educational, ethical, and practice competency standards for nurses.
- Nursing science developed a conceptual framework to guide future research and practice developments regarding ethical issues underlying genetic biobanking practices and research.

INTRODUCTION

Biobanking practices are now an integral component of genetic research, which often requires large disease- or population-based data sets and biospecimens to study complex or rare diseases. Data and biospecimens stored in genetic biobanks are used in studies to analyze genetic variations, which ultimately affect patient and population health. Genetic biobank resources provide epidemiologic findings that affect the well-being of populations, as well as genomic data tailored to personalized therapies.[1] Biobanks are designed to provide resources for translational research directed at moving scientific research from the laboratory into clinical practice. **Box 1** outlines the potential benefits of using a genetic biobank for translational research, including accelerated science that is translated into advances for clinical health care.[1,2] Fundamentally, genetic biobanks supply researchers with data to examine research questions geared toward advancing scientific knowledge.[1] Therefore, genetic biobanking efforts may result in the efficient use of research dollars, which often leads to

Dr. Williams is now with the College of Nursing, UAMS Little Rock Arkansas, University of Arkansas for Medical Sciences College of Nursing, 4301 W. Markham Street, Little Rock, AR 72205.
[a] School of Nursing, The University of Texas Health Science Center at Houston, 6901 Bertner Avenue, Suite 612, Houston, TX 77030, USA; [b] School of Nursing, The University of Texas Health Science Center at Houston, 6901 Bertner Avenue, Suite 548, Houston, TX 77030, USA; [c] School of Nursing, The University of Texas Health Science Center at Houston, 6901 Bertner Avenue, Suite 567, Houston, TX 77030, USA; [d] College of Nursing, Medical University of South Carolina, 99 Jonathan Lucas, Suite 423, Charleston, SC 29425, USA
* Corresponding author.
E-mail address: Jennifer.E.Sanner@uth.tmc.edu

Box 1
Benefits of using a genetic biobank for translational research

1. Provides an efficient, cost-effective way to accelerate the generation of scientific knowledge from data and biospecimens into practice, which ultimately benefits society

2. Enables researchers to study the combined impact of genetics and environment on large disease- or population-based biospecimens, essential for epidemiologic studies that require large sample sizes

3. Provides a resource of high-quality data and biospecimens on complex disorders and rare genetic conditions

4. May serve as an avenue for personalized medicine because medically relevant findings may be available to individual donors

5. Allows for the collection of data and biospecimens in the advancement of studies, essential for studies of rare genetic diseases that historically have been challenged in building sufficient sample sizes

---

interdisciplinary collaborations and the rapid generation of scientific knowledge from clinical data and biospecimens into clinical practice and personalized medicine.

These interdisciplinary collaborations often involve a wide range of health professionals, health policy makers, health industry delegates, potential research participants, and representatives of the public.[1] The integration of genetic biobanking practices into research and ultimately health care necessitates that all clinical disciplines actively participate in educating members of their discipline in genomics and engaging in genetic and genomic practices.[3] The nursing profession is no exception and has expanded and evolved as genetic biobanking practices have progressed from research to clinical settings.[4] Consequently, nurses should become familiar with genetic biobanking practices to

- Maintain professional competency when interacting with genetic biobanking activities in research and clinical settings
- Influence the development and management of high-quality genetic biobanks
- Apply genomics to clinical care, health promotion, and health outcomes
- Contribute to the development of genetics- and genomics-related standards and policies

To effectively use biobanking resources for advancing nursing research, it would be helpful for nurses to become familiar with genetic biobanking practices. The impact of nursing input and involvement is essential to develop biobanking resources that include the collection of data relevant to both medical genetics and nursing.[5] For all disciplines, including nursing, the existence of biobanks expedites the translational process to incorporate basic research findings into clinical practice. The nursing profession provides a vital component to genetic biobanking practices offering unique perspectives to the nursing discipline. This article (1) provides a general overview of genetic biobanking, (2) considers nursing roles and interdisciplinary collaboration in genetic biobanking, (3) discusses nursing competencies for ethical issues relative to genetic biobanking and health care, and (4) examines ethical responsibilities and issues of importance to nurses regarding genetic biobanking.

OVERVIEW OF GENETIC BIOBANKING

Simply defined, a biobank is a system established for data collection and future sharing. A biobank can be disease based or population based and can be governed by one specific site, a consortium, or a group of sites that agree to specific operating procedures and guidelines. Resources for establishing and maintaining a biobank may include the following:

- Infrastructure: office and laboratory space, clinical and biospecimen databases, and biospecimen storage space
- Personnel: director, research manager, laboratory manager and technicians, administrative assistants, bioinformatics personnel, research nurses, ethicists, and geneticists
- Business plan: funding, marketing, and cost recovery
- Standard operating procedures and guidelines

Further defined, a genetic biobank is the collection, processing, storage, management, and distribution of genetic material and associated clinical data.[2] **Box 2** provides a glossary of common genetic biobanking terms. Genetic biobanks may include the collection and storage of a wide variety of biospecimens, along with relevant clinical data that link personal and familial histories with human biospecimens for genetic research.[5] Detecting genetic contributions to disease requires careful collection and management of large data sets to obtain high-quality genetic biospecimens, as well as the collection of accurate corresponding clinical data. Examples of human biospecimens stored in biobanks for genetic research are provided in **Table 1**. The robustness and the reproducibility of research resulting from a genetic biobank depend greatly on the quality of the clinical data and biospecimens, which ultimately affect the quality of the research. Accordingly, accurate and standardized clinical and biospecimen data collection, processing, storage, management, and distribution are essential.[6]

To maximize research outcomes and fully reap societal benefits, genetic biobanks ideally involve the public, health care providers, industry, and legal and ethical strategists in their development, management, and utilization.[1] Specifically, engagement with potential participants and members of the public, as well as correspondence between genetic biobanks nationally and globally, is advantageous.[7] Involvement with

---

Box 2
Glossary of genetic biobank terminology

1. Biobank: a repository of human biologic material and corresponding clinical data

2. Complex diseases: diseases caused by the interaction of multiple genes and environmental factors

3. Translational research: research focused on moving knowledge and discovery gained from science to its application in health care, often summarized by the phrase "bench-to-bedside"

4. Population-based research: the study of a group of individuals defined by a set of common characteristics

5. Disease-based research: the study of a pathologic condition of a part, organ, or system of an organism resulting from various causes and is characterized by an identifiable group of signs or symptoms

6. Biologic material: a material that contains genetic information

7. Opt-out consent: individual must decline consent; if the individual does not clearly decline consent, then consent is granted

8. Opt-in consent: individual must expressly state or provide consent

Table 1
Examples of human biospecimens stored for genetic research

Biospecimens Type	Output	Biomarkers	Methods/Analysis
Whole blood/buffy coat/saliva	DNA	Genetic	Genotyping
Fresh frozen tissue	RNA	Genetic	Gene expression
Whole blood	Serum/plasma	Protein	Proteomics, metabolomics, biochemistry assays

potential participants and the public fosters research participation and is essential to establish diversity within genetic biobanks. This engagement hinges on the ability to educate potential participants and the public on genetic research and biobanking efforts. Engagement and correspondence between genetic biobanks is also essential to promote and expedite efficient scientific collaboration.[7] To examine data between genetic biobanks, standardization of data collection, handling, preservation, management, and distribution among genetic biobanks is imperative.[6] Resources available to promote best practices within genetic biobanking are provided in **Box 3**. These resources provide best practices and standard operating procedures for data collection, storage, retrieval, and distribution along with guidelines for the development of standardized operational procedures and informed consent examples. In summary, developing and implementing quality genetic biobanks include the following[7]:

- Clear governance regarding the utilization, access, and tracking of shared resources along with standardized operating procedures and guidelines
- Quality data collection, processing, storage, management, and distribution from both a laboratory and an informatics standpoint
- Potential participant and public engagement to encourage participation and diverse representation
- Engagement between genetic biobanks to promote scientific collaboration
- Complying with established best practices and ethical standards

NURSING ROLES IN GENETIC BIOBANKING

Patients in clinical settings are increasingly approached to contribute data to supply genetic biobanks, which signifies an increasing need for nursing to respond by developing and maintaining genetic and genomic knowledge along with implementing the best ethical practices to reduce risks and promote patient advocacy. The unique perspectives nursing discipline brings to genetic biobanks ensure that biobanking resources are designed with the protection and benefit of participants and members

Box 3
Best practices resources for genetic biobanks

1. 2012 Best Practices for Collection, Storage, Retrieval and Distribution of Biological Materials for Research from the International Society for Biological & Environmental Repositories, http://www.isber.org/bp/

2. Organisation for Economic Co-operation & Development Guidelines on Human Biobanks and Genetic Research Databases, http://www.oecd.org/dataoecd/41/47/44054609.pdf

3. National Human Genome Research Institute National Institutes of health informed consent form examples & model consent language, http://www.genome.gov/27526660

of the public in mind. Furthermore, the nursing component ensures the contribution of genetic biobank data that are meaningful to nursing-relevant research questions.[5] Moreover, translating science into clinical practice involves quality scientific endeavors drawing from a range of interdisciplinary viewpoints, including the nursing discipline.[1] Nurse scientists, research nurses, and clinical practice nurses have unique contributions to genetic biobanking, facilitating the use of genomic data in clinical practice and genetic research. **Table 2** provides an overview of each nursing role and potential interdisciplinary collaborations within genetic biobanks. Regardless of nursing roles, several key aspects are important for all nurses to implement as they interact with potential biobank participants:

- Exercise empathic honest communication
- Fully inform potential participants of the possible future use of biospecimens and clinical data, as well as the implications related to potential future results
- Ensure potential participants' autonomy in decision making is protected
- Ensure potential participants' respect for vulnerability
- Provide opportunities for potential participants to ask questions
- Understand and respect personal, religious, and cultural beliefs

Table 2
Examples of potential interdisciplinary collaborations with nursing roles in genetic biobanks

Title	Definition	Examples of Potential Interdisciplinary Collaborations
Nurse scientist	Nurse scientists who conduct independent research that improves nursing, clinical practice and health care. These scientists design studies, analyze data, and disseminate study results. Primary role within genetic biobanks focuses on development and administration or as a scientist using the data	Consultations with members of an Institutional Review Board for study protocol development. Consultations with an ethicist regarding ethical regulations and concerns. Collaboration with epidemiologists, geneticists, statisticians, laboratory managers, and informatics experts for data collection, handling, analysis, and interpretation
Research nurse	Nurses who are specialized in an area of research. These nurses support study implementation within the context of a research project	Consultations with members of an Institutional Review Board to maintain protocol and study integrity. Collaboration with laboratory managers and informatics experts to ensure the accuracy of data collection, handling, and recording
Clinical practice nurse	Nurses who provide direct patient care at primary, secondary, and tertiary health care settings	Collaboration with nurse scientists and research nurses to recruit patients for clinical studies, provide informed consent, and collect biospecimens. Consultations with members of an Institutional Review Board to maintain protocol and study integrity

Nurse Scientists

The National Institutes of Health (NIH)-supported Clinical and Translational Science Award (CTSA) program was launched in 2006 and has expanded to more than 60 academic institutions across the country.[8] The CTSA supports consortiums throughout the nation to maximize funding from NIH to advance research efforts. Many CTSA centers include a genetic biobank as one of their components to collect clinical and biospecimen data on large groups of human subjects. As one of the critical core components of the CTSA program, genetic biobanking is an important tool for the translational research process. These biobanks provide a platform to overcome barriers inherent to the research process such as difficulties in locating available, qualified clinical and translational investigators and challenges of conducting research in a silo.[8] With a large number of high-quality biospecimens already collected, genetic biobanks provide a plausible solution to funding restrictions.

Nurse scientists continue to participate in the application and development process of CTSA centers, and they are actively involved in various leadership positions within genetic biobanks across the nation.[9] More than 160 nurse scientists around the nation initiated a thematic special interest group to discuss ways to elevate nursing participation in clinical and translational science endeavors within the available CTSAs.[10] The CTSA initiative challenges nurse scientists to reconsider how they conduct research with greater emphasis on interaction and collaboration across disciplines. The school of nursing dean and associate dean for research are often members of centralized planning committees that provide advice on how to best involve nurse scientists in the CTSA initiative.[10] Among the first 12 funded CTSA centers, 9 had participating schools of nursing.[10] In addition, nurse scientists held leadership positions at 7 CTSA centers.[9] These CTSA leadership roles include memberships on the executive or leadership committees, acting as directors or codirectors of core programs such as genetic biobanks, as well as chairing major CTSA committees.[9] Nurse scientists continue to be actively involved in numerous community engagements or outreach programs of the CTSA centers and remain an integral part of the development, administration, contribution, and utilization of genetic biobanks.

Nurse scientists focus on scientific discoveries and translational studies; therefore, their professional roles also include generating new scientific knowledge from clinical and biospecimen data obtained from genetic biobanks. One of the priorities for genetic biobanks is to standardize the application process to facilitate utilization of genetic biobanks for all qualified researchers, including nurse scientists. In addition, as nurse scientists or collaborators, nurses may contribute genotypic and related clinical data to genetic biobanks; therefore, their input and involvement is imperative to developing genetic biobanking resources that include the collection of nursing relevant data, including nursing practice, behavioral variables, cost of care, and patient outcome data.[5]

Research Nurses and Clinical Practice Nurses

Research nurses are at the fulcrum of clinical research.[11] With the increase in genetic biobanking in clinical trials, it is critical for research nurses to keep abreast of the rising ethical, clinical, and regulatory research issues involving human subjects. Research nurses focus on essential genetic biobanking activities to support research efforts, including potential participant recruitment, informed consent, and educational needs. Therefore, research nurses need to have a comprehensive understanding of genetic biobanking practices related to ethical, clinical, and regulatory issues. Contrary to clinical studies not involving genetic biobanking, it is often difficult to explain to potential participants the future research that may occur using clinical and biospecimen data stored in a genetic biobank.[12] Research nurses are often involved in the development of informed consent and provide direction to ensure that participant rights are protected both legally and ethically. In general, potential participants involved in research should not be exposed to any risks without informed consent, and all potential participants must be well informed before obtaining any consent.[13] However, future research using banked clinical and biospecimen data may be unknown at the time of consent. Therefore, universal and standardized informed consent documents for future biobank-based research are gaining popularity among researchers for practical advantages.[13] Recontacting genetic biobanking participants to provide additional or new informed consent for every future research study can be time consuming, expensive, and even confusing for participants.

Initially, potential participants are approached to partake in a genetic biobank by a recruiter, often a research nurse. This process involves a dynamic and continuing exchange of information between the members of the research team and the potential participant throughout the research experience. Research nurses must understand and follow ethical guidelines specified by the governing Internal Review Board and Committee for the Protection of Human Subjects.

Recruitment efforts involve explaining the risks and the benefits associated with participating. Often cited as the greatest risk of genetic biobanking participation, loss of confidentiality is the unexpected release of personal health information; however, steps are taken to protect the privacy of information.[13] Often, no direct benefit is noted for the current health status of the participant, but the needs of larger future populations of interest may benefit from the knowledge gained using clinical and biospecimen data from a genetic biobank.[14] Therefore, participants frequently state altruistic reasons for genetic biobanking participation.[14]

Along with research nurses, clinical practice nurses are often involved with data collection; therefore, they directly influence the quality of genotypic and clinical data obtained for genetic biobanking. The quality of the data affects future use of banked data by researchers. Biospecimens must be maintained reliably with minimal deterioration over time, and they must be protected from physical damage, both accidental and intentional. The registration of each biospecimen entering and exiting the biobanking system is generally centrally stored, usually on a computer-based system.[7] Once the participant has acquiesced to become a part of the genetic biobank, research nurses and clinical practice nurses must understand and execute standardized techniques, essential for proper collection, handling, processing, and storage of biospecimens. Research nurses often collaborate with laboratory personnel to establish standardized biospecimen protocols for collection, handling, processing, and storage. When clinical and biospecimen data are received by the genetic biobank, standardized informatics systems should be in place to process and secure all data. Research nurses should be knowledgeable in these informatics processes to facilitate data entry in a secure manner into the genetic biobanking system. Overall, collaboration and cooperation with other components of genetic biobanks is crucial to continue successful research practices among genetic biobanks.[15] Potential collaborations between nurses and other components are outlined in **Table 2**.

Although the benefits and applications of biobanks are well anticipated, the utilization of biobanks for clinical practice is evolving at a much slower rate than the growth of biobanks. However, opportunities for clinical practice nurses to be involved in participant recruitment and clinical and biospecimen data collection have markedly increased. Frequently, it may be the clinical practice nurse who collects biospecimen data, reinforces participant education, and performs multiple functions at the point of contact with the research participant. Therefore, the clinical practice nurse often functions as an extension of the genetic biobanking research team.[4] It is the nurse scientists and research nurses' responsibility to confirm that clinical practice nurses are fully aware of the proper procedures to ensure quality and accuracy of clinical and biospecimen data collection. In acquiring data to deposit into genetic biobanks, the clinical practice nurse and research nurses have an obligation to obtain quality data and related documentation.

NURSING COMPETENCIES IN GENETIC BIOBANKING AND HEALTH CARE

New discoveries in genetics and genomics are being translated to nursing practice at a fast pace; therefore, understanding the ethical issues surrounding genetic biobanking and health care is an essential competency. The American Nurses Association and National League for Nursing adapted essentials that incorporate genetic and genomic knowledge and skills into all levels of nursing practice.[16] The essentials of genetic and genomic nursing competencies address specific professional responsibilities and practice domains.[16] Professional responsibilities refer to the ability to advocate for patients' access to genetic and genomic resources and their rights to privacy and informed decision making regarding genetic- and genomic-related care.[16] Under the professional practice domain, the essential competencies address the importance of nurses to identify ethical, ethnic, cultural, religious, legal, fiscal, and societal issues related to genetic and genomic information and technologies.[16]

As public awareness of genetic and genomic influences on health care increases, nurses are required to address genetic and genomic questions and related ethical issues. To explain the risks and benefits of participating in a genetic biobank, nurses need to fully understand genetic biobanking practices. For successful translation of genetic and genomic discoveries into practice and quality health care outcomes, the nursing workforce needs to be prepared to deliver genetically competent health.[17] To address these issues and challenges, genetic and genomic nursing competencies were established to build on existing scope and standards of nursing practice. Implementation of genetic and genomic nursing competencies into nursing education and nursing practice has been incorporated into essential competencies for all nurses regardless of practice levels.[17] These nursing competencies serve as guidelines for individual and professional continuing education, academic curriculum development, and specialty certification.[18]

ETHICAL RESPONSIBILITIES AND GENETIC BIOBANKING

Nursing science developed a conceptual framework to guide considerations of ethical issues at the interface of nursing and genetic biobanking. The conceptual framework includes participant and population outcomes regarding genetic biobanking initiatives. Ethical principles embedded in the framework are derived from multiple sources, including the Belmont Report and the international principles underlying the Human Genome Project.[4] The framework guides nursing research, education, and best practice measures for nurses involved with genetic biobanking.[4,19] Addressing ethical responsibilities is essential to the genomic competencies underscoring nursing best practice measures in clinical and research settings.[18] The following section highlights 2 examples of controversial areas in genetic biobanking, where nursing science and clinical practice must consider ethical implications.

Informed Decision Making and Consent

Reports studying public perceptions using focus groups and survey methods in hypothetical situations to assess participant "willingness to contribute" consistently conclude that the general public expresses willingness to participate in genomic research and biobanking.[20–23] However, studies have yet to determine whether trust expressed by the public in hypothetically proposed research contexts are predictive of factual, real-time considerations by potential participants in actual clinical settings.[24] More research is needed to better understand perceptions of actual patients making real decisions while in clinical settings.[20,25,26] One research participation issue to consider is the potential for therapeutic misconception. Therapeutic misconception occurs when a potential participant considers contributing to a genetic biobank without understanding the distinction between current treatment goals and future research benefits.[27,28] Therefore, the potential participant inaccurately attributes or anticipates direct therapeutic benefit by consenting to contribute clinical and biospecimen data designated to benefit future populations.[27] This therapeutic misconception has been observed in studies of public perception regarding contribution to genetic biobanks.[28,29] The role of the nurse in preventing therapeutic misconception by potential participants may be best supported by reinforcing education concerning what happens to clinical and biospecimen data after biobank collection and storage.

A recent trend in clinical and biospecimen data collection for genetic biobanks includes "opt in" or "opt out" disclosures to potential participants. Academic health science centers, hospitals, or other institutions may ask potential participants to "opt in" or "opt out" of their institutional genetic biobanking collection initiative. These institutions use a wide range of disclosure or permission models that do not conform to traditional notions of informed consent. These nontraditional models are supported by statutory language that exempts biospecimens from traditional human subjects' informed consent regulations.[24–26] The exception states that future use of clinical or biospecimen data may not be fully disclosed to the participant or the identity of the researchers who may ultimately use the data.[24–26] The models for disclosure and permission may or may not link the medical record of the participant to clinical and biospecimen data. Informed decision making involves nursing to ensure that the individual understands the possible future use of data, potential implications of data use and findings, and risks and benefits. Genetic biobanking practices generate distinct areas for nursing involvement in the informed decision-making and disclosure process.[30] To summarize, through the collection, storage, and future use of banked clinical and biospecimen data, concerns regarding the protection of the participant's rights to informed decision making and consent, confidentiality or privacy, and ability to withdraw from the genetic biobank ensue.[27]

Newborn Screening Genetic Testing

A recent controversial topic involving the collection of biospecimens from medical waste occurred with neonatal blood spots collected during newborn screening for rare genetic conditions. Recent studies determined that variable or absent disclosure to parents occurred regarding forwarding their newborn screening biospecimens to biobanks for future research.[31–33] Collecting blood spots is an example of biobanking where biospecimens may be collected from clinical settings and stored for future unspecified genomic research without disclosure to the participants' parents.[32] Despite scrutiny of this practice and its threat to public trust in newborn care, the Secretary's Advisory Committee on Heritable Disorders in Newborns and Children acknowledged that patient and public awareness of blood spot storage and future research use was not uniformly supported.[31] The committee recommended that public education should be regulated by the state and regional programs conducting the biobanking practices.[31] Once more, nurses may serve as an advocate for patients' and parental rights to informed decision making and consent regarding genetic- and genomic-related care and research.[16]

SUMMARY AND DISCUSSION

Research using genetic biobanking resources is becoming increasingly commonplace as scientists, including nurse scientists, recognize the demand for large amounts of quality biospecimens and corresponding clinical data to identify genetic susceptibility to complex and rare diseases. Genetic biobanks have become a major resource in understanding the interaction between genetic susceptibilities, environmental exposures, lifestyle factors, and individual treatment responses for complex disease.[2] Ultimately, these resources provide valuable data that will potentially affect the well-being of populations.[1] Provided proper development and maintenance, genetic biobanks enable translational research and multidisciplinary research collaborations. Challenges remain to maximize research outcomes and societal benefits, including limited collaboration between biobanks, in part due to legislation restrictions.[34] The present review provides a general overview of genetic biobanking practices and applications for translational research. Specifically, the involvement of nurses in genetic biobanks are presented, which include nursing roles in genetic biobanking, genetic competencies related to nursing practice, research, and ethics, as well as nursing considerations. The integration of genetic biobanking practices into research and health care necessitates that all health care disciplines actively participate in cultivating members of their discipline in genomics.[3] Consequently, the nursing profession has continued to expand and evolve as genetic biobanking practices have flourished.[4] The distinct perspectives the nursing profession affords to genetic biobanking practices guarantee that resources are designed with the protection and benefit of participants and the public in mind and ensures contribution of data relevant to answering nursing research questions. As public understanding of genetic and genomic influences on health care expands, the nursing profession is required to address genetics and genomics and related ethical issues. For the successful translation of genetic and genomic discoveries into clinical practice and quality health care outcomes, the nursing workforce, including nurse scientists, research nurses, and clinical practice nurses, needs to be skilled in participating and delivering genetically competent health care.[17] The role of the nursing profession and genetic responsibilities will become increasingly important as the breadth and scope of genetic biobanking increases. Undoubtedly, discoveries made possible through genetic biobanks will lead to innovative and highly significant advances in health care.

REFERENCES

1. Murtagh MJ, Demir I, Harris JR, et al. Realizing the promise of population biobanks: a new model for translation. Hum Genet 2011;130(3):333–45.
2. Zielhuis GA. Biobanking for epidemiology. Public Health 2012;126(3):214–6.
3. Greco KE, Tinley S, Seibert D. Development of the essential genetic and genomic competencies for nurses with graduate degrees. Annu Rev Nurs Res 2011;29: 173–90. Available at: http://www-ncbi-nlm-nih-gov.ezproxyhost.library.tmc.edu/pubmed/228915042011.
4. Williams PH, Schepp K, McGrath B, et al. The stewardship model: current viability for genetic biobank practice development. ANS Adv Nurs Sci 2010;33(1):E41–9.
5. Frazier L, Sparks E, Sanner JE, et al. Biobanks and biomarker research in cardiovascular disease. J Cardiovasc Nurs 2008;23(2):153–8.

6. Rogers J, Carolin T, Vaught J, et al. Biobankonomics: a taxonomy for evaluating the economic benefits of standardized centralized human biobanking for translational research. J Natl Cancer Inst Monogr 2011;42:32–8.

7. Macleod AK, Liewald DC, McGilchrist, et al. Some principles and practices of genetic biobanking studies. Eur Respir J 2009;33(2):419–25.

8. Clinical and translational science awards progress report 2009–2011. NIH and Department of Health and Human Services; 2011. Available at: http://www.ncats.nih.gov/ctsa_2011/. Accessed March 30, 2013.

9. Woods NF, Magyary DL. Translational research: why nursing's interdisciplinary collaboration is essential. Res Theory Nurs Pract 2010;24(1):9–24.

10. Knafl K, Grey M. Clinical translational science awards: opportunities and challenges for nurse scientists. Nurs Outlook 2008;56(3):132–7.

11. Poston RD, Buescher CR. The essential role of the clinical research nurse (CRN). Urol Nurs 2010;30(1):55–63, 77.

12. Shickle D. The consent problem within DNA biobanks. Stud Hist Philos Biol Biomed Sci 2006;37(3):503–19.

13. Budimir D, Polašek O, Marušić A, et al. Ethical aspects of human biobanks: a systematic review. Croat Med J 2011;52(3):262–79.

14. Sanner JE, Frazier L. Factors that influence characteristics of genetic biobanks. J Nurs Scholarsh 2007;39(1):25–9.

15. Zuvich RL, Armstrong LL, Bielinski SJ, et al. Pitfalls of merging GWAS data: lessons learned in the eMERGE network and quality control procedures to maintain high data quality. Genet Epidemiol 2011;35(8):887–98.

16. American Nurses Association. Essentials of genetic and genomic nursing: competencies, curricula guidelines, and outcome indicators. 2nd edition. Silver Spring (MD): American Nurses Association; 2008.

17. Calzone KA, Jenkins J, Prows C, et al. Establishing the outcome indicators for the essential nursing competencies and curricula guidelines for genetics and genomics. J Prof Nurs 2011;27(3):179–91.

18. Jenkins J, Calzone KA. Establishing the essential nursing competencies for genetics and genomics. J Nurs Scholarsh 2007;39(1):10–6.

19. Jeffers BR. Human biological materials in research: ethical issues and the role of stewardship in minimizing research risks. ANS Adv Nurs Sci 2001;24(2):32–46.

20. Lemke AA, Wolf WA, Hebert-Beirne J, et al. Public and biobank participant attitudes toward genetic research participation and data sharing. Public Health Genomics 2010;13(6):368–77.

21. Pulley JM, Brace MM, Bernard GR, et al. Attitudes and perceptions of patients towards methods of establishing a DNA biobank. Cell Tissue Bank 2008;9(1):55–65.

22. Simon C, L'Heureux J, Murray J, et al. Active choice but not too active: public perspectives on biobank consent models. Genet Med 2011;13(9):821–31.

23. Kaufman D, Murphy J, Erby L, et al. Veterans' attitudes regarding a database for genomic research. Genet Med 2009;11(5):329–37.

24. Johnsson L, Helgesson G, Rafnar T, et al. Hypothetical and factual willingness to participate in biobank research. Eur J Hum Genet 2010;18(11):1261–4.

25. Helft PR, Champion VL, Eckles R, et al. Cancer patients' attitudes toward future research uses of stored human biological materials. J Empir Res Hum Res Ethics 2007;2(3):15–22.

26. Melas PA, Sjöholm LK, Forsner T, et al. Examining the public refusal to consent to DNA biobanking: empirical data from a Swedish population-based study. J Med Ethics 2010;36(2):93–8.

27. Lidz CW, Appelbaum PS. The therapeutic misconception: problems and solutions. Med Care 2002;40(9):55–63.

28. Luque JS, Quinn GP, Montel-Ishino FA, et al. Formative research on perceptions of biobanking: what community members think? J Cancer Educ 2012;27(1):91–9.

29. Halverson CM, Ross LF. Incidental findings of therapeutic misconception in biobank-based research. Genet Med 2012;14(6):611–5.

30. Lea DH. Genetic and genomic health care: ethical issues of importance to nurses. Online J Issues Nurs 2008;13(1). Manuscript 4.

31. Secretary's Advisory Committee on Heritable Disorders in Newborns and Children. Briefing paper: Considerations and recommendations for national guidance regarding the retention and use of residual dried blood spot specimens after newborn screening. Mol Genet Metab 2010;101(2–3):93–4.

32. Haga SB. Analysis of educational materials and destruction/opt-out initiatives for storage and use of residual newborn screening samples. Genet Test Mol Biomarkers 2010;14(5):587–92.

33. Lewis MH, Goldenberg A, Anderson R, et al. State laws regarding the retention and use of residual newborn screening blood samples. Pediatrics 2011;127(4):703–12.

34. Scholtes VP, de Vries JP, Catanzariti LM, et al. Biobanking in atherosclerotic disease, opportunities and pitfalls. Curr Cardiol Rev 2011;7(1):9–14.

An Overview of Epigenetics in Nursing

Ashley Erin Clark, MSN, RN[a], Maria Adamian, ACNP-BC, CRNA[b],
Jacquelyn Y. Taylor, PhD, PNP-BC, RN[a],*

KEYWORDS

- Epigenetics • Nursing • Fetal • Metabolic syndrome • Cancer

KEY POINTS

- This article focuses on the emerging role of the practicing nurse and nurse researcher in epigenetics.
- Major epigenetic studies in nursing specific to childbirth, preeclampsia, metabolic syndrome, immunotherapy cancer, and pain are examined.
- Evaluation of epigenetics related to nursing, clinical practice, and research, with recommendations for future work, is discussed.

INTRODUCTION

The last 2 decades of ongoing work in science have suggested that there is a genetic/genomic basis for health, illness, disease risk, and treatment response in health care.[1] Nurses have an intimate knowledge of patient, family, and community perspectives on health, as well as basic science training, in some cases. The profession of nursing tends to focus on health promotion and disease prevention, which are both fundamental to genetic/genomic health care practice.[2] Many diseases and conditions that affect the population have a genetic/genomic element influenced by environment, lifestyle, and other factors directly affecting patient care and the nursing profession.[2] Epigenetic changes include biochemical alterations to DNA molecules that do not change the sequence but do influence gene expression.[3] Epigenetic-related diseases have the following characteristics: (1) a heritability that could not be fully explained by strict genetic inheritance patterns (single nucleotide polymorphisms, mutations); (2) evidence of the influence of imprinting (eg, maternal diet, or other in utero exposure to toxins,

Funding for this research was provided in part by the Robert Wood Johnson Foundation, Nurse Faculty Scholars Grant (JYT).
[a] Yale University, School of Nursing, 400 West Campus Drive, Orange, CT 06477, USA;
[b] Graduate School of Health Sciences, Seton Hall University, 400 South Orange Avenue, South Orange, NJ 07079, USA
* Corresponding author.
E-mail address: jacquelyn.taylor@yale.edu

pathogens, or drugs), which could influence the development of the disease in the offspring even into adulthood; and (3) an increase in prevalence with aging.[4] This last characteristic is based on an epigenetic model of complex disease. This finding suggests that with progressive accumulation of epimutations over the life span, a critical threshold is reached, beyond which the genome, cell, or tissue can no longer function normally, resulting in a diseased phenotype.[4–6] The 2 most commonly examined epigenetic mechanisms include histone modifications and methylation.[3] An epigenetic approach in research is used to examine complex, multifactorial diseases (eg, cancer, pain, cardiovascular diseases [CVDs], childbirth, immunotherapy) that have an environmental component associated with the condition or disease of interest. These technologies will soon become a driving force in patient management and care. The nursing profession, which bridges the interface of technology and nursing science, is prepared to conduct epigenetic-focused nursing research.[7] This article (1) discusses current epigenetic nursing research, (2) provides an overview of how epigenetic research relates to nursing in practice, (3) lists recommendations, and (4) provides epigenetic online resources for nursing research. Based on these purposes, major epigenetic studies in nursing found in the literature are discussed and recommendations on next steps are provided. Topics covered in this overview include childbirth studies, preeclampsia, metabolic syndrome, immunotherapy, cancer, and pain.

EPIGENETICS IN NURSING
Epigenetic Impact of Childbirth

A group of international nurses formed an interdisciplinary research collaboration investigating the state of the science concerning normal intrapartum epigenetic physiology. Their group, named the Epigenetic Impact of Childbirth (EICC), has expertise in genetics, physiology, developmental biology, epidemiology, midwifery, and nursing.[8] Based on years of research, clinical practice, and recent basic science evidence, these investigators hypothesized that events during the intrapartum period of pregnancy, specifically the use of synthetic oxytocin, antibiotics, and cesarean section, affect the epigenetic remodeling processes and subsequent health of the mother and offspring. Numerous studies have linked mode of birth (particularly cesarean section) to increasing rates of asthma, eczema, type 1 diabetes, infant bronchiolitis, multiple sclerosis, and obesity.[8–19] The EPIIC hypothesis indicates that physiologic labor and birth have a positive stress, known as eustress, on the fetus and that this process has an epigenetic effect on particular genes, specifically those that program immune responses, genes responsible for weight regulation, and specific tumor suppressor genes.[8] Reduced or increased levels of cortisol, adrenalin, and oxytocin produced during the labor process may lead to fetal epigenomic remodeling discrepancies, which exert effects on abnormal gene expression. Effects of environmental stress on epigenetic changes and exposure to chemical and environmental toxins have been shown to disrupt epigenetic regulation of gene expression in cells by altering DNA methylation patterns[20–24] and chromatin structure[20,25–27] and may also have direct implications for a variety of human diseases, including cancer, infertility, and neurodegenerative disorders.[28–31] The EPIIC group proposed a program of research to examine general patterns of epigenomic remodeling in neonates born after home births in the most familiar environment to the woman without medical interventions, compared with those born after elective cesarean section for breech presentation, when there are no underlying medical complications preceding the cesareans.[8] The investigators propose this research to include prospective longitudinal cohorts undergoing various methods of labor, diverse environments, multiple ethnic groups, gestational ages, maternal ages, socioeconomic backgrounds, and a range of interventions. This work should enhance our scientific and medical understanding of epigenetics related to the childbirth process and prolonged health of the mother and child.

Preeclampsia

Preeclampsia, a condition associated with pregnancy, is defined as an increased blood pressure coupled with excess protein in the urine of pregnant women after 20 weeks of pregnancy, who previously had normal blood pressure.[32] If left untreated, this condition could lead to serious, even fatal, complications for the mother or baby. Preeclampsia results from placental insufficiency leading to pregnancy-induced hypertension in the second half of the pregnancy, affecting 8% to 10% of women in the United States.[32] Nurse scientists have been studying the acute effects of preeclampsia and genetic origins of this disorder.[33,34] They have begun pilot work toward examining DNA methylation patterns, focusing on maternal nutrition status and placental programming through epigenetic alternations in DNA as a plausible explanation for maternal preeclampsia.[34] These nurses used genome-wide DNA methylation patterns, targeting genes producing proteins used specifically in vitamin D signaling. Their results suggest that vitamin D insufficiency in pregnancy is associated with increased blood pressure and risk for preeclampsia, further increasing risk for CVD in mothers and offspring. Placental DNA hypermethylation in the genes VDR and RXR was found to possibly reduce vitamin D binding and gene transcription, thereby reducing utilization during pregnancy and programming the fetal cardiovascular system for possible future risk of preeclampsia and hypertension. Other studies addressing immune function, endothelial function, thrombophilia variants, and other potential biomarkers for heritable risk of preeclampsia have been conducted by nurses, such as with examining maternal vitamin D as a determinant in gestational diabetes.[35,36] Although diet plays a role in determining gestational diabetes, nutrition also affects the genome in terms of epigenetics.

Metabolic Syndrome

Nurses are beginning to address the role of epigenetics in the development of CVD, obesity, and diabetes. Metabolic syndrome is a clustering of these conditions or risk factors, including hypertension, insulin resistance, and obesity.[37,38] In the case of CVD, although a family history of heart disease is an independent risk factor for the occurrence of heart disease, CVD does not follow a standard Mendelian pattern.[39] Nurse scientists have found that race and ethnicity, sex differences, age, and prenatal influences (such as maternal diet) point to an epigenetic role in the development of CVD.[40] Although obesity is also a risk factor for CVD, the cause, like CVD is difficult to pinpoint. Obesity is related to an energy imbalance of too many calories consumed combined with inadequate exertion of physical activity. This relationship may also be associated with heritability, behavior, lifestyle, and genetic predisposition of obesity.[37,38,41–44] Roundtable discussions among basic scientists, clinicians, and researchers to address the issue of epigenetics and obesity highlight the need to work collaboratively to better understand the relationship between obesity and epigenetic changes to the genome.[45] Complications of obesity over time lead to insulin resistance, which is associated with type 2 diabetes. Studies revealed commonality associated with gene-activated hyperglycemic events and chromatin modification as well as microRNAs, which have also been implicated in epigenetic mechanisms with insulin secretion and immune function.[4,46] Although this research has been explicated by basic scientists and researchers, the literature addresses the nursing profession as becoming aware of, interested in, and active in elucidating genetic and epigenetic mechanisms in the case of metabolic syndrome. A 2013 special genomics issue of the *Journal of Nursing Scholarship* highlighted work on metabolic syndrome,[37] CVD,[40] and other conditions, with accompanying Webinars to inform the nursing community and general public about genomics in health care.

Immunotherapy

Immunotherapy is yet another area of medicine that uses epigenetic research as a basis for evidence and to guide treatment effectiveness. Sometimes referred to as biological therapy or biotherapy, immunotherapy uses certain parts of the immune system to fight diseases, such as cancer. This process begins by stimulating the immune system to work harder and smarter to attack cancer cells, or by providing the immune system with components such as proteins to better target cancer cells and boost the immune system.[47] In the case of acute myeloid leukemia, antigen-specific immunotherapy has been applied in elderly patients, for instance, by allogeneic stem cell transplantation.[48,49] Nurses are at the forefront of caring for patients undergoing allogeneic stem cell transplants, including delivering immunosuppressive drugs, managing risk for infection, using protective isolation and particulate air filters, managing patient hygiene and oral care, and monitoring clinical indicators of febrile neutropenia, and frequent vital signs (the most important indicator of infection).[50] Care of these patients without nursing would not be possible, yet a gap exists whereby nurses have not extended the profession to include bench-to-bedside care in this domain.

Although clinical trials are being conducted on pharmacotherapy, only a small fraction of the profession is involved in this area of medicine. The drug 5-azacytidine (5-aza), a hypomethylating agent approved for use in myelodysplastic syndromes, has led to a significant epigenetic regulating of cytokine genes and transcription factors. This situation suggests that it may have the ability to be an effective immunotherapy treatment.[51–53] Although progress is being made, large prospective studies aimed at correlating the induction of an efficient immune response with clinical responses in patients are warranted, with nursing helping to recruit patients and being involved in the active process of clinical trials. The profession has the training background and knowledge to bridge the gap between bench science and bedside care. By becoming involved in greater basic science pursuits, clinical trials, and comparative effectiveness studies, nursing could extend their scope and build a foundation for enhanced translational medicine in this burgeoning field of immunotherapy.[51] Cancer has also been an area of interest for epigenetic research, because abnormal gene expression leading to cancer is, like immunotherapy, multifactorial in nature.[54]

Cancer

Cancer can stem from genetic, infectious, radiation, environmental, hormonal, or lifestyle factors that modify the structure of DNA. Nurses are involved in many aspects of cancer treatment, including tumor profiling, cancer risk assessment, pharmacogenomics, and targeted therapy.[54] In the progression of cancer, epigenetic methylation is observed in certain cancers, such as the RB1 gene associated with retinoblastoma.[55] This gene, which is turned off, means that gene expression is no longer possible. In other cancers, such as colon cancer, methylation testing aids the provider to differentiate between sporadic colon cancers and Lynch syndrome.[54] Because nurses are at the forefront of patient care, the initial step that the profession can take is in evaluating an individual or family through a cancer risk assessment. This assessment provides an evaluation to the individual or family regarding cancer risk based on health and family history, identifies individuals who may benefit from genetic testing, assesses the psychosocial and cultural implication of risk, and provides education counseling and psychosocial support.[54,56,57] Tumor profiling is the evaluation of genomic, proteomic, and epigenomic expression factors. Tumors differ not only histologically, requiring different treatments, but also molecularly. Tumor profiling techniques influencing clinical care include immunohistochemistry staining, microsatellite instability, and microarray analysis.[54] Each of these techniques differs but all are performed using a blood sample, and these results inform the direction of care, consideration of genetic counseling, treatment regimens, and risk-reduction strategies. Nurses are involved in all of these processes.

Single nucleotide polymorphisms combined with pharmacogenomics (the study of how genomic factors determine an individual's response to drugs) are important to oncology care. Genetic testing can be performed for specific variants identified as interfering with the metabolism of a drug. Nurses can educate individuals regarding drug interactions and help individuals to understand why they may be receiving a different treatment of the same disease compared with another individual.[54] Oncology has changed to include nursing care in all aspects of patient care from risk assessment and prevention to diagnosis and management. It is more important now than ever for the profession to be aware of developments in epigenetics, genetics, and genomics.

Pain

Pain management is a major concern in the area of cancer treatment and is an issue for other chronic diseases as well. Pain is a pervasive symptom aligned with nearly every health condition or disorder. The epidemic of chronic pain, not necessarily associated with an underlying condition or trait, affects more than 100 million Americans.[58,59] When comparing this number with 25.8 million Americans suffering from diabetes,[60] 16.3 million Americans suffering from coronary heart disease,[61] 11.9 million suffering from cancer,[62] and 7 million Americans suffering from stroke, it is clear that addressing pain in nursing care is essential. Nursing epigenetic research has focused on examining knowledge of nociceptive pathways and alterations that could lead to pathologic pain.[59] Epigenetic mechanisms have been identified in the transition to, maintenance of, and response to pain and analgesics.[59] Although nurse scientists did not map out the biochemical pathways identified in the literature, nurses have begun using epigenetic applications in response to pain management, including initially identifying patients at risk for pain, performing pharmacogenetic tests, and guiding the selection of therapeutic modalities to target pain.

NURSING
Clinical Practice

The knowledge that science and nursing has gained from epigenetics concerns data related to chemical modifications and structure of the DNA, which affect gene regulation.[63] The clinical value of epigenetic contributions to patient care are vast. Because this research encompasses chromatin structure, activities of noncoding RNAs and DNA methylation, these modifications have the potential to guide diagnostic testing. Nurses are at the pivotal edge of patient care, collaborating with a variety of health care providers, and managing evidence-based research. Epigenetics, unlike other genomic approaches, has a dual role in which epigenetic data can allow a better understanding of biological phenomena and thereby health conditions related to the biological phenomenon of interest.[64] For nurses, these data can aid the profession in enhanced understanding in terms of variability of patient outcomes, therapeutic responses, and patient signs and symptoms. Although there is potential for manipulating epigenetic gene regulation through the modification of environmental factors such as nutrition, nursing must be kept up to date with advancing knowledge, technologies, and understanding of disease mechanisms.[63] Nurses must also seek to educate patients and families on the state of the science, dealing with uncertainty, managing expectations, explaining treatment choices, and targeting treatment. Nursing is a profession fueled by a multiplicity of roles and responsibilities and nurses are the right group of medical professionals to take on the job of incorporating epigenetics into clinical care.

Research Practice

With the National Institute for Nursing Research's (NINR) Summer Genetics Institute (SGI),[65] a competitive, tuition-free, 1-month intensive research training program held at the National Institutes of Health, nurses are able to gain a foundation of knowledge in molecular genetics. This program is grounded in increasing nursing research capability among graduate students and faculty and seeks to develop and expand clinical practice in genetics. Most of the nurses highlighted have gone through this program or similar ones such as the 18-week Web-Based Genetics Institute, which used the SGI as a template for development, education, and research efforts.[66] Nurses are already using the tools from this program and others in biobehavorial research, to describe epigenetic trends and identify applications in the clinical setting for continued research. Details of epigenetic resources are provided in **Table 1**, with various online Web sites to aid the practicing nurse and nurse researcher in epigenetic tools, education modalities, and research/practice trends. Nurses can continue in this vein by recruiting patients into studies, building the evidence base for epigenetic health care in nursing practice, and by leading in the translation of new knowledge and understanding of health care practice and pathways in research.[63]

Recommendations

In 2012, a Genomic Nursing State of the Science Advisory Panel was convened to develop a blueprint for genomic nursing science.[67] This framework was created to further genomic nursing science and to improve health outcomes using the state of the science and the NINR strategic plan to create nursing research priority considerations. The panel suggested that research focused on the value of nursing in the delivery of effective genomics-based care for individuals, families, communities, and populations will accelerate the translation of evidence into practice, which this is critical for moving health care forward.[67] Increasing the capacity of nurse scientists in genetic, genomic, and epigenetic science will promote the application of research discoveries to benefit individuals. However, perhaps the most critical and greatest challenge to nursing science and research lies in nursing education. A prepared nursing workforce is essential to effective translation of genetic/genomic and epigenetic research to benefit patient care.[68] Nurses need to be able to explain to patients and families the implications of screening and testing and to explain risk in an individualized context, regarding treatment options. They also need to be able to appraise new developments, technologies, and research appropriate for use in the clinical setting. The profession should possess a basic understanding of molecular laboratory science and be competent to translate the knowledge of physiology into a scientific setting. The role of nursing is fundamental to improving patient care, clinically and with research, and the body of evidence-based epigenetic nursing is increasing. However, continued research is essential to health promotion, education, and disease management in order to drive clinical relevance and improved patient outcomes.

Table 1
Epigenetic resources

Name	Web Address	Description
Genetics Home Reference	http://ghr.nlm.nih.gov/	National Library of Medicine Web site containing information on genetic conditions, genes, and chromosomes
Talking Glossary of Genetic Terms	http://www.genome.gov/Glossary/	A glossary with audible function from scientists at the National Institutes of Health providing spoken definitions of terms. Illustrations and animations of genetic/genomic processes also provided
Understanding the Basics of Microarrays	http://www.ncbi.nlm.nih.gov/About/primer/microarrays.html	An overview from the National Center for Biotechnology Information on DNA microarrays, gene expression, the technology of microarrays, the importance of microarrays, and basic epigenetic microarray experiments
Serial Analysis of Gene Expression (SAGE)	http://www.sagenet.org	Allows for the analysis of overall gene expression patterns with digital analysis, also provides SAGE applications, publications, and resources
Gene Expression Omnibus	http://www.ncbi.nlm.nih.gov/geo	A public repository and online virtual resource center for storage and retrieval of gene expression data. This site maintains microarray and SAGE data on many model organisms
Histone Database	http://www.research.nhgri.nih.gov/histones	National Human Genome Research Institute histone database, with histone sequence information and posttranslational modifications
Chromatin Structure and Function	http://www.chromatin.us/chrom.html	A site dedicated to information on chromatin biology, histones, and epigenetics
Database for DNA Methylation and Environmental Epigenetic Effects	http://www.methdb.de/	A human DNA methylation database site, open to the public
CpG Island Searcher	http://www.uscnorris.com/cpgislands2/cpg.aspx	A site dedicated to searching for CpG islands; searching algorithms allows for selection of percentage methylation and length of (ISLAND) and gaps between islands
The Epigenome Network of Excellence	http://www.epigenome-noe.net/WWW/index.php	A network of epigenetic research, including protocols, an antibody database, and reference information on epigenetics

(continued on next page)

Table 1 (continued)		
Name	Web Address	Description
Human Epigenome Project	http://www.epigenome.org/	The Human Epigenome Project Research Consortium, a collaborative site created to catalog and interpret genome-wise methylation patterns of all human genes and major tissues
The Genes, Environment, and Health Initiative	http://www.genesandenvironment.nih.gov	Site for genes, environment, and health initiative
Functional Genomics Resources: Epigenetics	http://www.sciencemag.org/site/feature/plus/sfg/resources/res_epigenetics.xhtml#methl	An epigenetic section on the *Science* functional genomics site, on chromatin, methylation, imprinting, and other genetic topics, with an epigenetics bend
Epigenome Informally Informative	http://www.epigenie.com	The latest epigenetic and noncoding RNA research with special features, technology highlights, and conference information

Data from Baumgartel K, Zelazny J, Timcheck T, et al. Molecular genomic research designs. Annu Rev Nurs Res 2011;29:1–26; and Conley YP, Biesecker LG, Gonsalves S, et al. Current and emerging technology approaches in genomics. J Nurs Scholarsh 2013;45(1):5–14.

REFERENCES

1. Human genome project information: medicine and the new genetics [Internet]. 2011. Available at: http://www.ornl.gov/sci/techresources/Human_Genome/medicine/medicine.shtml. Accessed December 29, 2012.
2. Calzone KA, Cashion A, Feetham S, et al. Nurses transforming health care using genetics and genomics. Nurs Outlook 2010;58(1):26–35.
3. Baumgartel K, Zelazny J, Timcheck T, et al. Molecular genomic research designs. Annu Rev Nurs Res 2011;29:1–26.
4. Dwivedi RS, Herman JG, McCaffrey TA, et al. Beyond genetics: epigenetic code in chronic kidney disease. Kidney Int 2011;79(1):23–32.
5. Fire A, Xu S, Montgomery MK, et al. Potent and specific genetic interference by double-stranded RNA in *Caenorhabditis elegans*. Nature 1998;391(6669):806–11.
6. Bjornsson HT, Fallin MD, Feinberg AP. An integrated epigenetic and genetic approach to common human disease. Trends Genet 2004;20(8):350–8.
7. Loescher LJ, Merkle CJ. The interface of genomic technologies and nursing. J Nurs Scholarsh 2005;37(2):111–9.
8. Dahlen HG, Kennedy HP, Anderson CM, et al. The EPIIC hypothesis: intrapartum effects on the neonatal epigenome and consequent health outcomes. Med Hypotheses 2013;80(5):656–62.
9. Hyde MJ, Mostyn A, Modi N, et al. The health implications of birth by caesarean section. Biol Rev Camb Philos Soc 2012;87(1):229–43.
10. Cardwell CR, Stene LC, Joner G, et al. Caesarean section is associated with an increased risk of childhood-onset type 1 diabetes mellitus: a meta-analysis of observational studies. Diabetologia 2008;51(5):726–35.
11. Cook MB, Graubard BI, Rubertone MV, et al. Perinatal factors and the risk of testicular germ cell tumors. Int J Cancer 2008;122(11):2600–6.

12. Goldani HA, Bettiol H, Barbieri MA, et al. Cesarean delivery is associated with an increased risk of obesity in adulthood in a Brazilian birth cohort study. Am J Clin Nutr 2011;93(6):1344–7.
13. Hakansson S, Kallen K. Caesarean section increases the risk of hospital care in childhood for asthma and gastroenteritis. Clin Exp Allergy 2003;33(6):757–64.
14. Joffe TH, Simpson NA. Cesarean section and risk of asthma. The role of intrapartum antibiotics: a missing piece? J Pediatr 2009;154(1):154.
15. Maghzi AH, Etemadifar M, Heshmat-Ghahdarijani K, et al. Cesarean delivery may increase the risk of multiple sclerosis. Mult Scler 2012;18(4):468–71.
16. Pistiner M, Gold DR, Abdulkerim H, et al. Birth by cesarean section, allergic rhinitis, and allergic sensitization among children with a parental history of atopy. J Allergy Clin Immunol 2008;122(2):274–9.
17. Thavagnanam S, Fleming J, Bromley A, et al. A meta-analysis of the association between caesarean section and childhood asthma. Clin Exp Allergy 2008;38(4): 629–33.
18. McKay JA, Groom A, Potter C, et al. Genetic and non-genetic influences during pregnancy on infant global and site specific DNA methylation: role for folate gene variants and vitamin B_{12}. PLoS One 2012;7(3):e33290.
19. Huh SY, Rifas-Shiman SL, Zera CA, et al. Delivery by caesarean section and risk of obesity in preschool age children: a prospective cohort study. Arch Dis Child 2012;97(7):610–6.
20. Watson RE, McKim JM, Cockerell GL, et al. The value of DNA methylation analysis in basic, initial toxicity assessments. Toxicol Sci 2004;79(1):178–88.
21. Arita A, Costa M. Epigenetics in metal carcinogenesis: nickel, arsenic, chromium and cadmium. Metallomics 2009;1(3):222–8.
22. Poirier LA, Vlasova TI. The prospective role of abnormal methyl metabolism in cadmium toxicity. Environ Health Perspect 2002;110(Suppl 5):793–5.
23. Baccarelli A, Bollati V. Epigenetics and environmental chemicals. Curr Opin Pediatr 2009;21(2):243–51.
24. Takiguchi M, Achanzar WE, Qu W, et al. Effects of cadmium on DNA-(cytosine-5) methyltransferase activity and DNA methylation status during cadmium-induced cellular transformation. Exp Cell Res 2003;286(2):355–65.
25. Ballestar E, Esteller M. The epigenetic breakdown of cancer cells: from DNA methylation to histone modifications. Prog Mol Subcell Biol 2005;38:169–81.
26. Foster WG, McMahon A, Rice DC. Sperm chromatin structure is altered in cynomolgus monkeys with environmentally relevant blood lead levels. Toxicol Ind Health 1996;12(5):723–35.
27. Song C, Kanthasamy A, Anantharam V, et al. Environmental neurotoxic pesticide increases histone acetylation to promote apoptosis in dopaminergic neuronal cells: relevance to epigenetic mechanisms of neurodegeneration. Mol Pharmacol 2010;77(4):621–32.
28. Lahiri DK, Maloney B, Zawia NH. The LEARn model: an epigenetic explanation for idiopathic neurobiological diseases. Mol Psychiatry 2009;14(11): 992–1003.
29. Ren X, McHale CM, Skibola CF, et al. An emerging role for epigenetic dysregulation in arsenic toxicity and carcinogenesis. Environ Health Perspect 2011; 119(1):11–9.
30. Donkena KV, Young CY, Tindall DJ. Oxidative stress and DNA methylation in prostate cancer. Obstet Gynecol Int 2010;2010:302051.
31. Zawia NH, Lahiri DK, Cardozo-Pelaez F. Epigenetics, oxidative stress, and Alzheimer disease. Free Radic Biol Med 2009;46(9):1241–9.

32. Preeclampsia [Internet]. 2011. Available at: http://www.mayoclinic.com/health/preeclampsia/DS00583. Accessed December 29, 2012.

33. Anderson C. Fetal origins of hypertension: placental insufficiency linking cause and effect. Omaha (NE): Midwest Nursing Research Society; 2007.

34. Uthus EO, Anderson CM. Epigenetic patterns in placental programming of preeclampsia. Carefree (AZ): Western Institute of Nursing; 2010.

35. Wright ML, Anderson CM, Uthus EO, et al. Validation of DNA methylation patterns: potential biomarker for heritable risk of preeclampsia. West J Nurs Res 2012;34(8):1074–5.

36. Senti J, Thiele DK, Anderson CM. Maternal vitamin D status as a critical determinant in gestational diabetes. J Obstet Gynecol Neonatal Nurs 2012;41(3):328–38.

37. Taylor JT, Kraja AT, de las Fuentas L, et al. An overview of the genomics of metabolic syndrome. J Nurs Scholarsh 2013;45(1):52–9.

38. Clark AE, Taylor JY, Morrison H, et al. Alternative methods for measuring obesity in African American women. Yale J Biol Med 2013;86(1):29–39.

39. Corwin EJ. The concept of epigenetics and its role in the development of cardiovascular disease: commentary on "new and emerging theories of cardiovascular disease". Biol Res Nurs 2004;6(1):11–6 [discussion: 21–3].

40. Wung SF, Hickey KT, Taylor JY, et al. Cardiovascular genomics. J Nurs Scholarsh 2013;45(1):60–8.

41. Genomics Resources Diseases Knowing obesity and genetics [Internet]. 2010. Available at: http://www.cdc.gov/genomics/resources/diseases/obesity/obesknow.htm. Accessed January 19, 2013.

42. Taylor JY, Maddox R, Wu CY. Genetic and environmental risks for high blood pressure among African American mothers and daughters. Biol Res Nurs 2009;11(1):53–65.

43. Taylor JY, Caldwell CH, Baser RE, et al. Classification and correlates of eating disorders among blacks: findings from the national survey of American life. J Health Care Poor Underserved 2013;24(1):289–310.

44. Taylor JY, Caldwell CH, Baser RE, et al. Prevalence of eating disorders among Blacks in the National Survey of American Life. Int J Eat Disord 2007;40(Suppl):S10–4.

45. Rowen L, Ross S, Milner JA. Obesity, cancer, and epigenetics. Bariatr Surg Pract Patient Care 2010;5:275–83.

46. Poy MN, Eliasson L, Krutzfeldt J, et al. A pancreatic islet-specific microRNA regulates insulin secretion. Nature 2004;432(7014):226–30.

47. Immunotherapy [Internet]. 2012. Available at: http://www.cancer.org/treatment/treatmentsandsideeffects/treatmenttypes/immunotherapy/immunotherapy-what-is-immunotherapy. Accessed January 19, 2013.

48. Atanackovic D, Luetkens T, Kloth B, et al. Cancer-testis antigen expression and its epigenetic modulation in acute myeloid leukemia. Am J Hematol 2011;86(11):918–22.

49. Socie G, Stone JV, Wingard JR, et al. Long-term survival and late deaths after allogeneic bone marrow transplantation. Late Effects Working Committee of the International Bone Marrow Transplant registry. N Engl J Med 1999;341(1):14–21.

50. Brown M. Nursing care of patients undergoing allogeneic stem cell transplantation. Nurs Stand 2010;25(11):47–56 [quiz: 58].

51. Frikeche J, Clavert A, Delaunay J, et al. Impact of the hypomethylating agent 5-azacytidine on dendritic cells function. Exp Hematol 2011;39(11):1056–63.

52. Goodyear O, Agathanggelou A, Novitzky-Basso I, et al. Induction of a CD8+ T-cell response to the MAGE cancer testis antigen by combined treatment with azacitidine and sodium valproate in patients with acute myeloid leukemia and myelodysplasia. Blood 2010;116(11):1908–18.

53. Jabbour E, Giralt S, Kantarjian H, et al. Low-dose azacitidine after allogeneic stem cell transplantation for acute leukemia. Cancer 2009;115(9):1899–905.

54. Santos EM, Edwards QT, Floria-Santos M, et al. Integration of genomics in cancer care. J Nurs Scholarsh 2013;45(1):43–51.

55. Das PM, Singal R. DNA methylation and cancer. J Clin Oncol 2004;22(22): 4632–42.

56. Aiello-Laws L. Genetic cancer risk assessment. Semin Oncol Nurs 2011;27(1): 13–20.

57. Weitzel JN, Blazer KR, Macdonald DJ, et al. Genetics, genomics, and cancer risk assessment: state of the art and future directions in the era of personalized medicine. CA Cancer J Clin 2011;61:327–59.

58. AAPM facts and figures on pain [Internet]. 2013. Available at: http://www. painmed.org/patientcenter/facts_on_pain.aspx#incidence. Accessed January 19, 2013.

59. Starkweather AR, Pair VE. Decoding the role of epigenetics and genomics in pain management. Pain Manag Nurs 2011;12:1–10.

60. Diabetes statistics: data from the 2011 national diabetes fact sheet [Internet]. 2013. Available at: http://www.diabetes.org/diabetes-basics/diabetes-statistics/. Accessed February 13, 2013.

61. American Heart Association. Heart disease and stroke statistics–2011 update: a report from the American Heart Association. Circulation 2011;123:e18–209.

62. Cancer prevalence [Internet]. 2013. Available at: http://www.cancer.org/cancer/ cancerbasics/cancer-prevalence. Accessed February 13, 2013.

63. Conley YP, Biesecker LG, Gonsalves S, et al. Current and emerging technology approaches in genomics. J Nurs Scholarsh 2013;45(1):5–14.

64. Hill VK, Ricketts C, Bieche I, et al. Genome-wide DNA methylation profiling of CpG islands in breast cancer identifies novel genes associated with tumorigenicity. Cancer Res 2011;71(8):2988–99.

65. Summer Genetics Institute [Internet]. 2011. Available at: http://www.ninr.nih.gov/ Training/TrainingOpportunitiesIntramural/SummerGeneticsInstitute/. Accessed February 20, 2013.

66. Prows CA, Hetteberg C, Hopkin RJ, et al. Development of a web-based genetics institute for a nursing audience. J Contin Educ Nurs 2004;35(5):223–31.

67. Genomic Nursing State of the Science Advisory Panel, Calzone KA, Jenkins J, et al. A blueprint for genomic nursing science. J Nurs Scholarsh 2013;45(1): 96–104.

68. Jenkins JF, Calzone KA. Are nursing faculty ready to integrate genomic content into curricula? Nurse Educ 2012;37(1):25–9.

Integrating Genetics and Genomics into Nursing Curricula
You Can Do It Too!

Sandra Daack-Hirsch, PhD, RN[a],*, Barbara Jackson, PhD[b],
Chito A. Belchez, MSN, RN-BC[c], Betty Elder, PhD, RN[d],
Roxanne Hurley, MS, RN[e], Peg Kerr, PhD, RN[f],
Mary Kay Nissen, ARNP-BC, MSN, COHN-S[g]

KEYWORDS

- Nursing education • Genetics • Genomics • Case study • Undergraduate curriculum

KEY POINTS

- Rapid advances in knowledge and technology related to genomics cross health care disciplines and touch almost every aspect of patient care—assessment, screening, diagnosis, and treatment.
- Nurses are key to bridging the gap between genomic discoveries and the human experience of illness.
- There is a critical need for genetics and genomics in nursing education.
- Strategies and recourses exist to enable nursing faculty to successfully integrate genetics and genomics into curricula.

INTRODUCTION

Three billion base pairs code for an entire human genome and hold the key to regulating biologic processes that are fundamental to our lives, and slight variations across the genome are responsible for our differences. Health care professionals can no longer categorize disorders and characteristics as either genetic or nongenetic.

This project was funding by The Heartland Genetic and Newborn Screening Collaborative.
[a] The University of Iowa College of Nursing, 364 CNB, Iowa City, IA 52242, USA; [b] Munroe-Meyer Institute, University of Nebraska Medical Center, 985450 Nebraska Medical Center, Omaha, NE 68198-5450, USA; [c] School of Nursing, The University of Kansas Medical Center, 2053 School of Nursing, Mail Stop 4043, 3901 Rainbow Boulevard, Kansas City, KS 66160, USA; [d] School of Nursing, Wichita State University, 1845 Fairmount Street, Box 41, Wichita, KS 67260-0041, USA; [e] College of Nursing, University of North Dakota, Room 311, 430 Oxford Street, Stop 9025, Grand Forks, ND 58202-9025, USA; [f] Department of Nursing, University of Dubuque, 2000 University Avenue, Dubuque, IA 52001, USA; [g] Department of Nursing, Briar Cliff University, 3303 Rebecca Street, Sioux City, IA 51104, USA
* Corresponding author.
E-mail address: sandra-daack-hirsch@uiowa.edu

Rather, they must consider what the genetic and genomic contributions are to susceptibility and predisposition to illness as well as responses to pharmacologic and nonpharmacologic therapies when caring for patients.

The Human Genome Project has accelerated discovery, expanded understanding of how genomes work, invigorated a wave of new technology resulting in the ability to sequence a single human genome for just thousands of dollars (the cost continues to drop), and revolutionized health care.[1] This ever-evolving knowledge and technology related to genomics is unique in that it crosses health care disciplines and touches almost every aspect of patient care—assessment, screening, diagnosis, and treatment. The ability to sequence a genome holds the promise that health care can be personalized based on a unique genome sequence and treatments tailored on a profound understanding of how their unique genetic characteristics interacts with their physical environment—leading to more-effective treatments and preventative care.[1,2]

Health care professionals, including nurses, are faced with a gap in the ability to use the rapidly expanding technology and knowledge related to genomics in practice.[3,4] Yet, nurses are key to bridging the gap between genomic discoveries and the human experience of illness because nurses care for patients, families, and communities with an intimate knowledge of their perspectives. Nurses are skilled communicators; are knowledgeable about the biologic, social, and psychological implications of illness; and have the public's trust.[5] Unfortunately, many practicing nurses do not have educational training in genetics. Recent studies show that nurses have low genetic literacy.[6–10] Furthermore, nursing faculty are not prepared to teach genetics/genomics in their curricula, thus perpetuating the problem.[6,11,12] To that end, professional groups have endorsed the need for genetics and genomics in nursing education.[13–17] Two seminal examples of professional endorsement in the United States include the *Essentials of Baccalaureate Nursing Education for Professional Nursing Practice*[13] and *Essentials of Genetic and Genomic Nursing: Competencies, Curricula Guidelines, and Outcome Indicators*.[14] Central to these documents is the understanding that nurses are crucial to the provision of health care that incorporates genetic and genomic information.[7,18]

Several articles have been published on how to go about planning for and integrating genetics and genomic content into nursing programs.[18–20] Likewise, several faculty resources and strategies to prepare faculty to integrate genomics into education programs exist.[21–24] There is, however, little documentation and evaluation of the process of integrating genetics and genomics into programs. The purpose of this article is to present a case study documenting the experience of five schools/colleges of nursing as they work to integrate genetics and genomics into their curricula.

OVERVIEW

The Genomic Nursing Education in the Heartland Initiative was developed to provide consultation to nursing education programs to support their integration of genetics and genomics into the nursing curriculum. This consultation provided practical assistance to faculty teaching in undergraduate programs as they prepared for accreditation or reaccreditation by the Commission on Collegiate Nursing Education. The consultant was a nurse academician who is a content expert in clinical genetics. Description of the five colleges/universities that completed the consultation is provided in **Table 1**. Deans or department heads from each nursing program identified a faculty member to serve as a site coordinator and change agent. In preparation for the consultation site visit, faculty completed a self-study; details of the self-study are presented in **Table 2**.

Table 1
Description of nursing programs that participated in the Genomic Nursing Education in the Heartland Initiative

Nursing Program	Number of Undergraduate Students	Total Number of Faculty Teaching in the Undergraduate Nursing Program
Briar Cliff University Department of Nursing	184	7
University of Dubuque Department of Nursing	64	7
University of Kansas School of Nursing	262	38
Wichita State University School of Nursing	325	27
University of North Dakota College of Nursing	326	41

The self-study was followed by a 1-day, on-site consultation, which addressed (1) information on the background and significance of integrating genetics into curricula; (2) models or examples of how genetics and genomics is placed in curriculum; (3) faculty teaching resources; and (4) faculty resources for acquiring skills and knowledge in genetics and genomics.

An evaluation of the process was competed to determine the extent the consultation was beneficial to faculty, if curricular changes were made to reflect an infusion of genetic material, and if preparations completed by faculty resulted in accreditation or reaccreditation. The evaluation included a series of interviews with designated change agents, the faculty who coordinated the consultation at each site, and the consultant. A total of five faculty were interviewed across 2 time periods, first shortly after the consultation and second after their accreditation visit. The initial interview questions focused on a description of the consultation process at each site and reflections on the quality and benefits of the consultation. The follow-up interviews focused on a discussion of system and curricular changes that occurred as a result of the consultation as well as barriers encountered and the impact of curricular changes on the program (eg, accreditation).

Table 2
Self-study process completed before the consultation

Activity	Purpose	Reference
Take the GLAI	• To assist faculty members to assess their own genetic literacy	Bowling et al,[25] 2008; Daack-Hirsch et al,[7] 2012
Complete a self-study of the current curriculum	• Create a matrix that displays current or planned course by baccalaureate essential	AACN,[13] 2008
	• Identify where genetics content is currently taught	Daack-Hirsch et al,[18] 2011
	• Identify where genetic and genomic content could be enhanced or added	Daack-Hirsch et al,[18] 2011

Data from Refs.[7,13,18,25]

FINDINGS

All five programs had support from their respective administration, and by the end of the consultation faculty at each site who participated were fully supportive of the process. The results of the interviews are summarized across two primary areas, the quality of the consultation process and the programmatic outcomes. The results are summarized.

Quality of the Consultation Process

Timing and preparation matter

Strategically, this consultation was positioned to support colleges and universities that were preparing for reaccreditation. The value of timing the consultation in this fashion was confirmed by the faculty. Because genetics was a new component of accreditation, focusing the work of the faculty in this area was a top priority, so there was a readiness to focus attention in this area. One site indicated that the consultation helped jump-start their work because prior to the consultation, genetics and genomics were on the back burner. All the programs were already in a planning process in preparation for their accreditation visit and they reported that the content greatly helped to facilitate that process in the area of genetics. As part of the consultation process, faculty in the departments were asked to complete a self-assessment. Structuring the faculty's preparation in this way prior to the consultation visit was viewed as invaluable. Not only did taking the Genetic Literacy Assessment Instrument (GLAI) help faculty members assess their own genetic literacy but also they reported that taking the GLAI reassured them that they knew something about genetics and genomics.[25]

In addition to identifying courses where genetic and genomic content could be added, the self-assessment process provided a framework for faculty to review the extent to which they were currently integrating the genetic and genomic content. Many were not aware that they already had a foundation to build on—that they already had some genetics content in their curriculum. Identifying existing content made faculty view the task as "doable" and feel less overwhelmed.

Effective consultation helped sites generate a plan of action

Three key components of the consultation were viewed as contributing to the success of the consultation: the characteristics of the consultant, the planning process, and access to evidence-based resources. All faculty commented positively on the quality of the consultation that was provided. The characteristics of the consultant were identified as important to the success of the review and planning process accomplished with the core faculty. Knowledgeable, adept consultation skills, resourceful, affirming, and expert in this area were all terms used to describe the consultant. As one site commented, "The consultant helped faculty become excited about working in this area—it was extraordinary."

> The Consultation helped to de-mystify "genomics" and helped us to see how we could incorporate this content into our courses.
> —Faculty Member

The process was viewed as important because it helped identify both the strengths and gaps of their existing curriculum. Specifically, several commented that the individualization of the consultation fit their needs that in their view enhanced the process. The process also included concrete examples of practical strategies to present the information (eg, activities for students, objectives, and PowerPoint presentations). This information could easily be translated into teaching plans. The evidence-based resources that were provided were helpful and the faculty accessed many of the resources to review as they began to plan the content for their courses (**Table 3** lists resources).

The process had unexpected secondary outcomes

The format of the consultation process provided a template to design and build curricular processes for other content areas, such as informatics, culture, interprofessional education, and mass casualty. The process provided a dialog base for teams to discuss other areas of curriculum and to assist in leveling genetic and genomic content across programs (eg, undergraduate to graduate). New faculty were actively involved in the curricular development process and could be mentored by more-experienced faculty in the process of incorporating new required content into ongoing

Table 3
Resource guide

Resource Name	Description	URL
Genetics/Genomics Competency Center for Education (G2C2)	A freely available, open source repository of curricular materials designed to provide nursing educators the tools with which to prepare their students to meet the discipline-specific genetic and genomic competencies of health care.	http://www.g-2-c-2.org/
National Coalition for Health Professional Education in Genetics	Core Principles in Family History is a module to promote an understanding of how to take and interpret a family health history.	http://www.nchpeg.org/
National Human Genome Research Institute	Provides on-line genetic education resources on • Family history • Genetics 101 • The Genetic Information Nondiscrimination Act • The Human Genome Project	www.genome.gov
Genetics Home Reference: Your Guide to Understanding Genetic Conditions	Provides consumer-friendly information about the effects of genetic variations on human health.	http://ghr.nlm.nih.gov/
The PharmGenEd™ Program	Funded by the Centers for Disease Control and Prevention and the American Society of Health-System Pharmacists, this site provides educational materials on pharmacogenomics.	http://pharmacogenomics.ucsd.edu
Online Mendelian Inheritance in Man (OMIM)	A comprehensive and authoritative compendium of human genes and genetic phenotypes.	http://www.ncbi.nlm.nih.gov/omim
GeneTests	A medical genetics information resource on genetic testing developed for health care providers and researchers.	http://www.ncbi.nlm.nih.gov/sites/GeneTests/

classes. An unexpected outcome of the consultation for one program was that for new faculty there was increased understanding of the accreditation process. For some, the faculty developed a "sense of community." One faculty member commented: "…together we are responsible for the education of students in this area."

Programmatic Outcomes

Genetics content was integrated in nursing coursework

As a result of the consultation, all sites indicated that concrete changes occurred. Not only did the consultation support curricular changes but also overall it was reported that nursing faculty from each of the nursing programs had increased confidence in their ability to integrate genetic and genomic content into their courses. For all, the changes included integrating genetics and genomics across the curriculum rather than creating a freestanding genomics course.

Integrating content, however, takes a considerable amount of collaboration in order to avoid unnecessary repetition of content, and teamwork was key to each program's ability to integrate genetics throughout the curricula. In order to avoid unnecessary repetition of content, faculty in one of the programs developed a table for the undergraduate curriculum to identify which course would "introduce" or "reinforce/apply" each essential nursing competency for genetic and genomics content. Four of the five programs made changes throughout the curriculum within the first year after the consultation by either adding or strengthening genetic or genomic content in four or more of the follow courses: pathophysiology, health assessment, therapeutic intervention, health communication, foundations courses, community or population-based health care, maternal child nursing, obstetrics, medical/surgical, and pharmacology. The extent to which integration took place was faculty driven based on the program needs and comfort level of the faculty. The programs intend to increase the amount and complexity of the genetic and genomic content as the faculty become increasingly confident in their knowledge of genetics and genomics. Faculty brought up the need to focus on legal, social, and cultural implications of genetic testing. Ideas for future genetic and genomic–related topics included genetic and genomic implications to health care cost, pedigrees and the electronic health record, and roles of genetics in addressing a multicultural mixed race patient care delivery system.

At one of the programs, the faculty expressed a sense of overload related to the amount of genetic and genomic content that needs to be covered in the curriculum. They thought that in order to make the change successful, it was important to develop the genomics content incrementally rather than expecting wholesale incorporation of content that the faculty were still trying to understand themselves. In consideration of this, the faculty developed one goal statement for the new academic year:

> Faculty will individually evaluate their courses, and based on this evaluation incorporate content related to genetics by adding to unit-level objectives for a minimum of one course this academic year. Outcomes will be assessed either in test or assignment format. Faculty will share their work at the convening Nursing Faculty meeting in the fall.

The first step in their process was the decision to establish a foundation for the incorporation of genetics and genomics for nursing core courses to build on. It seemed evident to faculty in this program that a first-semester course, pathophysiology and applied pharmacology, was the obvious place to do this. The faculty who team teach this course conducted an appraisal of their existing course content outline; then, based on this assessment, the decision was made to add genomic content to the unit that addresses the concept of altered cell and tissue biology.

This approach proved successful, so the following year the faculty made the decision to continue this goal as part of the nursing department's assessment plan action items for improvement in the next year. In this way, they are adding genomics content to the curriculum in a manner that faculty do not find overwhelming yet still demonstrates progress toward addressing the American Association of Colleges of Nursing (AACN) essentials related to genomics.

All sites received accreditation or reaccreditation
One program was reviewed for accreditation and four programs were under reaccreditation review. All five programs were successful in receiving accreditation or recommended for reaccreditation. The follow-up interviews suggested participation in the Heartland Initiative helped their university/college to receive their accreditation or reaccreditation. Many cited that the students will benefit from these changes in the curriculum content because the will have increased knowledge of genetics and genomics.

Challenges and areas for improvement
Challenges to the process included lack of knowledge in genetics and genomics, difficulty keeping up with rapid changes in genetics, time constraints, and crowded curriculum. Faculty at one university shared that there is still limited discussion on genetics in nurse educator continuing education conferences. Many of the sites indicated that a 3- to 6-month follow-up session would be helpful. This would provide for an opportunity to bring the faculty together to review what they have planned and have a consultant to join them in this review. This follow-up would help assure accountability to the individual action plans that were developed at each institution.

SUMMARY

These schools and colleges of nursing faculty were able to face the challenges that make incorporating genetics and genomics difficult by working with a content expert and, more importantly, through collaboration and teamwork. By mapping existing and new courses to AACN guidelines, faculty were able to identity where genetics content already existed and where gaps occurred. Faculty from each program tailored a plan to incrementally integrate their curriculum with genetics and genomics content that built on their strengths at a pace that accommodated faculty readiness. In turn, faculty reported increasing confidence and comfort in their ability to apply genetics and genomics content within their curriculum.

REFERENCES

1. Green ED, Guyer MS. Charting a course for genomic medicine from base pairs to bedside. Nature 2011;470(7333):204–13. http://dx.doi.org/10.1038/nature09764.
2. Calzone KA, Jenkins J, Nicole N, et al. Relevance of genomics to healthcare and nursing practice. J Nurs Scholarsh 2013;45(1):1–2. http://dx.doi.org/10.1111/j.1547-5069.2012.01464.x.
3. Lea DH, Skirton H, Read CY, et al. Implications for educating the next generation of nurses on genetics and genomics in the 21st century. J Nurs Scholarsh 2011;43(1):3–12. http://dx.doi.org/10.1111/j.1547-5069.2010.01373.x.
4. Thompson HJ, Brooks MV. Genetics and genomics in nursing: evaluation essentials implementation. Nurse Educ Today 2011;31(6):623–7. http://dx.doi.org/10.1016/j.nedt.2010.10.023.

5. Calzone KA, Cashion A, Feetham S, et al. Nurses transforming health care using genetics and genomics. Nurs Outlook 2010;58(1):26–35. http://dx.doi.org/10.1016/j.outlook.2009.05.001.

6. Collins CA, Stiles AS. Predictors of student outcomes on perceived knowledge and competence of genetic family history risk assessment. J Prof Nurs 2011; 27(2):101–7. http://dx.doi.org/10.1016/j.profnurs.2010.09.007.

7. Daack-Hirsch S, Driessnack M, Perkhounkova Y, et al. A practical first step to integrating genetics into curriculum. J Nurs Educ 2012;51(5):294–8. http://dx.doi.org/10.3928/01484834-20120309-02.

8. Dodson CH, Lewallen LP. Nursing students' perceived knowledge and attitudes towards genetics. Nurse Educ Today 2011;31(4):333–9. http://dx.doi.org/10.1016/j.nedt.2010.07.001.

9. Kiray Vural B, Tomatir AG, Kuzu Kurban N, et al. Nursing students' self-reported knowledge of genetics and genetic education. Public Health Genomics 2009; 12(4):225–32. http://dx.doi.org/10.1159/000197972.

10. Maradiegue A, Edwards QT, Seibert D, et al. Knowledge, perceptions, and attitudes of advanced practice nursing students regarding medical genetics. J Am Acad Nurse Pract 2005;17(11):472–9. http://dx.doi.org/10.1111/j.1745-7599.2005.00076.x.

11. Edwards QT, Maradiegue A, Seibert D, et al. Faculty members' perceptions of medical genetics and its integration into nurse practitioner curricula. J Nurs Educ 2006;45(3):124–30.

12. Secretary's Advisory Committee on Genetics, Health, and Society (SACGH). Genetics education and training; 2011. Available at: http://oba.od.nih.gov/oba/SACGHS/reports/SACGHS_education_report_2011.pdf. Accessed February 24, 2013.

13. American Association of Colleges of Nursing. The essentials of baccalaureate education for professional nursing practice. Washington, DC: Author; 2008.

14. Consensus Panel on Genetic/Genomic Nursing Competencies. Essentials of genetic and genomic nursing: competencies, curricula guidelines, and outcome indicators. 2nd edition. Silver Spring (MD): American Nurses Association; 2009.

15. Grady PA, Collins FS. Genetics and nursing science: realizing the potential. Nurs Res 2003;52(2):69.

16. Jenkins J, Grady PA, Collins FS. Nurses and the genetics revolution. J Nurs Scholarsh 2005;37(2):98–101. http://dx.doi.org/10.1111/j.1547-5069.2005.00020.x.

17. National Coalition for Health Professional Education in Genetics [NCHPEG]. Available at: http://www.nchpeg.org. Accessed April 2, 2013.

18. Daack-Hirsch S, Dieter C, Quinn Griffen MT. Integrating genomics into undergraduate nursing education. J Nurs Scholarsh 2011;43(3):223–30. http://dx.doi.org/10.1111/j.1547-5069.2011.01400.x.

19. Read CY, Dylis AM, Mott SR, et al. Promoting integration of genetics core competencies into entry-level nursing curricula. J Nurs Educ 2004;43(8):376–80.

20. Hetteberg C, Prows CA. A checklist to assist in the integration of genetics into nursing curricula. Nurs Outlook 2004;52(2):85–8. http://dx.doi.org/10.1016/j.outlook.2004.01.007.

21. Calzone KA, Jerome-D'Emilia B, Jenkins J, et al. Establishment of the genetic/genomic competency center for education. J Nurs Scholarsh 2011;43(4):351–8. http://dx.doi.org/10.1111/j.1547-5069.2011.01412.x.

22. The Genetics/Genomics Competency Center [G2C2]. Available at: http://www.g-2-c-2.org/. Accessed April 2, 2013.

23. Tonkin E, Calzone K, Jenkins J, et al. Genomic education resources for nursing faculty. J Nurs Scholarsh 2011;43(4):330–40. http://dx.doi.org/10.1111/j.1547-5069.2011.01415.x.
24. Williams JK, Prows CA, Conley YP, et al. Strategies to prepare faculty to integrate genomics into nursing education programs. J Nurs Scholarsh 2011;43(3):231–8. http://dx.doi.org/10.1111/j.1547-5069.2011.01401.x.
25. Bowling BV, Acra EE, Wang L, et al. Development and evaluation of a genetics literacy assessment instrument for undergraduates. Genetics 2008;178(1): 15–22. http://dx.doi.org/10.1534/genetics.107.079533.

Cytochrome p450, Part 1
What Nurses Really Need to Know

Stephen D. Krau, PhD, RN, CNE

KEYWORDS

- Adverse drug reactions • Adverse drug events • Pharmacogenetics
- Cytochrome p450 • Medication variation • Pharmacokinetics • Pharmacodynamics

KEY POINTS

- The purpose of this first article in a series of three is to describe the cytochrome p450 (CYP), to familiarize nurse practitioners with the nomenclature, and to explain the basis for variations in drug metabolism at it relates to the CYP family of enzymes.
- Because more pharmaceutical companies are including this information on their products, it is imperative that a thorough understanding of the meaning and function of the enzymes be included when prescribing medications.
- It is important to consider patients' classifications with regard to their ability to metabolize drugs based on variants in the enzyme system and the genetic basis for the distinctions.
- Gender and race considerations are demonstrable factors in the effect of medications and the levels of efficacy and toxicity or no effect.
- Through understanding the information that is available, and using the information in clinical practice, nurse practitioners will be more effective prescribers, have fewer adverse events, and have overall faster and better patient outcomes.

An abundance of literature and recent studies describes the impact of the CYP enzyme system and its impact on patient pharmacokinetics and pharmacodynamics as more pharmaceutical companies are including CYP information on their products. This important information has not translated, however, in practice, resulting in under-medicating patients, overmedicating patients, and treating patients with medications that simply do not work for those patients. In the absence of this information, or more accurately, not using or understanding the information that is available, clinicians prescribe medications in a trial-and-error approach, hoping for the desired outcome. Nurses administering medications must be vigilant for common side effects and for evaluating the efficacy of the medication, which can vary tremendously. In current clinical practice, when the desired results are not achieved by a specific medication, a different medication is prescribed, and then another and another until a desired outcome is reached. Each time this occurs, the patient becomes an experiment in

The author has nothing to disclose.
Vanderbilt University Medical Center, School of Nursing, 461 21st Avenue South, Nashville, TN 37240, USA
E-mail address: steve.krau@vanderbilt.edu

Nurs Clin N Am 48 (2013) 671–680
http://dx.doi.org/10.1016/j.cnur.2013.09.002
0029-6465/13/$ – see front matter © 2013 Elsevier Inc. All rights reserved.

finding the right medication for the situation. In the meantime, although patients are not experiencing therapeutic effects of medications, they may experience drug events that are harmful and in some cases even lethal. This is largely due to the genetic variations and drug interactions mediated by the CYP enzyme family.

Although well understood and enlightened by scientific research, the clinical application of the CYP enzyme family in nursing and in medicine remains embryonic. This is the first article in a series of 3 articles that hopes to provide nurses with an overview of the CYP family of enzymes, to describe their impact on drug metabolism, and to provide nurses at the bedside and nurses that prescribe with the tools needed to incorporate existing information about the enzymes into their practices to safely achieve effective patient outcomes.

INTERINDIVIDUAL VARIATION IN DRUG RESPONSE

Interindividual variation in drug response poses a serious problem in the management of patients who are receiving medications to treat or prevent any disease or illness. Bioavailability of drug concentrations can vary more than 600-fold between two individuals with the same weight and using the same drug dosage.[1] Genetic variants can make a difference between two people even when treated with the same medications and same dose. Additionally, due to individual variations in response to drug therapy, this variability can result in toxicity and adverse drug reactions (ADRs). There are many factors that may account for differences in drug response, such as lifestyle choices or cultural practices, that inherently have the potential for alteration and change and, thus, are to some extent modifiable. Factors, such as gender, genetic makeup, and race, cannot be easily altered, if at all, and warrant consideration when determining which medication and dosage will provide appropriate treatment. Persons who are administering or prescribing medications can make the best decisions with regard to the most effective medication regimen when they understand fundamental aspects of interindividual variations at the cellular level that account for the disparities in drug responses. It is important for patient-centered care for nurses to have fundamental knowledge about the human CYP system, its impact on variant medications, current considerations in the management of specific clinical outcomes, and the ability to incorporate this information into nursing practice.

ADVERSE DRUG REACTIONS

Nurses who administer medications have known for years that substantial interindividual variability occurs in clinical responses to drug treatments of acute and chronic diseases. The proportion of patients who respond to medications as intended is, on average, only approximately 50%, with a range of 25% to 60%.[2,3] This not only contributes to the incidence of ADRs but also poses a delay in reaching an appropriate therapeutic level of another drug and in achieving beneficial outcomes for patients. A landmark meta-analysis suggested that ADRs ranked between the fourth and sixth leading causes of death in the United States in 1994, having an impact on more than an estimated 2 million patients.[4–6] A more recent study identifies ADRs as the seventh leading cause of death[7]; there is evidence to support that fatal ADRs occur in approximately 0.32% of hospitalized patients.[6] Approximately 2 days of prolonged hospitalization are attributed to ADRs in the United States, and 100,000 deaths annually are estimated due to ADRs.[8,9]

Although ADRs have not been studied in the pediatric population to the same extent as in adults, the significance of the problem is a major concern. ADRs have been reported as the cause of 4.3% of pediatric hospital admissions in children under 2 years of age.[4,10] The incidence of ADRs is even higher for infants in intensive care units who are suffering from multiple system failure.

RACE AND GENDER DISPARITIES IN CLINICAL DRUG TRIALS

The importance of understanding the impact of the CYP family of enzymes on human drug metabolism becomes more apparent when considering the subjects in clinical drug trials. Although considered one of the rigorous forms of research and reliable evidence, it is important to look at the gender and ethnic background of the participants in these studies. For example, in a review by Umarjee and colleagues,[11] from the Food and Drug Administration (FDA), of cardiovascular drug trials reviewed by the FDA from 2007 to 2008, 78% of the subjects enrolled were white, 7% black, 6% Asian, and 6% Hispanic. Furthermore, in drug trials related to hypertension, which is of high incidence among blacks in the United States, the composition of the drug trials from 2007 to 2008 were white (73%), black (11%), Asian (3%), Hispanic (7%), and other (7%).[11] For medications related to arrhythmias that were reviewed from 2007 to 2008, 93% of the participants were white.[11] Using clinical trials to determine dosing strategies for all patients of all ethnic backgrounds is clearly problematic.

Umarjee and colleagues[11] also identified gender disparities among the subjects in drug trials related to cardiovascular medications from 2007 to 2008. With the high incidence of mortality among women with cardiovascular diseases, it should be apparent that women do not present with the symptoms that are typical of men, so physiologic gender differences are apparent in symptoms, just as they are in drug metabolism. With the clinical drug trials related to these medications, however, overall the participants were identified as 62.99% men and 34.88% women.[11] For specific cardiac drugs, such as drugs used for acute coronary syndrome, the participants were 70.7% men, and for drugs used in heart failure, 72.79% were men.[11]

The FDA Adverse Event Reporting System (AERS) is a voluntary database of adverse events. Based on an analysis of AERS data and other data resources, women experience more adverse events than men, and, for the most part, these adverse events are of a more serious nature.[12–16] There are additional data that support the negative effects of approved medications on women. Ten drugs that were withdrawn from the market between January 1, 1997, and December 2000 were reviewed by the US Government Accountability Office, which found that 8 of the 10 were withdrawn due to greater risks of ADRs in women.[17]

It is apparent that the current evidence based on clinical drug trials and of the potential impact of medications on a variety of patients is lacking. Current medication protocols and dosing strategies based on predominant subject groups do not represent society as whole and do little to consider genetic differences. The vulnerability of the system is detrimental to the health of patients, in particular those not included in the clinical drug trial. The current paradigm of medication prescription is based on diagnosis, then prescription based on the meager evidence that exists, and then observing patient response. When what is prescribed is not working, or there is an adverse effect, the medication is changed and changed again until the desired outcome is achieved. The current paradigm is little more than trial and error based on limited information. Pharmacogenetics is the basis for a change in the paradigm where after diagnosis, based on patient genetics, the correct medication is prescribed for a patient.

THE CONTEXT OF PHARMACOGENETICS

Genomics is a science that is central to all health care providers because essentially all diseases, disorders, and conditions have a genetic or genomic component. In order to understand the genetic variants that occur with medication administration, it is essential to understand the components and concepts from the perspective of pharmacogenetics. Additionally, clarification of terms helps clarify the concept and aids in common discussion among health care providers. Pharmacogenetics is the study of single gene variations that result in altered drug response. Pharmacogenetics originated in the 1950s as a result of many discoveries, including the sensitivity to primaquine, slow isoniazid acetylation, and butyrylcholinesterase deficiency—all of which indicated the influence of genetics on drug response. Subsequent pharmacogenetic studies focused on characterizing the effects of variation in drug-metabolizing enzymes on pharmacokinetics and have considered primarily type A ADRs. Type A ADRs are those that are commonly dose dependent and are predictable exaggerations of the known actions of the drug. Type B ADRs, in contrast, are idiosyncratic and typically show no apparent dose-response relationship.[1] In the past decade, there has been a concerted effort to broaden genetic variation and to sequence the entire human genome. This has been the focus of the Human Genome Project completed in 2003. Additionally there have been efforts to identify and map genomic variability through such projects as the HapMap Project, which is ongoing. These projects have opened the venue for linking phenotypes with genetic variation in previously unknown drug targets, such as those responsible for type B ADRs.

These efforts have resulted in the newer term, *pharmacogenomics*, which is essentially an extension of pharmacogenetics to the study of the drug response–related polymorphisms at the genomic level.[1] This field advances the goal of personalized medicine through identifying patients who should not receive certain medications and those who should receive modified dosing. There has been a dramatic increase in the body of literature related to pharmacogenomics in the past decade. The extensive body of literature provides many examples of noteworthy alterations in drug metabolism, drug transport, and drug interactions as a result of gene polymorphisms. These advances parallel advances in medical technology and the completion of the Human Genome Project; however, they have yet to find a strong base in clinical practice.

CYTOCHROME p450 ENZYME SYSTEM

The CYP enzyme family constitutes a superfamily of heme-thiolate enzymes, of which more than 2700 individual members are known. They are associated with oxidative metabolism of a large number of both endogenous and exogenous organic compounds. Although absent in some species of bacteria, CYP enzymes have been found in all 5 biologic kingdoms.[18] There are 57 varieties of CYP in *Homo sapiens* with a majority of these enzymes present in the families of CYP1 to CYP4. It is well known that CYP1, CYP2, and CYP3 have a major role in the metabolism of exogenous compounds, whereas CYP4 has its main role on endogenous processes. In addition to the aforementioned impact on exogenous drug metabolism, there is an endogenous functionality of CYP that centers on the biosynthesis of steroid hormones, prostaglandins, fatty acids, eicosanoids, and vitamin D_3.[19,20]

CYP is a cellular chromophore that was named as such because the pigment has a 450-nm spectral peak when reduced and bound to carbon monoxide.[21] At first glance, the numbering nomenclature of these enzymes may seem daunting, but the organization of the families and subfamilies is based on the percentage of amino acid sequence identity. The enzymes that share greater than or equal to 40% sequence identity are assigned to a particular family designated by an Arabic numeral. Enzymes that share more than or equal to 55% identity make up a subfamily identified by a letter. Nebert and Russell[20] pose that this example, the sterol 27-hydroxylase enzyme and the vitamin D 24-hydroxylase enzyme, are both assigned to the CYP27 family because they share more than 40% of the sequence identity. Sterol hyroxylase is further assigned to the CYP27A subfamily, and the vitamin D 24-hydroxylase is assigned to the CYP27B family because their protein sequences are less than 55% identical. In the event that an additional enzyme is discovered that shares greater than or equal to 55% identity with the sterol 27-hydroxylase, it would be classified as CYP27A2.[20] This logical system of nomenclature has eliminated much of the confusion that is frequently associated with other gene family nomenclatures. A more comprehensive view of the nomenclature is available on the cytochrome allele Web site (http://www.cypalleles.ki.se/criteria.htm).[9]

The CYP family of enzymes represents the most important phase I drug-metabolizing enzymes, which oxidize a large number of endogenous substances, such as eiconsanoids, steroids, and a large number of xenobiotics, mostly therapeutic drugs and environmental compounds, into more hydrophilic compounds. More than 90% of human drug oxidation can be attributed to the CYP enzyme family.[22] A breakdown of the percentages for the salient enzyme subfamilies is conveyed in **Fig. 1**. It is the variability in the CYP content and activities that have a profound influence on the response of humans to drugs.

Although much of this discussion is related to drug metabolism, advances in biology and genomics have revealed several processes associated with the CYPs. Once believed to only metabolize drugs in the liver, current data indicate that the CYPs also act on a variety of endogenous substrates that are not necessarily medication related by introducing oxidative, perioxidative, and reductive changes into small molecules of a variety of chemicals.[20] Some of these substrates include saturated and unsaturated fatty acids, vitamin D derivatives, sterols and steroids, bile acids, retinoids, and uroporphyrinogens. It is now also known that CYPs metabolize not only drugs but also a variety of exogenous compounds, including environmental chemicals and pollutants as well as natural plant products. The implications of this function have only just

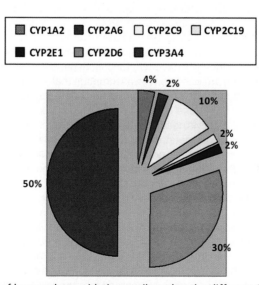

Fig. 1. Percentage of human drug oxidation attributed to the different CYP enzymes. (*Data from* Zhou SF. Polymorphism of human cytochrome p450 2D6 and its clinical significance: part 1. Clin Pharmacokinet 2009;48(11):689–723.)

begun to be uncovered. Additionally, metabolism of foreign chemicals usually results in the detoxification of an irritant; however, the metabolites that are generated from this process can also contribute to increased risks of cancer, birth defects, and other toxic effects.[20] The wide range of CYP functions has clear significance for patients and warrants consideration at every level. The prescriptive role of nurse practitioners focuses the discussion of the CYPs toward medication; however, when considering patients in holistic terms, all aspects of the impact of the CYPs mandate deliberation.

DRUG-METABOLIZING VARIANTS

In humans, the CYP genes are highly polymorphic, which means that they occur in different forms and have variant mutations. These variant forms can produce enzymes with altered, reduced, increased, or no enzyme activity in the total amount of the enzyme that is expressed. It is these variants that may produce drug levels that are higher or lower than anticipated, resulting in an ADR or a decreased efficacy of the drug. The enzymatic activity of the CYP provides the basis for the classification levels of metabolization. Individuals are classified phenotypically as poor metabolizers (PMs), intermediate metabolizers (IMs), extensive metabolizers (EMs), or ultrarapid metabolizers (UMs).[21] The variations are the results of differences in a person's genetics, particularly as related to their alleles. An allele is one member of a pair of genes occupying a specific spot on a particular chromosome that determines a trait.[23] In humans, simple traits are the result of the interaction between one pair of alleles, whereas more complex traits are often the result of interactions among a series of alleles. The interactions between a pair of alleles when they are the same are considered homozygous and when they are different are referred to as heterozygous. In lay terms, people often refer to genes that are accompanied by a trait that is actually a phenotype. For example, people may say they have "tall genes," in which case the phenotype is tall; however, the more scientific term for genes is *allele*.[23]

Persons who are PMs are either compound heterozygous for different inactivating alleles or homozygous for an inactivating variant and may display functional enzyme deficiencies. In either case, persons who are PMs deviate dramatically from what is expected when administered a drug specific to that enzyme. IMs carry one allele that is functional and one allele that is nonfunctional but may demonstrate a great deal of variation in enzyme activity. EMs have two functional gene copies. In general, current strategies for drug dosing are based on the assumption that a patient is an EM. Persons who are EMs usually comprise the largest proportion of the population. UMs have more than 2 functional genes from gene duplication resulting in ultrarapid metabolism.[22]

The clinical relevance of this is necessary to this discussion. Dosing based on normal concentrations are based on metabolism exhibited by EMs. For PMs, the targeted medication is metabolized slowly or not at all, which increases the risk of side effects, some which might even be lethal. PMs more than likely require lower doses of the target medication compared with standard EMs. IMs break down the targeted medication at a slower rate than EMs, possibly requiring a lower than normal dose of the medication. EMs are the identified as metabolizers at a normal rate and provide the basis for most standard dosaging. For polymorphisms to be clinically important, the effect of the polymorphism must be identified and separated from other factors that might cause variance in the drug effect. UMs metabolize a targeted medication rapidly, resulting in decreased bioavailability of the drug, which can result in a poor therapeutic response, possibly mandating a dose higher than the standard for that medication.[24,25]

Additionally, the therapeutic index, which is the space between the efficacy of a drug and its toxicity, of each drug warrants consideration. For example, if a drug has a high therapeutic index and is safe over a wide range of concentrations that encompasses the variations caused by genetics, then it might not be necessary to consider polymorphisms in the context of therapeutics. If a drug, such as warfarin, however, has a low therapeutic index, minor variations in concentrations as the result of polymorphisms may be extremely important.[22]

As a clear consequence, drug adverse effects or lack of drug effect can occur when standard dosing is applied. For example, 30% of human drug oxidation can be attributed to CYP2D6. Typical substrates for the metabolism of largely lipophilic bases include several antidepressants, antipsychotics, antiarrythmics, β-blockers, opiods, and antiemetics.[22] Phenotypically, among whites, UMs comprise 3% to 5% of the population whereas EMs comprise 70% to 80%, IMs comprise 10% to 17%, and 5% to 10% are PMs.[26] Among Chinese, PMs of the CYPD26 enzyme account for approximately 1% of the population, whereas 0% to 19% of African Americans are PMs.[22,27,28] Additionally, 1% to 2% of Swedish whites[29] and 16% of black Ethiopians[30] have more than extrafunctional allele resulting in an UM phenotype. The PM phenotype is the result of the presence of 2 nonfunctional, or null, alleles, whereas the EM phenotype is due to 1 or 2 alleles with normal function.

The rate of metabolism of a drug is important in discerning the therapeutic regimen of that drug. This point is illustrated in two cases concerning persons who are UMs of codeine related to the CYP2D6. Codeine is activated into morphine exclusively by the CYP2D6 enzyme. In one case, a person was receiving prescribed cough medicine containing codeine. Due to the excessive activation of the enzyme, the patient experienced life-threatening opioid intoxication.[31] In another case, a breastfeeding mother was prescribed codeine as an analgesic postdelivery. Thirteen days after delivery, the baby died. Postmortem analysis of the breast milk showed levels of morphine 4 times higher than expected. The mother was found to have CYP2D6 gene duplication, which explains higher than normal morphine levels in the breast milk; however, the baby was an EM.[32] Studies have also shown that in administration of codeine to healthy volunteers of known CYP2D6 genotype, UMs are significantly more likely than EMs metabolizers to suffer sedation.[33] There is also current evidence suggesting that babies of mothers with UM CYP2D6 genotypes who use codeine as an analgesic are more likely to experience central nervous system depression than other babies.[34,35]

GENDER DIFFERENCES IN DRUG METABOLISM

There are significant differences in the drug responses between men and women. The importance of these differences has put women at higher risk for adverse drug events. It is known that women are more frequently overdosed than men and that pharmadynamically women are more sensitive to medications than men, and, related to issues of drug interactions, it is known that women take more medications than men.[36] There are many physiologic differences between men and women that influence absorption, and there are body composition differences that influence drug distribution. There are CYP enzymes that are coded by autosomal chromosomes that account for differences in certain enzymes, but furthermore it is plausible that gender-related disparities in drug metabolism could be the result of endogenous hormonal influences.[36] In spite of efforts to include women in clinical studies, there remain many gaps in knowledge relating to appropriate dose, dosing schedule, and treatment intervals for not only pregnant women but also women in general.[37]

Differences in the pharmacokinetics-related CYP enzymes are conclusive for certain enzymes. For example, it is known that there is a higher activity level of CYP3A in women than in men.[38] Typical substrates for this enzyme include midazolam, dapsone, cortisol, lidocaine, nifedipine, and erythromycin. Additionally, the activity level of CYP1A is more active in men than in women.[39] Model substrates of this enzyme include caffeine, nicotine, and paracetamol (acetaminophen). The CYP2D6 enzyme is less active in men than in women, and model substrates of this enzyme include dextromethorphan, debrisoquine, and spartene.[36] The CYP2E1 enzyme is more active in men than in women because the model substrate for this enzyme is chlorzoxazone. This is just a formative list of how the enzyme is different between genders.

Although some of these enzymes were discovered more than 30 years ago, and there has been genetic testing to determine some of these nuances for more than 20 years, genetic testing has failed to move into clinical practice on a routine basis.[35] There are several potential reasons for this, which include the general difficulty of introducing genetic tests into clinical settings, the fact that several key substrates for some of these enzymes have been taken off the market because of issues with PMs, and the changes in medication and ever-improving pharmaceutics. Additionally, there is a current lack of knowledge among providers about genetics and pharmacogenetics, and there is a lack of solid clear evidence in large conclusive studies related to improvement as a result of genotyping.[40] There is increasing evidence, however, that these enzymes are relevant to the outcomes of treatments with commonly used medications.[35]

SUMMARY

The purpose of this first article in a series of three is to describe the CYP, to familiarize nurse practitioners with the nomenclature, and to explain the basis for variations in drug metabolism at it relates to the CYP family of enzymes. Because more pharmaceutical companies are including this information on their products, it is imperative that a thorough understanding of the meaning and function of the enzymes be included when prescribing medications. It is important to consider patients' classifications with regard to their ability to metabolize drugs based on variants in the enzyme system and the genetic basis for the distinctions. Gender and race considerations are demonstrable factors in the effect of medications and the level of efficacy, toxicity, or no effect. Through understanding the information that is available and using the information in clinical practice, nurse practitioners will be more effective prescribers, have fewer adverse events, and have overall faster and better patient outcomes.

REFERENCES

1. Sim SC, Ingelman-Sundberg M. The Human Cytochrome p450 Allele Nomenclature Committee web site. Cytochrome P450 Protocols. In: Phillips IR, Shepard EA, editors. Methods in molecular biology, vol. 320, 2nd edition. Totowa (NJ): Humana Press Inc; 2006. p. 183–9.
2. Squassina A, Manchia M, Vangelis G, et al. Realities and expectations of pharmacogenics and personalized medicine: impact of translating genetic knowledge into clinical practice. Pharmacogenomics 2010;11(8):1149–67.
3. Spear BB, Heath-Chiozzi M, Huff J. Clinical application of pharmacogenetics. Trends Mol Med 2001;7:201–4.
4. Becker ML, Leeder JS. Identifying genomic and developmental causes of adverse drug reactions in children. Pharmacogenomics 2010;11(11):1591–602.
5. Lazarou J, Pameranz BH, Corey PN. Incidence of adverse drug reactions in hospitalized patients. JAMA 1998;279:1200–5.
6. Davies EC, Green CF, Mottram DR, et al. Adverse drug reactions in hospitals: a narrative review. Curr Drug Saf 2007;2:79–87.

7. Wester K, Johnson AK, Sigset O, et al. Incidence of fatal adverse drug reactions: a population based study. Br J Clin Pharmacol 2008;65:573–9.
8. Eichelbaum M, Ingelmann-Sunberg M, Evans WE. Pharmagogenomics and individualized drug therapy. Annu Rev Med 2006;57:119–37.
9. Sim SC, Ingelman-Sunberg M. The human cytochrom P450 (CYP) Allele nomenclature website: a peer-reviewed database of CYP variants and their associated effects. Hum Genomics 2010;4(4):278–81.
10. Martinez-Mir I, Garcia-Lopez M, Palop V, et al. A prospective study of adverse drug reactions in hospitalized children. Br J Clin Pharmacol 1999; 47:681–8.
11. Umarjee S, Lemtouni S, Fadiran E, et al. Enrollment of women in cardiovascular drug trials reviewed by the FDA from 2007 to 2008. Office of Women's Health, Office of the Commissioner, Food and Drug Administration. Available at: http://www.docstoc.com/docs/75241529/US-Food-and-Drug-Administration-Home-Page. Accessed August 1, 2011.
12. Zopf Y, Rabe C, Neubert A, et al. Risk factors associated with adverse drug reactions following hospital admission: a prospective analysis of 907 patients in two German university hospitals. Drug Saf 2008;31(9):789–98.
13. Tran C, Knowles SR, Liu BA, et al. Gender differences in adverse drug reactions. J Clin Pharmacol 1998;38(11):1003–9.
14. Gray J. Why can't a woman be more like a man? Clin Pharmacol Ther 2007;82(1): 15–7.
15. Schwartz JB. The current state of knowledge on age, sex, and their interactions on clinical pharmacology. Clin Pharmacol Ther 2007;82(1):87–96.
16. Aarnoudse AL, Dieleman JP, Stricker BH. Age- and gender-specific incidence of hospitalisation for digoxin intoxication. Drug Saf 2007;30(5):431–6.
17. Heinrich J. Drug safety: most drugs withdrawn in recent years had greater health risks for women. 2001. Available at: http://www.gao.gov/new.items/d01286r.pdf. Accessed August 1, 2011.
18. Lewis DF. 57 varieties: the human cytochrome p450. Pharmacogenomics 2004; 5(3):305–18.
19. Rendic S. Summary of information on the human CYP enzymes; human p450 metabolism data. Drug Metab Rev 2002;34:83–448.
20. Nebert DW, Russell DW. Clinical importance of the cytochrome p450. Lancet 2002;360:1155–62.
21. Jaja C, Wylie B, Thummel K, et al. Cytochrome P450 enzyme polymorphism frequency in indigenous and native American populations: a systematic review. Community Genet 2008;11:141–9.
22. Zhou S. Polymorphism of the human cytochrome P450 D26 and its clinical significance: part I. Clin Pharmacokinet 2009;48(11):689–723.
23. Available at: http://www.biology-online.org/dictionary/Allele. Accessed August 1, 2011.
24. Pestka EL, Hale AM, Johnson BL, et al. Cytochrome p450 testing for better psychiatric care. Psychopharmacology 2007;45(10):15–8.
25. Gardiner SJ, Begg EJ. Pharmacogenetics, drug metabolizing ensymes, and clinical practice. Pharmacol Rev 2006;58(3):521–90.
26. Sachse C, Brockmoller J, Bauer S, et al. Cytochrome p450 2D6 variants in a Caucasian population: allele frequencies and phenotypic consequences. Am J Hum Genet 1997;60:284–95.
27. Bradford LD. CYP2D6 allele frequency in European Caucasians, Asians, African and their descendants. Pharmacogenomics 2002;3:229–43.

28. Johansson I, Yue QY, Dahl ML, et al. Genetic analysis of the interethnic difference between Chinese and Caucasians in the polymorphic metabolism of debrisoquine and codeine. Eur J Clin Pharmacol 1991;40:553–6.

29. Dahl ML, Johansson I, Bertilsson L, et al. Ultrarapid hydroxylation of debrisoquine in a Swedish population: analysis of the molecular genetic basis. J Pharmacol Exp Ther 1995;274:516–20.

30. Aklillu E, Persson I, Bertilsson L, et al. Frequent distribution of ultrarapid metabolizers of debrisoquine in an Ethiopian population carrying duplicated and multi-duplicated functional CYP2D6 alleles. J Pharmacol Exp Ther 1996;278:441–6.

31. Gasche Y, Daali Y, Fathi M, et al. Codeine intoxication associated with ultrarapid CYP2D6 metabolism. N Engl J Med 2004;351:2827–31.

32. Koren G, Cairns J, Chitayat D, et al. Phramacogenetics of morphine poisoning in a breastfed neonate of a codeine prescribed mother. Lancet 2006;368:704.

33. Kirchheiner J, Schmidt H, Tzvetkov M, et al. Pharmacokinetics of codeine and its metabolite morphine in ultra-rapid metabolizers due to CYP2D6 duplication. Pharmacogenomics J 2006;7:257–65.

34. Madadi P, Ross CJ, Hayden MR, et al. Pharmacogenetics of neonatal opioid toxicity following maternal use of codeine during breastfeeding: a case-control study. Clin Pharmacol Ther 2009;85:31–5.

35. Daly AK. Pharmacogenetics and human genetic polymorphisms. Biochem J 2010;429:435–49.

36. Soldin OP, Mattison DR. Sex differences in pharmacokinetics and pharmacodynamics. Clin Pharmacokinet 2009;48(3):143–57.

37. Marrocco A, Steward DE. We've come a long way, maybe: recruitment of women and analysis of results by sex in clinical research. J Womens Health Gend Based Med 2001;10(2):175–9.

38. Anderson GD. Sex differences in drug metabolism: cytochrome P-450 and uridine disphosphate glucurononsyltransferase. J Gend Specif Med 2002;5(1):25–33.

39. Lane HY, chang YC, Chang WH, et al. Effects of gender and age on plasma levels of clozapine and its metabolites: analyzed by critical statistics. J Clin Psychiatry 1999;60(1):36–40.

40. Inglelman-Sundberg M. Pharmacogenetics of Cytochrome p450 and its application in drug therapy: the past present and future. Trends Pharmacol Sci 2004;25(4):193–200.

Cytochrome p450 Part 2
What Nurses Need to Know About the Cytochrome p450 Family Systems

Stephen D. Krau, PhD, RN, CNE

KEYWORDS

- Cytochrome p450 • Enzyme families • CYP1 • CYP2 • Drug metabolism
- Pharmacokinetics • Pharmacogenomics

KEY POINTS

- Over the period from 1957 to 1997, pharmacogenetics evolved into pharmacogenomics.
- Since 1997 there has been considerable progress in the scientific understanding of genetic effects on drug metabolism, but the translation of well-validated and clinically relevant information has been slow to translate into patient care.
- There have been numerous predictions of moving prescriptive guidelines and protocols toward more personalize approaches, but this has not happened to any great extent.
- There are many barriers to this movement, including lack of understanding by prescribers about some of the genetic issues.
- The discussion on cytochrome p450 among nurse practitioners has moved toward a more individualized approach to prescribing medications for patients, with the promise of better outcomes.

The cytochrome p450 (CYP) enzyme system comprises the most important enzyme system in the process of phase I drug metabolism. In addition to many physiologic functions that are mediated by these enzymes, it is estimated that 90% of all prescribed drugs undergo oxidation reactions catalyzed by these enzymes.[1] The major families responsible for the oxidative metabolism of drugs and environmental chemicals are CYP1, CYP2, and CYP3.[2] To provide the best patient care related to medication administration and prescription, an understanding of the specific enzymes is essential. The enzymes have a clear impact on the metabolizing of most medications that nurses administer and that nurse practitioners and physicians prescribe on a regular basis. More specifically, the most important p450 enzymes in drug metabolism are CYP1A2, the CYP2C family, CYP2D6, and CYP3A4.[2–5]

The author has nothing to disclose.
Vanderbilt University Medical Center, School of Nursing, 461 21st Avenue South, Nashville, TN 37205, USA
E-mail address: steve.krau@vanderbillt.edu

Nurs Clin N Am 48 (2013) 681–696
http://dx.doi.org/10.1016/j.cnur.2013.09.003
0029-6465/13/$ – see front matter © 2013 Elsevier Inc. All rights reserved.

CYP1 GENE FAMILY

Expression of the CYP1 family of enzymes is induced by the aryl hydrocarbon receptor (AHR). The AHR mediates the carcinogenic and other toxic effects of environmental pollutants by binding to polycyclic aromatic hydrocarbons such as those found in cigarette smoke, industrial incineration, and charcoal-grilled food.[5] CYP1A1 also inactivates prostaglandin G_2[6]; CYP1A2 and CYP1B1 hydroxylate estrogen; CYP1A2 oxidizes uroporphyrinogen, which is involved in heme synthesis, as well as melatonin. There are several medications that are metabolized completely or in part by members of the CYP1 family, especially CYP1A2, because CYP1A1 and CYP1B1 do not seem to have a major role in the metabolism of drugs. Drugs metabolized by the CYP1 gene family are presented in **Table 1**.

The CYP1A1 and CYP1A2 enzymes have been studied at length because of their roles in the activation of carcinogens. They are at least 70% identical in their amino acid sequences; however, CYP1A1 is expressed at only low levels in the human liver and is essentially an extrahepatic enzyme.[7] There is a large interindividual variation of the CYP1A enzyme that for years scientists thought suggested that there is a causative role of the induction of this enzyme in cancer in certain populations. Now there is evidence showing that increased levels of CY1A2 can be a predisposing factor to colon cancer.[8] Evidence suggests that the classic activities of CYP1A metabolism

Table 1	
Substrates metabolized by the CYP1 family	
Therapeutic Class or Indication	**CYP1 Substrate**
Analgesic	Phenacetin (nonopioid)
Antiarrhythmics	Mexiletine (class 1B), Verapamil (calcium channel blocker and class IV)
Anticholinesterase	Tacrine (also parasympathomimetic)
Anticoagulant	R-warfarin
Antidepressants	Tricyclic: amitriptyline, clomipramine, imipramine N-DeMe Selective serotonin uptake inhibitor: fluvoxamine
Antiemetic	Ondansetron
Antipsychotics	Clozapine, haloperidol, olanzapine
β-Blockers	Propranolol
Hormones	Estradiol
Muscle relaxants	Cyclobenzaprine, tizanidine (alpha-2 adrenergic agonist)
Environmental toxins	Polycyclic aromatic hydrocarbons: cigarette smoke, car exhaust, charbroiled meats and vegetables Chlorinated benzines, solvents
Local anesthetic	Ropivacaine (amino amide group)
Nonsteroidal Antiinflammatory	Naproxen
Selective serotonin receptor agonist	Zolmitriptan, used for migraine headaches
TTX-sensitive Na channel blocker	Riluzole (Rilutek), Used to treat amyotrophic lateral sclerosis
Toxic by-products	Acetaminophen (N-acetyl-p-benzoquinone imine is a toxic by product of acetaminophen)
Xanthines	Caffeine, theophylline
5-Lipoxygenase inhibitor	Zileuton (antiasthmatic)

and activation of exogenous toxic and carcinogenic xenobiotics are only a part of what these enzymes do. With exposure to many chemicals and environmental challenges that can activate AHR, it is hypothesized that CYP1A may be instrumental in providing normal physiologic homeostatic regulation.[7]

The major groups of compounds shown to be metabolized by CYP1B1 enzymes include polycyclic aromatic hydrocarbons, aromatic amines, and several steroid hormones including estradiol and to a lesser extent testosterone. There are studies that show that CYP1B1 metabolically inactivates a large range of structurally diverse anticancer drugs including docetaxel, doxorubicin, paclitaxel, mitoxantrone, and tamoxifen.[9] Related to disease processes, there is an unusually high expression of CYP1B1 in solid cancer tumors, which might have significance for the creation of drugs for chemotherapeutic intervention.[10] CYP1B1 is now widely acknowledged as a promising target for prodrug anticancer therapy because it enhances selective activation in tumor cells without toxicity in normal cells.

CYP1B1 seems to be a developmentally regulated gene. Mutations in the CYP1B1 gene have been associated with primary congenital glaucoma, or buphthalmos. It follows that during embryogenesis there is probably an important substrate in the development of the anterior chamber of the eye that warrants metabolism by this enzyme.[11]

CYP2 GENE FAMILY

CYP2 is the largest p450 in mammals, because CYP2C8, CYP2C9, CYP2C18, and CYP2C19 together metabolize greater than half of frequently prescribed medications, arachidonic acid, and some steroids.[10] Although most of this article focuses on drug metabolism, a beta-naphthoflavone–inducible CYP2C enzyme is thought to be instrumental in the synthesis of a potent vasodilator by the human vascular epithelium. This association presumably indicates a recurrent theme in much of the literature related to CYP products in vertebrates: that they probably first evolved for important life functions, before plant-metabolite degradation, and drug metabolism abilities.[10]

CYP2A Subfamily

There has only been negligible attention given to the CYP2A subfamily of enzymes because these enzymes have restricted substrate specificities. However, once CYP2A6 and CYP2A13 enzymes were shown to be high-affinity metabolizers of nicotine and several other carcinogens, interest in CYP2A forms increased considerably.[12] Many of the CYP2A genes are regulated by several physiologic conditions such as gender, circadian rhythm, and nutrition.

There are only a few drugs that are cleared solely or mainly by this subfamily, coumarin and nicotine being the exceptions. Some of the other drugs that are partially metabolized by this subfamily include the anesthetics halothane and methoxyflurane; the antiepileptics losigamone and valproic acid; anticancer drugs tegafur and doxifluridine; and disulfiram, used for alcohol withdrawal. A more complete list of the substrates metabolized by the CYP2A6 subfamily is presented in **Table 2**.

Genetic studies have shown that individuals with deficient CYP2A6 alleles may have slower rates of nicotine activation.[13] Studies have shown that individuals who are slow activators of nicotine are approximately 2 times less likely to be current adult smokers. Those who do smoke, smoke 7 to 10 fewer cigarettes a day than those individuals with normal metabolic rates. In addition, slow nicotine metabolizers smoke for a shorter time before quitting, are found more frequently among former smokers, and are more successful in quitting during clinical trials.[14] Fast metabolizers, those with CYP2A6 allele duplications, smoke more.

Table 2
Substrates of the CYP2A6 subfamily

Therapeutic Use or Indication	Substrates for CYP2A6
Alcohol withdrawal	Disulfiram
Anesthetics	Methoxyflurane, halothane
Anticancer	Tegafur, doxifluridine
Antiepileptic	Losigamone, valproic acid
Aromatase inhibitor	Letrozole (used for hormone-responsive breast cancer)
Experimental antithrombotic	SM-12502, 3,5-dimethyl-2-(3pyridyl)thiazolidin-4-one hydrochloride (antagonist of platelet activating factor, not currently in clinical use)
Herbal constituent	Coumarin
Smoking withdrawal preparations	Nicotine

Despite the considerable amounts of information available about the members of the CYP2A subfamily, there is still little known about the physiologic function of these enzymes. Because there are many species that lack these enzymes, it is reasonable to assume that these enzymes are not essential to life. In humans, functional CYP2A6 is missing in about 50% of some populations.[12] CYP2A6 has a clear role in nicotine elimination, and there is a suspected association between poor metabolizers (PMs) of CYP2A6 and a decreased risk of tobacco smoke–induced cancer.

CYP2B Subfamily

CYP2B enzymes are versatile catalysts with a broad range of substrates, including environmental pollutants, endobiotics such as steroids, and several drugs. Some of the drugs that are metabolized by CYP2B include antitumor drugs such as cyclophosphamide and ifosfamide, analgesics such as pethidine, and some anesthetics such as propofol and ketamine. In addition, the antidepressant bupropion, the antiviral efavirenz, and the monoamine oxidase inhibitor selegiline are metabolized by this enzyme.[15] More recently, studies have shown that CYP2B6 is a metabolizer of methadone.[16] A comprehensive list of pharmacologic substrates metabolized by the CYP2B6 subfamily is presented in **Table 3**.

In addition to their metabolic contributions, the importance of CYP2B enzymes depends on the variations in their level of expression, which seems to be in part a function

Table 3
Substrates metabolized by the CYP2B subfamily

Therapeutic Class or Indication	CYP1 Substrate
Antidepressant and smoking cessation aid	Bupropion
Nitrogen mustard alkylating agents (anticancer)	Cyclophosphamide, ifosfamide
Non-nucleoside reverse transcriptase inhibitor	Efavirenz (highly active antiretroviral therapy, used in human immunodeficiency virus type 1)
Synthetic opioid	Methadone

of gender, inducibility, and the differences in the allele compositions. These variations have certain implications for pharmacogenetic-based and pharmacogenomic-based approaches to individualized drug treatments. At present, this subfamily is the focus of much research related to cancer therapy, only because of the ability of the enzyme to metabolize chemotherapeutic drugs but also because of the correlation of specific natural allelic forms of CYP2Bs with better outcomes for cancer treatment. This subfamily could one day be part of the cancer chemopreventative approach in some patients.[15]

The CYP2C Subfamily

The CYP2C subfamily of metalloenzymes is considered the second most pharmacologically important group of CYP450s (after CYP3A) because of its prominent role in drug metabolism.[17] The CYP2C subfamily is involved in the metabolism of many frequently prescribed drugs of clinical importance, such as omeprazole, warfarin, mephenytoin, and paclitaxel. In addition, this subfamily is important in the metabolism of several endogenous substrates needed for physiologic processes such as cell signaling. These endogenous substances include arachidonic acid and retinoic acid.[18] In humans, the CYP2C family is composed of 4 enzymes (CYP2C8, CYP2C9, CYP2C18, and CYP2C19), each of which is located on a single gene cluster of chromosome 10.[17] CYP2C9 is thought to be the most pharmacologically important enzyme because of its high expression in human liver and its impact on numerous drugs. CYP2C8 and, to a lesser extent, CYP2C19 are expressed in the liver and have important roles in drug metabolism.[17] At present, CYP218 has not been shown to be highly expressed, does not seem to play an important role in drug metabolism, and is not be discussed here.[19,20] A more complete summary of the drugs metabolized to some extent by this subfamily, along with clinical indications, is presented in **Table 4**. It is important to consider some of the substrates that are affected by the CYP2C family.

CYP2C8

This enzyme is increasing in importance with regard to its impact on drug metabolism. One of the most notable substrates of CYP2C8 is paclitaxel (Taxol), which is a miotic inhibitor that is currently used as a leading drug treatment of soft tumors (sarcoma) in tissues such as breast, ovary, and lung, as well as in brain tumors. It is also been used as an antiproliferative agent to minimize scar tissue formation, for example in coating shunts used for cardiac and other disorders.[21]

Several type II diabetes medications are metabolized by CYP2C8, as are several antimalarial medications, even though the chemical structures of these drugs are different from the chemical structure of paclitaxel. This enzyme is also important in physiologic processes because of its impact on arachidonic acid. Because of the more recent importance and impact of this enzyme on medically prescribed therapeutics, the 2006 US Food and Drug Administration (FDA) *Draft Guidance for Drug-Drug Interactions* now includes CYP2C8 for in vitro consideration for drug developers marketing new drugs.[17,22]

CYP2C9

CYP2C9 is considered to be the most pharmacologically important of the CYP2C enzymes and is the most abundant in the human liver, because it comprises approximately one-third of the total hepatic p450 content.[17,23,24] It is involved in the metabolism of more than 100 different approved drugs, but most notably the anticoagulant warfarin, which is among the most dangerous drugs for humans

Table 4
Substrates of the CYP2C subfamily

Enzyme	Classification or Therapeutic Indication	Substrates
CYP2C8	Anticancer agents	Paclitaxel
	Loop diuretic	Torsemide
	Antimalarial/antiinflammatory	Amodiaquine
	Lipid lowering agent	Cerivastatin
	Oral hypoglycemic agent	Repaglinide
CYP2C9	Anticancer agents	Tamoxifen
	Anticoagulants (coumarin)	Acenocoumarol, phenprocoumon, warfarin
	Antidepressants	Amitriptyline, fluoxetine
	Antiepileptics	Phenytoin-4-OH2
	Angiotensin II blockers	Candesartan, irbesartan, losartan
	Lipid lowering agents	Fluvastatin
	NSAIDs	Celecoxib, diclofenac, ibuprofen, lornoxicam, meloxicam, S-naproxen, piroxicam, tenoxicam, suprofen
	Oral hypoglycemic agents	Nateglinide, glipizide, tolbutamide
	Sulfonylureas	Glibenclamide, gliclazide, glipizide, glimepiride, glyburide, tolbutamide
	Thiazolidinediones (insulin sensitizer)	Rosiglitazone
CYP2C19	Antidepressants	Amitriptyline, citalopram, clomipramine, imipramine, moclobemide
	Anticancer agent	Cyclophosphamide, nilutamide, teniposide
	Anticoagulant	R-warfarin → 8-OH
	Anticonvulsant	Primidone
	Antiepileptics	Diazepam → Nor, phenytoin(O), 5-mephytoin, phenobarbitone
	Antimalarial	Proguanil
	Antimicrobial	Chloramphenicol
	Antiretroviral	Nelfinavir
	Barbiturate	Hexobarbital, R-mephobarbital
	Benzodiazepines	Diazepam, flunitrazepam, quazepam, clobazam
	β-Blocker	Propranolol
	Muscle relaxant	Carisoprodol
	NSAIDs	Indomethacin
	Proton pump inhibitors	Lansoprazole, omeprazole, pantoprazole, rabeprazole
	Steroid hormone	Progesterone

Abbreviation: NSAIDs, nonsteroidal antiinflammatory drugs.

because of its narrow therapeutic index, resulting in dosing dilemmas for prescribers. There are several studies that support the use of genetic testing for this enzyme for people receiving warfarin, and evidence that shows CYP2C9 genotype–guided dosing is more efficient and safer than routine dosing protocols.[25,26]

In addition to numerous medications, CYP2C9 also metabolizes numerous endogenous substrates. Along with CYP2C8, the 2C9 enzyme also contributes to the metabolism of arachidonic acid, producing compounds that are instrumental in vasodilation as well as cell signaling functions such as hormone secretion, modulation of electrolyte transport, vascular tone, inflammatory responses, and inhibition of Na/K ATPase. These also function as endothelial-derived hyperpolarizing factors.[27–33]

CYP2C19

As the third member of the CYP2C subfamily, this enzyme is important in the metabolism of many and frequently prescribed drugs. One of the most prominent drugs metabolized by this enzyme is the antiulcer drug omeprazole. As a proton pump inhibitor, omeprazole is one of the most frequently prescribed/administrated drugs and a popular over-the-counter medication. Omeprazole, like other proton pump inhibitors, irreversibly blocks the terminal stage of gastric acid secretion. PMs experience more effective acid suppression and healing of duodenal and gastric ulcers when treated with omeprazole and lansoprazole compared with extensive metabolizers (EMs).[34] Another well-known substrate of CYP2C19 is the S-enantiomer of the anticonvulsant mephenytoin.[17] CYP2C19 is a metabolizer of many anticonvulsants, as shown in **Table 4**.

Another important medication metabolized by the CYP2C19 enzyme is clopidogrel, which combined with aspirin is a standard treatment of acute coronary syndrome (ACS). Dual antiplatelet therapy reduces the risk of subsequent ACS events and death compared with aspirin alone.[35] Neurovascular patients are frequently on dual antiplatelet therapy as well, because of the coincident probability of cardiac disease, whereas persons with aspirin allergies or suspected aspirin ineffectiveness are prescribed clopidogrel as secondary prophylaxis of stroke. The importance of the genetic impact on the metabolism of this medication is recognized by the FDA, who in March 2010 announced that clopidogrel would require a new black box warning regarding reduced effectiveness in persons who are PMs, recommending the testing of the CYP2C19 genotype to help guide clinical management.[35] In addition, because both clopidogrel and proton pump inhibitors (PPIs) use this enzyme, as a result of this and other mechanisms there is evidence that, when administered with clopidogrel, PPIs (especially omeprazole) decrease the antiplatelet effect.[36]

In many cases, the variations in the alleles of this enzyme result in the inactivation of the enzyme. For example, a genetic polymorphism of CYP219, CYP219*2, is associated with a decrease in the ability to hydroxylate mephenytoin. It is estimated that about 3% of the white population are PMs of mephenytoin because of this allele, whereas 20% of Japanese and 15% to 17% of Chinese are PMs. The frequency in Koreans is about 12% to 16% more than in white people.[37]

Understanding the polymorphisms of the CYP2C subfamily is essential in understanding the interindividual variations in drug metabolism modulated by this enzyme family. A case example of this is seen in the anticancer agent indisulam. Patients who express the CYP2C9*3 allele, the CYP2C19*2 allele, and CYP219*3 allele, had a lower rate of elimination than those carrying the normal allele (the *1 allele), which increases their risk of severe toxicity.[38] This finding supports the practice of screening for CYP2C polymorphisms for people taking this medication because failure to consider the metabolic capacity of the patient can lead to ineffective bioavailability or, conversely, toxic levels of this medication, or even death.[17]

CYP2D6

The most widely studied enzyme in relation to polymorphisms that affects the elimination of about 20% to 30% of the drugs that are prescribed is the CYPD26.[1,2,19,39] This enzyme has a role in more than 50 prescribed drugs, most of them acting on the central nervous system or on the heart.[40] Many of the medications that are metabolized by this enzyme family have a narrow therapeutic index.[41] These percentages are related to the number of medications and do not necessarily reflect the frequency of prescription. The human cytochrome D26 was the first CYP to be identified for which the classic polymorphism had an impact on pharmacology. As a result of observations of the antiarrhythmic and oxytocic drug sparteine and the antihypertensive debrisoquine, CYP2D6 was discovered. To date there are 128 different CYP2D6 variants identified by the human CYP allele nomenclature committee (http://www.imm.ki.se/CYPalleles).[42] The reader is encouraged to examine the table of medications metabolized by the CYPD26 family of enzymes (**Table 5**) to determine the relevance of the enzyme activity in relation to the medications that are prescribes. For example, polymorphism has been found in the CYP2D6 family, which primarily metabolizes most of the medications used in palliative care.[43,44] In psychiatry and geriatrics, 52% of psychiatric, 49% of psychogeriatric, and 46% of geriatric patients are consumers of at least one drug metabolized by CYPD26, of which 62% are classified as either an antidepressant or an antipsychotic.[45]

Table 5
List of medications metabolized by CYP2D6

Classification or Therapeutic Use	Specific Medications
Antitussive	Dextromethorphan
Antiarrhythmic	Encainide (no longer used because of proarrhythmic side effects); sparteine (not approved in the United States as an antiarrhythmic, has been used to stimulate uterine contractions during labor)
β-Blockers	Alprenolol, bufuralol, carvedilol, metoprolol, nebivolol, propafenone, propranolol, timolol
Tricyclic antidepressants	Amitriptyline, imipramine, clomipramine, doxepin, desipramine, nortriptyline
Selective serotonin reuptake inhibitors	Fluoxetine, paroxetine, fluvoxamine, venlafaxine, duloxetine
Other antidepressants	Maprotiline, mianserin, venlafaxine, minaprine
Antipsychotics	Chlorpromizine, haloperidol, perphenazine, thioridazine, zuclopenthixol, risperidone, aripiprazole
Antiarrhythmics	Propafenone, flecainide, mexiletine
Opioid analgesics	Codeine, dihydrocodeine, tramadol, oxycodone
Analgesics	Phenacetin (removed from market in United States because of kidney damaging properties and carcinogenic effects)
Antiemetics	Tropisetron, ondansetron, dolasetron, metoclopramide
Antihistamines	Promethazine, azelastine, chlorpheniramine
Antihypertensive	Debrisoquine (guanethidine type)
Noradrenergic uptake inhibitor	Atomoxetine
Antianginal	Perhexiline, lidocaine
Antihyperglycemic	Phenformin
Anticholinergic	Tolterodine
Anticancer (hormone receptor)	Tamoxifen
Psychostimulant	Amphetamine, methoxyamphetamine
Serotoninergic anorectic	Dexfenfluramine

There is a large interindividual variation in the enzyme activity of CYP2D6, mainly because of genetic polymorphisms, which frequently results in a barrier to reaching optimal therapeutic concentrations of medications metabolized by this family.[46] Among persons of various ethnic backgrounds, the patterns of CYP2D6 polymorphisms have striking differences. Approximately 5% to 10% of white people can be classified as PMs by lacking CYP2D6 activity and 1% to 10 % as ultrarapid metabolizers because of the gene duplication that results in an increased enzyme activity.[47] Frequencies up to 29% have been observed in Saudi Arabians and Ethiopians.[48,49] Because of the polymorphism of this enzyme, there are data to support and explain the low frequency of the PM phenotype among Asian and African populations,[50] which would result in the need for lower doses of a medication in Asian and African patients compared with white patients. There is little to no influence on the expression of CYP2D6 by other factors such as age and gender, which makes it an excellent example of a drug-metabolizing enzyme under genetic control.[40]

In order to determine the clinical importance of cytochrome 2D6 and the relevance of genetic testing, there are several criteria that warrant consideration. As suggested by Gardiner and Begg,[2] these criteria include (1) the dramatic effects of the polymorphism on the total concentration of all the active moieties (ie, genotyping would predict desired effect), (2) the clear association of concentration with desired effect (ie, genotyping would predict desired effect), (3) the significant concentration-related adverse effects, and (4) the drug's low therapeutic index.[2]

Based on these criteria and several studies, a strong case can be made to genetically test patients who are going to receive codeine. There is evidence to show there is a gene-concentration effect for the prodrug to covert to morphine in PMs and in phenocopied EMs. As a result, there is a predictable failure but a less clear relationship with adverse effects. The high therapeutic index for codeine and the familiarity of codeine with many prescribers make genetic testing for this drug less imperative.

Because CYP2D6 is absent in a large percentage of the human population, it does not have an important role in endogenous metabolic pathways. However, numerous studies have shown that differences in neurotransmitters or neuromodulatory amines account for differences in personalities among individuals with different CYP2D6 phenotypes. There are variant expressions of CYP2D6 in the human brain[51] and a clinical association of CYP2D6 phenotypes with Parkinson disease.[52]

CYP2E Subfamily

Although first identified in the liver, CYP2E has been found in many extrahepatic tissues including the brain, nasal mucosa, lungs, kidneys, breast, ovary, and stomach.[53–55] One of the salient issues with this subfamily of enzymes is that it is altered in response to xenobiotics as well a variety of physiologic and pathophysiologic conditions, including those affected by nutrition, such as starvation, fasting, obesity, and diets that are high in fat.[56] Some of the other conditions that alter response include metabolic and endocrine disorders (diabetes, metabolic syndrome), inflammation, viral infections, and carcinoma.[56] When considering the medications that this subfamily metabolizes, as indicated in **Table 6**, high risk associated with surgical and other procedures requiring anesthetics is apparent. There are a variety of hormonal regulators of CYP2E1 expression that have been the focus of many studies. Among those examined have been thyroid hormone and growth hormone, but the most salient has been the relationship between insulin and the regulation of CYP2E1, in which investigators have reported an increase in human lymphocyte CYP2E1.[57,58]

CYP2E seems to be developmentally regulated.[56] In humans, the activity of CYP2E1 increases with age for both genders, with 81% greater activity for men more than

Table 6
Substrates of the CYP2E subfamily

Classification or Therapeutic Use	Substrate
Anesthetics	Enflurane, halothane, isoflurane, methoxyflurane, sevoflurane, ethers (diethyl ether, methyl t-butyl ether, 1,1,2,3,3,3,-hexafluoropropyl methyl ether)
Environmental compounds	Benzene (hydrocarbon), aniline2 (dye base), N,N-dimethyl Formamide (solvent)
Muscle relaxant	Chlorzoxazone
Alcohol and ketone	Acetone, acetoacetate, acetaldehyde, butanol, ethanol, glycerol, isopropanol, pentanol
Bronchodilator	Theophylline 8-OH
By-products of metabolism	Acetaminophen N-acetyl-p-benzoquinone imine is a toxic byproduct of paracetamol
Fatty acids	Arachidonic acid, lauric acid

50 years of age, and 87% more activity for women more than 50 years of age compared with individuals 30 to 35 years old.[59] There is also a gender difference in the expression of this subfamily, with men having higher expression of CYP2E1 than women, making the substrates metabolized by this subfamily gender dependent.[60]

THE CYP3 FAMILY

The CYP3A enzymes have an important role in human biology and clinical therapeutics.[61–63] They are the most abundant group of CYP enzymes in the liver and the only CYPs in significant amounts in the mucosa of the human gastrointestinal tract. The substrate specificity is broad because CYP3A mediates the biotransformation of numerous environmental chemicals that have toxicologic importance, as well as numerous endogenous substances, and has a role in the metabolizing of a large variety of medications, as shown in **Table 7**.

The dual locations of CYP3A in the mucosa and in the liver give humans 2 chances for protection against potentially toxic environmental chemicals before entry into the systemic circulation. In addition, there is not a null phenotype of the enzyme as there is with CYP2D6, which constitutes the PM for that enzyme, which supports the idea that CYP3A is essential to human life.[61] Several endogenous steroid hormones, particularly those required for sexual maturation and reproduction, depend on CYP3A.[64,65] A large number of substrates for CYP3A are derived from plants and fungi as natural resources, including opiates, aflatoxins, cinchona alkaloids, and the immunosuppressants cyclosporine, tacrolimus, and sirolimus.

There are 4 encoding alleles of CYP3A: CYP3A4, CYP3A5, CYP3A7, and CYP3A43. CYP3A7 is a fetal enzyme and is not expressed after birth. CYP3A43 is an adult enzyme and is localized in the prostate.[66,67] To date, there is no clear functional significance of CYP3A43. CYP3A4 is the dominant isoform in humans, and along with CYP3A5 is the only CYP of functional importance in the gastrointestinal tract. The levels expressed at the hepatic and gastrointestinal sites are not correlated, and the regulation between the two sites is not coordinated.[61] They are often considered collectively as CYP3A because of their promiscuous substrate specificity and the difficulty discerning the role of each in the metabolism of drugs.

Because of the variety and number of substrates metabolized by the CYP3A enzyme (see **Table 7**), the possible influence of age and gender on the modulation

Table 7
Substrates of the CYP3A subfamily (CYP3A4, CYP3A5, CYP3A7)

Classification or Therapeutic Use	Substrate
Aldosterone antagonist	Eplerenone
Antiandrogen	Finasteride
Antiarrhythmics	Quinidine, lidocaine
Anticancer	Docetaxel, Gleevec, irinotecan, tamoxifen, taxol, vincristine
Antidepressant	Aripiprazole, trazodone, nefazodone
Antiemetic	Aprepitant, ondansetron
Antiepileptic	Carbamazepine
Antihistamine	Terfenadine
Antimicrobials	Clarithromycin, erythromycin, telithromycin, dapsone
Antipsychotic	Haloperidol, pimozide, quetiapine, risperidone, ziprasidone
Antihistamines	Astemizole, chlorpheniramine, terfenadine
Antitussive	Dextromethorphan
Antivirals	Indinavir, nelfinavir, ritonavir, saquinavir
Anxiolytic	Buspirone
Benzodiazepine	Alprazolam, diazepam 3OH, midazolam, triazolam
β-Blockers	Propranolol
β2-Adrenergic agonist	Salmeterol
Calcium channel blockers	Amlodipine, diltiazem, felodipine, lercanidipine, nifedipine, nisoldipine, nitrendipine, verapamil
Erectile dysfunction	Sildenafil, tadalafil, vardenafil
Glucocorticoids	Betamethasone
HMG CoA reductase inhibitors	Atorvastatin, cerivastatin, lovastatin, simvastatin
Immune modulators	Cyclosporine, tacrolimus, sirolimus
Migraines	Cafergot, eletriptan
Opioids natural and synthetic	Alfentanil, codeine demethylation, fentanyl, LAAM, methadone
Oral hypoglycemics	Nateglinide
Phosphodiesterase inhibitor	Cilostazol
Prokinetic	Cisapride, domperidone
Sedative/hypnotic	Zaleplon, zolpidem
Serotonin-norepinephrine-dopamine reuptake inhibitor	Cocaine
Steroids	Estradiol, hydrocortisone, progesterone, testosterone
Xanthine	Caffeine TMU

Abbreviations: HMG CoA, 3-hydroxy-3-methylglutaryl-coenzyme A; LAAM, levo-α-acetylmethadol; TMU, trimethyluric acid.

of the activity of the enzyme is of both scientific and public health importance.[61] Numerous studies have been done in vivo on human liver samples, but they are inconclusive with regard to age or gender. However, clinical studies have indicated that the effects of age and gender are not independent.[61] In many studies, the clearance of substrates in women of increasing age was higher than for men of increasing age. After a thorough review, and considering a variety of issues related to measurement differences and physiologic differences in aging, Greenblatt and colleagues[61] concluded that, "The net clinical implication is that lower doses of most CYP3A substrate drugs are recommended for the elderly."

Because of the location of this enzyme in the gastrointestinal tract, there have been numerous studies on the impact of foods and other drugs that inhibit or enhance the metabolism of the target substrate. The individual variability in the phenotype metabolic activity of the CYP3A enzymes continues to be enigmatic, and continues to pose a challenge for researchers and clinicians. There are some sources of the variability that can be indentified and explained but, for the most part, the individual variation remains unexplained. To that end, the approach to therapeutic dosing for substrates of this enzyme continues to be an initial dose estimation followed by monitoring and adjustments based on clinical response and plasma levels.[61]

SUMMARY

Over the period from 1957 to 1997 pharmacogenetics evolved into pharmacogenomics.[3] Since 1997 there has been considerable progress in the scientific understanding of genetic effects on drug metabolism, but the well-validated and clinically relevant information has been slow to translate into patient care. There have been numerous predictions of moving prescriptive guidelines and protocols toward more personalize approaches, but this has not happened to any great extent. There are numerous barriers to this movement, including lack of understanding by prescribers about some of the genetic issues. The discussion on CYP among nurse practitioners is moving toward a more individualized approach to prescribing medications for patients, with the promise of better outcomes.

REFERENCES

1. Zhou S. Polymorphism of the human cytochrome P450 D26 and its clinical significance: part I. Clin Pharm 2009;48(11):689–723.
2. Gardiner SJ, Begg EJ. Pharmacogenetics, drug metabolizing enzymes and clinical practice. Pharmacol Rev 2006;58:521–90.
3. Daly AK. Pharmacogenetics and human genetic polymorphisms. Biochem J 2010;429:435–49.
4. Gregg CR. Cytochrome p450, encyclopedia of gastroenterology. St. Louis (MO): Elsevier; 2004. p. 542.
5. Hankinson O. Role of coactivators in transcriptional activation by the aryl hydrocarbon receptor. Arch Biochem Biophys 2005;433(2):379–86.
6. Plastaras JP, Guengerich FP, Nebert DW, et al. Xenobiotic-metabolizing cytochrome p450 convert prostaglandin endoperoxide to hydroxyhepadecatrienoic acid and mutagen, malondialdehyde. J Biol Chem 2000;275: 11784–90.
7. Moorthy B. The CYP1A subfamily. In: Ioannides C, editor. Cytochromes p450: role in the metabolism and toxicity of drugs and other xenobiotics. Cambridge (United Kingdom): Royal Society of Chemistry; 2008. p. 97–135.
8. Lang NP, Butler MA, Massengill M, et al. Rapid metabolic phenotypes for acetyltransferase and cytochrome P4501A2 and putative exposure to food-borne heterocyclic amines increase the risk for colorectal cancer or polyps. Cancer Epidemiol Biomarkers Prev 1994;3(8):675–82.
9. McFadyen MC, Murray GI. The CYP1B subfamily. In: Ioannides C, editor. Cytochromes p450: role in the metabolism and toxicity of drugs and other

xenobiotics. Cambridge (United Kingdom): Royal Society of Chemistry; 2008. p. 136–49.

10. Nebert DW, Russell DW. Clinical importance of cytochrome p450. Lancet 2002; 360:1155–62.

11. Vasiliou V, Gonzalez FJ. Role of CYP1B1 in glaucoma. Annu Rev Pharmacol Toxicol 2008;48:333–58.

12. Raunio H, Hakkola J, Pelkonen O. The CYP2A subfamily. In: Ioannides C, editor. Cytochromes p450: role in the metabolism and toxicity of drugs and other xenobiotics. Cambridge (United Kingdom): Royal Society of Chemistry; 2008. p. 150–77.

13. Xu C, Goodz S, Sellers EM, et al. CYP2A6 genetic variation and potential consequences. Adv Drug Deliv Rev 2002;54:1245–56.

14. Malaiyandi V, Sellers EM, Tyndale RF. Implications of CYP2A6 genetic variation for smoking behaviors and nicotine dependence. Clin Pharmacol Ther 2005; 77(3):145–58.

15. Corcos L, Berthou F. The CYP2B subfamily. In: Ioannides C, editor. Cytochromes p450: role in the metabolism and toxicity of drugs and other xenobiotics. Cambridge (United Kingdom): Royal Society of Chemistry; 2008. p. 178–99.

16. Totah RA, Sheffels P, Roberts T. Role of CYP2B6 in stereoselective human methadone metabolism. Anesthesiology 2008;108(3):363–74.

17. Ferguson SS, Black K, Jackson JP. The CYP2C subfamily. In: Ioannides C, editor. Cytochromes p450: role in the metabolism and toxicity of drugs and other xenobiotics. Cambridge (United Kingdom): Royal Society of Chemistry; 2008. p. 200–40.

18. McSorley LC, Daly AK. Identification of human cytochrome P450 isoforms that contribute to all-trans-retinoic acid 4-hydroxylation. Biochem Pharmacol 2000; 60(4):517–26.

19. Gardiner SJ, Begg EJ. Pharmacogenetic testing for drug metabolizing enzymes: is it happening in practice? Pharmacogenet Genomics 2005;15: 365–9.

20. Lapple F, von Richter O, Fromm MF, et al. Differential expression and function of the CYP2C isoforms in human live and intestines. Pharmacogenetics 2003; 13(9):565–75.

21. Marx SO, Totary-Jain H, Marks AR. Vascular smooth muscle cell proliferation in restenosis. Circ Cardiovasc Interv 2011;4:104–11.

22. Food and Drug Administration. Draft guidance for industry on drug interactions studies–study design, data analysis, and implications for dosing and labeling. Available at: http://www.fda.gov./Cder/drug/drugInteractions/guidance.htm. Accessed August 1, 2011.

23. Lasker JM, Wester MR, Aramsombatdee E, et al. Characterization of CYP2C19 and CYP2C9 from human liver: respective roles in microsomal tolbutamide, S-mephenytoin, and omeprazole hyroxylations. Arch Biochem Biophys 1998; 353:16–28.

24. Goldenstein JA, de Morais SM. Biochemistry and molecular biology of the human CYP2C subfamily. Pharmacogenetics 1994;4(6):285–99.

25. Caraco Y, Blotnick S, Muszkat M. CYP2C9 genotype-guided warfarin prescribing enhances the efficacy and safety of anticoagulation: a prospective randomized controlled study. Clin Pharmacol Ther 2008;83:460–70.

26. Wadelius M, Chen LY, Lindh JD. The largest prospective warfarin-treated cohort supports genetic forecasting. Blood 2009;113(4):784–92.

27. Falck HM, Westermark P. Protein AA in primary and myeloma associated amyloidosis. Clin Exp Immunol 1983;54(1):259–64.
28. Chen JK, Falck JR, Reddy KM, et al. Epoxyeicosatrienoic acids and their sulfonimide derivatives stimulate tyrosine phosphorylation and induce mitogenesis in renal epithelial cells. J Biol Chem 1998;273(44):29254–61.
29. Harder DR, Campbell WB, Roman RJ. Role of cytochrome p450 enzymes and metabolites of arachidonic acid in the control of vascular tone. J Vasc Res 1995;32(2):79–92.
30. Zou AP, Fleming JT, Falck JR, et al. 20-HETE is an endogenous inhibitor of the large-conductance Ca(2+)-activated K+ channel in renal arterioles. Am J Physiol 1996;270(1 part 2):R228–37.
31. Bauersachs J, Christ M, Ertl G, et al. Cytochrome P450 2C expression and EDHF-mediated relaxation in porcine coronary arteries is increased by cortisol. Cardiovasc Res 2002;54(3):669–75.
32. Campbell WB, Harder DR. Endothelium-derived hyperpolarizing factors and vascular cytochrome P450 metabolites of arachidonic acid in the regulation of tone. Circ Res 1999;84(4):484–8.
33. Dai D, Zeldin DC, Blaisdell JA, et al. Polymorphisms in human CYP2C8 decrease metabolism of the anticancer drug paclitaxel and arachidonic acid. Pharmacogenetics 2001;11(7):597–607.
34. Klotz U. Clinical impact of CYP2C19 polymorphism on the action of proton pump inhibitors: a review of a special problem. Int J Clin Pharmacol Ther 2006;44(7):297–302.
35. Anderson CD, Biffi A, Greenberg SM, et al. Personalized approaches to clopidogrel therapy: are we there yet? Stroke 2010;41:2997–3002.
36. Li XQ, Andersson TB, Ahlstrom M, et al. Comparison of inhibitory effects of the proton pump inhibiting drugs omeprazole, esomeprazole, lansoprazole, pantoprazole, and rabeprazole on human cytochrome p450 activities. Drug Metab Dispos 2004;32:821–7.
37. Ruas JL, Lechner MC. Allele frequency of CYP2C19 in a Portuguese population. Pharmacogenetics 1997;7(4):333–5.
38. Zandvliet AS, Huitema AD, Copalu W, et al. CYP2C9 and CYP2C19 polymorphic forms are related to increased indisulam exposure and higher risk of severe hematologic toxicity. Clin Cancer Res 2007;13(10):2970–6.
39. Ingelman-Sundberg M. Genetic polymorphisms of cytochrome P450 2D6 (CYP2D6): clinical consequences, evolutionary aspects and functional diversity. Pharmacogenomics J 2005;5:6–13.
40. Zanger UM. The CYPD2D subfamily. In: Ioannides C, editor. Cytochromes p450: role in the metabolism and toxicity of drugs and other xenobiotics. Cambridge (United Kingdom): Royal Society of Chemistry; 2008. p. 241–75.
41. Cascorbi I. Pharmacogenetics of cytochrome p4502D6: genetic background and clinical implications. Eur J Clin Invest 2003;33(Suppl 2):17–22.
42. Home page of the Human Cytochrome P450 (CYP) Allele Nomenclature Committee. Available at: http://www.imm.ki.se/CYPalleles. Updated September 2008. Accessed August 1, 2011.
43. Kuebler K, Verga J, Mihelic RA. Why there is no cookbook approach to palliative care: implications of the p450 enzyme system. Clin J Oncol Nurs 2003;7(5):569–72.
44. Davis M, Homsi J. The importance of cytochrome P450 monooxygenase CYP2D6 in palliative medicine. Support Care Cancer 2001;9:442–51.

45. Mulder H, Heerdink ER, van Iersel EE, et al. Prevalence of patients using drugs metabolized by cytochrome p450 in different populations, a cross-sectional study. Ann Pharmacother 2007;41(3):408–13.

46. Zhou S, Di YM, Chan E, et al. Clinical pharmacogenetics and potential application in personalized medicine. Curr Drug Metab 2008;9:738–84.

47. De Leon J, Armstrong SC, Cozza KL. Clinical guidelines for psychiatrists for the use of pharmacogenetic testing for CYP450 2D6 and CYP450 2C19. Psychosomatics 2006;47:75–85.

48. McLellan RA, Oscarson M, Seidegard J, et al. Frequent occurrence of CYPD6 gene duplication in Saudi Arabians. Pharmacogenetics 1997;7(3):187–91.

49. Aklillu E, Persson I, Bertilsson L, et al. Frequent distribution of ultrarapid metabolizers of debrisoquine in an Ethiopian population carrying duplicated and multiduplicated functional CYP2D6 alleles. J Pharmacol Exp Ther 1996;278: 441–6.

50. Wang SL, Lai MD, Huang JD. G169R mutation diminishes the metabolic activity of CYP2D6 in Chinese. Drug Metab Dispos 1999;27:385–8.

51. Fonne-Pfister R, Bargetzi MJ, Meyer UM. MPTP, the neurotoxin inducing Parkinson's disease, is a potent competitive inhibitor of human and rat cytochrome P450 isozymes (P450bufl, P450db1) catalyzing debrisoquine 4-hydroxylation. Biochem Biophys Res Commun 1987;148(3):1144–50.

52. Barbeau A, Cloutier T, Roy M, et al. Ecogenetics of Parkinson's disease: 4-hydroxylation of debrisoquine. Lancet 1985;2(8446):1213–36.

53. Tsutsumi M, Lasker JM, Shimizu M, et al. The intralobular distribution of ethanol-inducible P450IIE1 in rat and human liver. Hepatology 1989;10(4):437–46.

54. Raucy JL, Lasker JM, Lieber CS, et al. Acetaminophen activation by human liver cytochromes P450IIE1 and P450IA2. Arch Biochem Biophys 1989;271(2): 270–83.

55. Watkins PB, Wrighton SA, Maurel P, et al. Identification of an inducible form of cytochrome P-450 in human liver. Proc Natl Acad Sci U S A 1985;82(18):6310–4.

56. Overton LC, Hudder A, Novak RF. The CYP2E subfamily. In: Ioannides C, editor. Cytochromes p450: role in the metabolism and toxicity of drugs and other xenobiotics. Cambridge (United Kingdom): Royal Society of Chemistry; 2008. p. 276–308.

57. Wang Z, Hall SD, Maya JF, et al. Diabetes mellitus increases the in vivo activity of cytochrome p450 2E1 in humans. Br J Clin Pharmacol 2003;55(1):77–85.

58. Hauford V, Ligocka D, Buysschaert M, et al. Cytochrome P4502E1 (CYP2E1) expression in peripheral blood lymphocytes: evaluation in hepatitis C and diabetes. Eur J Clin Pharmacol 2003;59(1):29–33.

59. Bebia Z, Buch SC, Wilson JW, et al. Bioequivalence revisited: influence of age and sex on CYP enzymes. Clin Pharmacol Ther 2004;76(6):618–27.

60. Kim RB, O'Shea D. Inter-individual variability of chlorzoxazone 6-hydroxylation in men and women and its relationship to CYP2E1 genetic polymorphisms. Clin Pharmacol Ther 1995;57(6):645–55.

61. Greenblatt DJ, He P, Von Moltke LL, et al. The CYP3 family. In: Ioannides C, editor. Cytochromes p450: role in the metabolism and toxicity of drugs and other xenobiotics. Cambridge (United Kingdom): Royal Society of Chemistry; 2008. p. 354–83.

62. Guengerich FP. Pharmacogenomics of cytochrome P450 and other enzymes involved in biotransformation of xenobiotics. Drug Dev Res 2000;49:4–16.

63. Guengerich FP. Cytochrome P450: what have we learned and what are the future issues? Drug Metab Rev 2004;36(2):159–97.

64. Tsuchiya Y, Nakajima M, Yokoi T. Cytochrome P450-mediated metabolism of estrogens and its regulation in human. Cancer Lett 2005;227(2):115–24.
65. Yu AM, Fukamachi K, Krausz KW, et al. Potential role for human cytochrome P450 3A4 in estradiol homeostasis. Endocrinology 2005;146(7):2911–9.
66. Gellner K, Eiselt R, Hustert E, et al. Genomic organization of the human CYP3A locus: identification of a new, inducible CYP3A gene. Pharmacogenetics 2001; 11(2):111–21.
67. Westlind A, Malmebo S, Johansson I, et al. Cloning and tissue distribution of a novel human cytochrome p450 of the CYP3A subfamily, CYP3A43. Biochem Biophys Res Commun 2001;281(5):1349–55.

Cytochrome p450 Part 3: Drug Interactions
Essential Concepts and Considerations

Stephen D. Krau, PhD, RN, CNE

KEYWORDS

- Cytochrome p450 • Inducers • Inhibitors • Drug interactions • Cancer therapy
- Grapefruit juice • Medication administration

KEY POINTS

- The most important consideration related to understanding cytochrome p450 enzymes is the appreciation that all drug effects vary among individuals and are strongly influenced by genes.
- The same enzyme may display a variety of functions and alterations, which can range from ultrarapid activity, to no activity.
- The science exists to improve patient outcomes and to improve understanding of drug response; however, clinical progress in implementing pharmacogenomics is lacking.
- The main challenges for the future are to identify among all of the polymorphisms those that contribute to idiosyncratic effects and adverse drug reactions.
- Technological efforts should also be focused on the development of tests that can easily be done in the clinic or at the bedside, which would remove one of the barriers to the use of pharmacogenomics in routine practice.

Cytochrome p450 enzymes have an important role in the metabolism of medications, and a critical function when it comes to drug-drug interactions. This is not just the result of administering the medications at the same time, but rather the physiologic effects of the medications on the enzymes caused by the bioavailability that can last for hours to months. This dynamic is not limited to prescribed or over-the-counter medications but also takes into account different foods or beverages the patient eats or drinks during drug therapy. Just as it is well known that many green leafy vegetables block the action of Coumadin, or drinking beverages with vitamin C enhances the absorption of oral iron preparations, there are food sources that affect the function of the cytochrome p450 (CYP) enzymes. For example, the effect of many

Disclosure: The author has nothing to disclose.
Vanderbilt University Medical Center, School of Nursing, 461 21st Avenue South, Nashville, TN 37240, USA
E-mail address: steve.krau@vanderbilt.edt

Nurs Clin N Am 48 (2013) 697–706
http://dx.doi.org/10.1016/j.cnur.2013.09.004
0029-6465/13/$ – see front matter © 2013 Elsevier Inc. All rights reserved.
nursing.theclinics.com

medications is altered when taken with grapefruit juice (GJ). The explanation given here will help nurses who administer medications, prescribe medications, and teach patients about their medications to understand how knowledge of CYP enzymes can ameliorate the incidence of adverse drug-drug interactions.

Two essential concepts in understanding the role of CYP in drug-drug interactions focus on the functional roles of the enzymes as inducers and/or inhibitors. Exposure to certain substances or drugs can induce the synthesis of the cytochrome p450 enzymes. This induction results in an acceleration of the metabolism of drugs that are substrates for the enzyme. Inducers increase the enzyme levels, increasing the metabolism of the drug. Depending on the drug, an inducer can decrease the effect of the drug and/or lead to toxic buildup of metabolites.[1] With a decrease in the therapeutic effect of a drug, a common practice is to increase the dose of the drug, which has the potential to increase toxic metabolites. The induction process is presented in **Fig. 1**.

Along with the allele phenotype that relates to the individual variation in the enzymes, it is important to consider polypharmacy and the impact that one medication may have on the enzyme that is the substrate of another. Some of the most important inducers of p450 enzymes include cigarette smoking, anticonvulsants, rifampin, glucocorticoids, and chronic alcohol consumption. As such, following cytochrome p450 induction, the enhanced metabolism of other drugs can impede the pharmacologic activity of the substrate and these effects may persist for a long time following cessation of the inducer drug.

In contrast, there are drugs that inhibit specific cytochrome p450 enzyme metabolism, which can result in an immediate decrease in the metabolism of the substrate, resulting in an accumulation and potential toxicity.[1] Inhibiting compounds for the specific enzyme blocks the activity of that enzyme. Depending on the drug, inhibition can lead to reduced therapeutic effects, or a buildup of unmetabolized compounds. The conundrum is that, when there is not a therapeutic effect, there can follow an increase in dosing, which results in a higher probability of toxicity. This process is shown in **Fig. 2**.

Some of the clinically important drugs for which there have been clinical toxicities caused by inhibitory drug interactions have included theophylline, warfarin, carbamazepine, benzodiazepines, phenytoin, cyclosporine, psychotropic drugs, calcium channel blockers, tacrolimus, and hydroxymethylglutaryl coenzyme A (HMG-CoA). Potent inhibitors for many medications are the furanocoumarins, which are found in GJ. A more complete list of inducers and inhibitors for the specific enzyme subfamilies is presented in **Table 1**. A cytochrome p450 inhibitor is not necessarily metabolized by the enzyme it is inhibiting. The mechanism of inhibiting is the result of competitive binding at the site of the enzyme, as conveyed in **Fig. 2**. The beginning and the ending

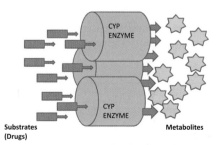

Fig. 1. Inducers of drug metabolism. Inducers increase the cytochrome p450 enzyme activity, resulting in increased drug metabolism. This process can lead to increase in toxic metabolites, and reduced therapeutic effect of the substrate.

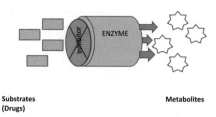

Substrates
(Drugs)   Metabolites

Fig. 2. Inhibitors of drug metabolism. Inhibitors block the cytochrome p450 enzymes. Inhibition can lead to decreased therapeutic effects and/or toxic accumulation of unmetabolized drugs.

of the inhibition is the result of the half-life of the inhibitor. For example, cimetidine has a half-life of about 2 hours, and is a known inhibitor of CYP1A2. Cimetidine inhibits drug metabolism of CYP12A within 24 hours of a single dose, but then, because of the half-life, the inhibitory effect disappear within 24 hours of discontinuation.[2] In contrast, a medication such as amiodarone, which inhibits CYP2C9, has a half-life of 30 to 60 days. The inhibitory action of amiodarone may not take place for months because of its long half-life, and the inhibitory effect may continue for months after amiodarone is discontinued.[2]

An inducer that increases the activity of the CYP450 enzyme may not necessarily be metabolized by the enzymes. The onset of enzyme induction depends on the half-life of the inducer agent. In addition, the time trajectory of induction also depends on the time required for new enzyme production as well as the patient variants such as age, general health, and liver function.[2] So now the issue is not just the two medications but also the phenotype of the enzyme metabolizing the drugs, which dictates whether the patient is an ultrarapid metabolizer, extensive metabolizer, intermediate metabolizer, or a poor metabolizer, as discussed in the first part of this series. To minimize adverse effects of concomitantly administered medications, knowledge of the relationship of target drugs to their potential inducers and/or inhibitors is essential for prescribers and for nurses monitoring patient responses to medications.

DRUG-DRUG INTERACTIONS

There are many known drug-drug interactions that are modulated by the effect that different drugs have on the different enzyme subfamilies. Drugs that are inducers can deactivate the effect of a substrate and its intended effect, as seen with the use of rifampin. Rifampin is a potent inducer of several of the subfamilies of the enzymes, as shown in **Table 1**. When rifampin is given with other medications, there can be a reduction of up to 95% of the other drug that is administered. Drugs that are metabolized by the CYP3A subfamily of enzymes are particularly sensitive to inducers. As an example of induction by rifampin, consider a situation in which a female patient is on estrogen oral contraceptives. Because of an infection, she is begun on rifampin while on the contraceptives. Because rifampin has not only an impact on the CYP enzymes but also on other physiologic processes, the interaction begins. The rifampin induces the CYP enzymes, which results in an increased metabolism of the estrogens. While this is occurring, the rifampin decreases the microflora in the intestine, preventing enterohepatic circulation of estrogens. The result is contraceptive failure. This process is presented in **Fig. 3**.

A class of medications that are often inhibited by other medications via the effect the CYP enzyme families is HMG-CoA reductase inhibitors (statins). Statins are frequently

---

Table 1
Cytochrome p450 subfamily with known inhibitors and inducers

Enzyme	Inhibitor	Inducer
CYP1A2	Fluvoxamine, ciprofloxacin, cimetidine, amiodarone, fluoroquinolones, furafylline, interferon, methoxsalen, mibefradil	Broccoli, Brussels sprouts, char-grilled meat, insulin, methylcholanthrene, modafinil, nafcillin, beta-naphthoflavone, omeprazole, rifampin, tobacco
CYP2B6	Thiotepa, ticlopidine	Phenobarbital, rifampin
CYP2C8	Gemfibrozil, trimethoprim, glitazones, montelukast, quercetin	Rifampin
CYP2C9	Fluconazole, amiodarone, fenofibrate, fluvastatin, fluvoxamine, isoniazid, lovastatin, phenylbutazone, probenicid, sertraline, sulfamethoxazole, sulfaphenazole, teniposide, voriconazole, zafirlukast	Carbamazepine, phenytoin, rifampin, secobarbital
CYP2C19	Lansoprazole, omeprazole, pantoprazole, rabeprazole, chloramphenicol, cimetidine, felbamate, fluoxetine, fluvoxamine, indomethacin ketoconazole, modafinil, oxcarbazepine, probenicid, ticlopidine, topiramate	Carbamazepine, norethindrone, prednisone, rifampin
CYP2D6	Bupropion, fluoxetine, paroxetine, quinidine, duloxetine, terbinafine, amiodarone, cimetidine, sertraline, celecoxib, chlorpheniramine, chlorpromazine, citalopram, clemastine, clomipramine, cocaine, diphenhydramine, doxepin, doxorubicin, escitalopram, halofantrine, histamine H1 receptor antagonists, hydroxyzine, levomepromazine, methadone, metoclopramide, mibefradil, midodrine, moclobemide, perphenazine, ranitidine, reduced haloperidol, ritonavir, ticlopidine, tripelennamine	Dexamethasone, rifampin
CYP2E1	Diethyldithiocarbamate, disulfiram	Ethanol, isoniazid
CYP3A4, CYP3A5, CYP3A7	Indinavir, nelfinavir, ritonavir, clarithromycin, itraconazole, ketoconazole, nefazodone, saquinavir, telithromycin, aprepitant, erythromycin, fluconazole, GJ, verapamil, diltiazem, cimetidine, amiodarone, chloramphenicol, ciprofloxacin, delaviridine, diethyldithiocarbamate, fluvoxamine, gestodene, imatinib, mibefradil, mifepristone, norfloxacin, norfluoxetine, star fruit, voriconazole	Efavirenz, nevirapine, barbiturates, carbamazepine, eefavirenz, glucocorticoids, modafinil, nevirapine, ocarbazepine, phenobarbital, phenytoin, pioglitazone, rifabutin, rifampin, St John's wort, troglitazone

Data from Flockhart DA. Drug interactions: cytochrome P450 drug interaction table. Indiana University School of Medicine. 2007. Available at: http://medicine.iupui.edu/clinpharm/ddis/table.aspx. Accessed August 2, 2011; and Spriet I, Meersseman W, de Hoon J, et al. Mini-series II. Clinical aspects. Clinically relevant CYP450-mediated drug interactions in the ICU. Intensive Care Med 2009;35:603–12.

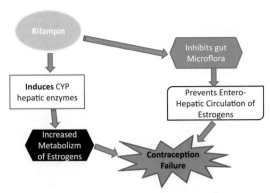

Fig. 3. Inductive properties of rifampin on a patient who is taking oral contraceptives.

prescribed hypolipidemic agents that are used to decrease cardiovascular morbidity and mortality in both primary and secondary prevention. For the most part, side effects and adverse reactions to these medications are rare; however, one of the most important adverse effects is the development of myopathy in which there is necrosis of the muscle cells (rhabdomyolysis), which leads to myoglobinuria and renal failure, and possibly death.[3,4]

The subfamily CYP3A4 metabolizes several statins including lovastatin, simvastatin, and atorvastatin. There are many widely used drugs that inhibit CYP3A4, including erythromycin, clarithromycin, itraconazole, and ketoconazole. When these medications are part of the same medication regimen, the inhibitors lead to an increase in the bioavailability of the statin drug along with reduced elimination of the statin drug, which increases the chances for the development of myotoxicity.[4–6] The inhibiting effect of fluconazole on simvastatin is presented in **Fig. 4.**

REPORT OF A CASE

Hazin and colleagues[7] described a case of a 79-year-old African American man with a variety of medical issues, but presenting with what seemed to be a mild stroke 3 weeks earlier, with progressive weakness. Among the patient's medical regimen were

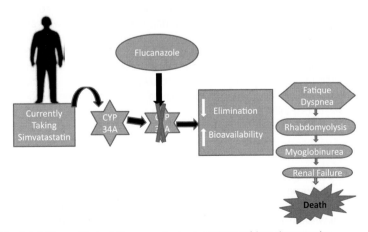

Fig. 4. The inhibition effect of fluconazole on a patient taking simvastatin.

fluconazole and simvastatin. A thorough examination showed no other deficits, and normal vital signs. Laboratory evaluation revealed a white blood cell count of $8.6 \times 10^3/\mu L$, hemoglobin of 10.6 g/dL, platelet count of $370 \times 10^3/\mu L$, creatinine of 3 mg/dL and a creatine phosphokinase (CPK) level of 24,000 units/L.[7] Computed tomography scans were used to rule out neurologic pathophysiologies, and troponin was used to rule out myocardial involvement.

The diagnosis of rhabdomyolysis was based on increased CPK levels, with evidence of acute renal failure and myoglobinuria. On diagnosis, the patient was transferred to the intensive care unit (ICU), where fluconazole, lisinopril, and simvastatin were withdrawn. In addition, the patient was started on intravenous hydration and bicarbonate for urine alkalinization. Two weeks after being admitted to the ICU, with subsequent evaluation revealing normal ranges for both CPK (165) and creatinine (0.9), the rhabdomyolysis was resolved.[2]

Nurses administering medications should be aware, and prescribers must be cautious, when prescribing a drug known to be a cytochrome p450 inhibitor or inducer. With this information, the target drug may warrant substitution with another drug, or the dose may need to be adjusted to account for potential variations in metabolism. Information about a drug's cytochrome p450 properties, including its metabolism and potential to act as an inhibitor or inducer, can be found on the drug label, accessed through the US Food and Drug Administration (FDA), or the manufacturer's Web sites. The FDA has mandated this information for every drug since 1997.[8]

INTERACTION OF MEDICATIONS WITH GJ

Because more than 50% of the CYP3A is located in the intestinal mucosa, it is particularly vulnerable to the substances that people ingest. Among the best known dietary interactions between ingested substances and the cytochrome enzymes is GJ. Even the ingestion of 1 cup of GJ can cause interactions that could last for days,[9] caused by suppression of the CY3A enzyme in the intestinal wall. The furanocoumarin derivative 6′,7′-dihyroxybergamottin is thought to be the principal component in GJ accounting for the inhibitory effect.[10] The mechanism of suppression is 2-fold. Not only does the GJ quickly inhibit the enzyme but it also can cause irreversible damage as it destroys the CYP3A4 protein.[11] GJ has no effect on the liver, and inhibits only those medications that are taken orally. A list of medications that interact with GJ is presented in **Table 2**.

Considering the wide-ranging effects of GJ on the pharmacokinetics of various drugs, nurse practitioners should be kept informed of these interactions, and the ongoing research related to these interactions. This information will enhance their ability to advise and educate their patients regarding potential consequences of concomitant ingestion of GJ with these medications. The elderly are at particular risk because studies have shown they are more prone to GJ-drug interactions.[12] In the future, nurse practitioners might be able to use these effects to patients' advantage and potentially reduce the dosage requirements of certain drugs. However, further research is required into the mechanism of action of GJ, so it is premature to recommend GJ as an adjunctive booster with other drugs.[13]

GENETIC TESTING

Even without genetic testing, knowledge of the interactions between medications as mediated by cytochrome p450 should alert the cautious nurse practitioner to potential problems in a patient's medical regimen. At present, with the exception of some hospitals, patients who have difficulty achieving a therapeutic level of drug bioavailability, or patients who pose particular challenges, genetic testing is not done on a routine

Table 2
Drugs that interact with GJ

Classification	Definite Interaction	Possible Interaction
Immunosuppressants	Cyclosporine	Tacrolimus
Calcium channel blockers	Amlodipine, felodipine, nifedepine, nimodipine, nisoldipine, nitrendipine, pranidipine	—
Antiarrhythmic	Amiodarone	—
HMG-CoA-reductase inhibitors	Atorvastatin, lovastatin, simvastatin	Cerivastatin
Benzodiazepines	Diazepam, midazolam, triazolam	—
Anticancer agents	Etoposide	—
Psychotropics	Buspirone, carbamazepine, clomipramine, sertaline	Zalepion
Corticosteroids	Ethinyl-estradiol	Progesterone
Antiparasitic	Artemether, praziquantel, albendazole	—
Prokinetics	Cisapride	—
Protease inhibitors	Saquinavir	—
Antihistamine	Terfenadine	Ebastine
Other	—	Cilostazol, losartan, methadone, sildenafil

Data from Kiani J, Imam SZ. Medical importance of grapefruit juice and its interaction with various drugs. Nutr J 2007;6:33; and Kane GC, Lipsky JJ. Drug-grapefruit juice interactions. Mayo Clin Proc 2000;73:933–42.

basis. However, a thorough and updated medical history might illuminate problems by considering them through a perspective informed about cytochrome p450 enzymes and the issues of induction and inhibition. At present, there is a clear lack of prospective hypothesis-driven evidence supporting widespread pharmacogenomic testing. The need for more studies, especially with the possibility of health and economic advantages, is evident.

There are a variety of pharmacogenomic tests that have been approved by regulatory agencies. These tests are designed to reveal information related to a certain drug, or for a certain class of drugs, and for identifying individual phenotypes particularly as they relate to CYP2D6, and CYP2C19.[14] For the most part, these tests have to be processed through an accredited laboratory and the time between testing and receiving the results may cause delays. This delay would be problematic in situations in which a drug is indicated immediately, such as clopidogrel during a suspected myocardial infarction. Some drugs might be introduced before the results are delivered, especially if the drug has a long half-life, such as warfarin. In Bicêtre Hospital, in the suburbs of Paris, France, patients with end-stage renal failure who are placed on the renal transplant registry are genotyped for CYP3A5. The results are available in about 2 to 3 weeks and indicate, once the transplant is complete, the ideal initial dose of tacrolimus based on the patient's genotype.[14]

Some CYP genetic testing is available as direct-to-consumer (DTC) tests. As with all genetic tests, there are considerations that the nurse practitioner must take into account in order to properly inform and counsel patients. Whether DTC or from a clinical laboratory, these tests do not detect all the known variants, and the absence of an analyzed variant does not eliminate the possibility of an adverse drug reaction. Also, drug metabolism is affected by factors other than genetic makeup, so prescription and monitoring decisions should consider those environmental, lifestyle, physiologic (and/or pathophysiologic) factors and drug interactions as well.[15] There are numerous ethical, bioethical, legal, and policy issues related to genetic testing that are beyond the scope of the discussion here; however, as these discussion take place, they should include the perspectives of nurse practitioners.

CYTOCHROME p450 IN CANCER THERAPEUTICS

There is much to be said for the cytochrome p450 family of enzymes, but no discussion would be complete without addressing the developments in cytochrome p450–based cancer therapeutics. There are many scientific and research venues that currently focus on these enzymes, and all warrant discussion, but the exemplar that seems the most progressive currently relates to the area of gene-directed enzyme prodrug therapy (GDEPT). Some of the currently available anticancer medications are substrates for various drugs involved in drug biotransformation. Some of these medications require enzymatic activity in order to produce metabolites that are pharmacologically active, which is where the cytochromes, particularly CYP1, CYP2, and CYP3, play a significant role.

Current standard treatment modalities available to patients with cancer are radiation, surgery, and chemotherapy. The discovery and development of new cytotoxic pharmaceutics has been a priority for many pharmaceutical companies and researchers, but chemotherapy for cancer, especially as it relates to solid tumors, has essentially not changed in the last couple of decades. A major issue with chemotherapeutic agents is that they are not tumor selective, and, because they have a narrow therapeutic index, adverse symptoms are often severe and dose limiting.[16] Because these medications are not tumor selective, they are administered systemically, or have a strong systemic effect with severe side effects. At first, it was thought that there was a lack of cytochrome p450 expression in the tumor sample. However, based on more current data, as conveyed by Chang,[16] the CYP1, CYP2, and CYP3 proteins have been identified in specific tumors. **Table 3** shows the different subfamilies that are associated with different tumors, but with the collective finding that the expression of CYP1B1 seems to be commonly expressed in all examined tumors. This information is foundational to understanding the basis of GDEPT.

The presence of these enzymes in tumoral tissues has certain implications related to tumoral metabolism of cancer therapeutic agents. The presence of these enzymes in different tumors might lead to a pathway in chemotherapy in which the local bioactivation of the drug can yield a pharmacologically active metabolite. Although the levels of cytochrome p450 expression are less than the expression that takes place in the liver, there are those who think that there is sufficient catalytic capability in the tumor microsomes to activate cytochrome p450–mediated anticancer drug metabolism.[16] To overcome the major limitations of traditional chemotherapy agents and to improve drug efficacy while minimizing systemic toxicity to the patient, there has emerged gene therapy, or gene transfer, which specifically targets tumor cells and increases tumor sensitivity to other chemotherapeutic agents.

Some of the genes that are suitable for this pathway are those that encode prodrug activation enzymes. This form of cancer gene therapy embodies the idea behind GDEPT. Instead of the prodrug activation occurring in the liver, or another site distant from the tumor, the bioactivation of the pharmacologically inactive prodrug occurs in the tumor cells transduced with the prodrug activation enzyme.[16]

Table 3 Cytochrome p450 enzymes detected in solid malignant tumors	
Tumor Location	**Enzymes Identified**
Bladder	CYP1B1, CYP2C8, CYP2C9, CYP2J2
Brain	CYP1B1
Breast	CYP1A1, CYP1A2, CYP1B1, CYP2B6, CYP2C8, CYP2C9, CYP2D6, CYP2E1, CYP3A4
Colon	CYP1B1, CYP2C8, CYP2C9, CYP2D6, CYP2E1, CYP3A4, CYP3A5, CYP3A7
Esophageal	CYP1A, CYP1B1, CYP3A
Renal	CYP1B1, CYP2C8, CYP2C9, CYP3A
Hepatic	CYP1A, CYP2A6, CYP2C9, CYP3A
Pulmonary	CYP1A, CYP1B1, CYP2C8, CYP2C9, CYP2E1, CYP3A
Ovarian	CYP1B1, CYP2C8, CYP2C9, CYP2D6, CYP2E1, CYP3A4, CYP3A5
Prostate	CYP1A, CYP1B1, CYP2C8, CYP2C9, CYP3A
Stomach	CYP1A, CYP1B1, CYP2C9, CYP3A
Testicular	CYP1B1, CYP2C8, CYP2C9

Data from Chang TK. Cytochromes P450 in cancer therapeutics. In: Ioannides C, editor. Cytochromes p450: role in the metabolism and toxicity of drugs and other xenobiotics. Cambridge (United Kingdom): Royal Society of Chemistry; 2008. p. 480–508.

Investigational studies indicate that cytochrome p450–based GDEPT is a viable strategy to mitigate patient toxicity of prodrugs and improve chemotherapy efficacy. There are other pathways that are being explored in cancer therapy that involve the CYP enzymes, such as cytochrome P-450 based cancer immunotherapies and antisense oligmers. These intiatives are new, and currently prospective research studies are lacking. However, there are advances in cytochrome p450–based experimental cancer therapeutics that hold great promise for new ways of treating cancer.

SUMMARY

The most important considerations related to understanding cytochrome p450 enzymes is the appreciation that all drug effects vary among individuals and, although there are multiple causes of these variations, drug effects are strongly influenced by genes. Related to this family of enzymes, it is clear that the same enzyme may display a variety of functions and alterations, which can range from ultrarapid activity to no activity. Each cytochrome p450 subfamily is instrumental in the metabolism of numerous drugs.

The science exists to improve patient outcomes and to improve understanding of drug response. However, clinical progress in implementing pharmacogenomics is lacking.

The main challenges for the future are to identify among all of the polymorphisms those that contribute to idiosyncratic effects and adverse drug reactions. Although new pathways for known diseases are explored using cytochrome p450 enzymes, technological efforts should also be focused on the development of tests that can easily be done in the clinic or at the bedside, which will remove one of the barriers to the use of pharmacogenomics in routine practice.

One day pharmacogenomics will allow clinicians to prescribe medications based on the patient's genotype, without regard to the proxy classifications of gender or race.

REFERENCES

1. Gregg CR. Drug interactions and anti-infective therapies. Am J Med 1999;106(2): 227–37.
2. Cheng JW, Frishman WH, Aronow WS. Updates on cytochrome P450-mediated cardiovascular drug interactions. Am J Ther 2009;16:155–63.
3. Thompson PD, Clarkson P, Karas RH. Statin-associated myopathy. JAMA 2003; 289:1681–90.
4. Omar MA, Wilson JP, Cox TS. Rhabdomyolysis and HMG-CoA reductase inhibitors. Ann Pharmacother 2001;35:1096–107.
5. Williams D, Feely J. Pharmacokinetic-pharmacodynamic drug interactions with HMG-CoA reductase inhibitors. Clin Pharmacokinet 2002;41:343–70.
6. Omar MA, Wilson JP. FDA adverse event reports on statin-associated rhabdomyolysis. Ann Pharmacother 2002;36:288–95.
7. Hazin R, Abuzetun JY, Suker M, et al. Rhabdomyolysis induced by simvastatin-fluconazole combination. J Natl Med Assoc 2008;100(4):444–6.
8. Lynch T, Price A. The effect of cytochrome p450 metabolism on drug response, interactions, and adverse effects. Am Fam Physician 2007;76(3):391–6.
9. Bojanic ZZ, Bojanic NZ, Bojanic VV. Drug interactions with grapefruit. Med Pregl 2010;63(11–12):805–10.
10. Mertens-Talcott SU, Zadezensky I, De Castro WV, et al. Grapefruit-drug interactions: can interactions with drugs be avoided? J Clin Pharmacol 2006;46(12): 1390–416.
11. Guo LQ, Fukuda K, Ohta T, et al. Role of furanocoumarin derivatives on grapefruit juice-mediated inhibition of human CYP3A activity. Drug Metab Dispos 2000;28: 766–71.
12. Saito M, Hirata-Koizumi M, Matsumoto M, et al. Undesirable effects of citrus juice on the pharmacokinetics of drugs: focus on recent studies. Drug Saf 2005;28: 677–94.
13. Kiani J, Imam SZ. Medicinal importance of grapefruit juice and its interaction with various drugs. Nutr J 2007;6:33.
14. Becquemont L. Pharmacogenomics of adverse drug reactions: practical applications and perspectives. Pharmacogenomics 2009;10(6):961–9.
15. Lea DH, Skirton H, Read CY, et al. Implications for educating the next generation of nurses on genetics and genomics in the 21st century. J Nurs Scholarsh 2010; 43(1):3–12.
16. Chang TK. Cytochromes P450 in cancer therapeutics. In: Ioannides C, editor. Cytochromes p450: role in the metabolism and toxicity of drugs and other xenobiotics. Cambridge (United Kingdom): Royal Society of Chemistry; 2008. p. 480–508.

Index

Note: Page numbers of article titles are in **boldface** type.

Nurs Clin N Am 48 (2013) 707–714
http://dx.doi.org/10.1016/S0029-6465(13)00109-6
0029-6465/13/$ – see front matter © 2013 Elsevier Inc. All rights reserved.